Handbook of Culture
and Mental Illness:
An International Perspective

Handbook of Culture and Mental Illness: An International Perspective

Edited by

Ihsan Al-Issa

International Universities Press, Inc.
Madison   Connecticut

Second Printing, 1996

Copyright © 1995, International Universities Press, Inc.

INTERNATIONAL UNIVERSITIES PRESS and IUP (& design) ® are registered trademarks of International Universities Press, Inc.

Library of Congress Cataloging-in-Publication Data

Handbook of culture and mental illness : an international perspective
/ edited by Ihsan Al-Issa.
  p. cm.
Includes bibliographical references and index.
ISBN 0-8236-2288-6
  1. Psychiatry, Transcultural. 2. Cultural Psychiatry. I. Al
-Issa, Ihsan.
  [DNLM: 1. Mental Disorders. 2. Cross-Cultural Comparison.
3. Psychiatry. 4. Ethnic Groups. WM 100 H233665 1995]
RC455.4.E8H36 1995
616.89—dc20
DNLM/DLC
for Library of Congress   94-41857
                                          CIP

Manufactured in the United States of America

Contents

Contributors

Ihsan Al-Issa, Department of Psychology, University of Calgary Alberta, Canada.

Yoram Bilu, Department of Psychology; Department of Sociology and Anthropology, Hebrew University, Jerusalem, Israel.

Béla Buda, Chief of Department, Department of Psychotherapy, National Institute of Sporthygiene, Budapest, Hungary.

Subho Chakrabartl, Department of Psychiatry, Postgraduate Institute of Medical Education and Research, Chandigarh, India.

Raymond Cochrane, Professor, School of Psychology, The University of Birmingham, Edgbaston, Birmingham, United Kingdom.

René Collignon, Chargé de Recherche au Centre National de la Recherche Scientifique, Laboratoire d'Ethnologie et de Sociologie Comparative, Université de Paris-X, Nanterre, France.

Yubarandt Bespali de Consens, Ex-Presidenta Sociedad de Psiquiatria del Uruguay, Montevideo, Uruguay.

Mason H. Durie, Professor of Maori Studies, Massey University, Palmerston North, New Zealand.

M. S. A. El-Gawad, Professor of Psychiatry, Cairo University, Cairo, Egypt.

A. Fernandez-Doctor, Departmento de Historia de la Medicina, Universidad de Zaragoza, Zaragoza, Spain.

János Füredi, President, Hungarian Psychiatric Association; Professor and Chairman, Department of Psychiatry and Postgraduate Medical University Clinical Psychology, Budapest, Hungary.

Momar Gueye, Maître de Conférence Agrégé Université de Dakar, Centre Hospitalier Universitaire de Fann-Dakar, Clinique Psychiatrique Moussa Diop, Dakar-Fann, Sénégal.

Kwang-iel Kim, Department of Neuropsychiatry, School of Medicine, Hanyang University, Seoul, Korea.

Wolfgang Krahl, Department of Psychological Medicine, Faculty of Medicine, University of Malaya, Kuala Lumpur, Malaysia.

Kok Lee-Peng, Consultant Psychiatrist, Gleneagles Medical Center, Singapore.

Inge Lynge, Former Chief Psychiatrist in Greenland; Consultant for the Health Service of Greenland, Snekkersten, Denmark.

Spero M. Manson, Professor and Director, National Center for American Indian and Alaska Native Mental Health Research, Colorado Psychiatric Hospital, Denver, Colorado.

I. H. Minas, Associate Professor of Transcultural Psychiatry, University of Melbourne; Director, Victorian Transcultural Psychiatry Unit, St. Vincent's Hospital, Melbourne, Australia.

N. K. Ndosi, Neuropsychiatrist, Senior Lecturer, Department of Psychiatry, Muhimbili University College of Health Sciences, Dar-es-Salaam, Tanzania.

A. Seva, Departmento de Psiquiatria Psychologia Medica, Universidad de Zaragoza, Zaragoza, Spain.

James H. Shore, Professor and Chairman of Psychiatry; Superintendent, Colorado Psychiatric Hospital, Denver, Colorado.

O. A. Sijuwola, Provost and Medical Director, Neuropsychiatric Hospital ARO; WHO Collaborating Centre for Research and Training in Mental Health, Ogun State, Nigeria.

Ctirad Skoda, Psychiatric Demography Unit, Prague Psychiatric Center, WHO Collaborating Center for Research and Training, CZ-18103 Prague, Czech Republic.

Philip D. Somervell, Assistant Professor, Department of Psychiatry, National Center for American Indian and Alaska Native Mental Health Research, Denver, Colorado.

Luh Ketut Suryani, Head of Department of Psychiatry, Faculty of Medicine, Udayana University, Denpasar, Indonesia.

Leslie Swartz, Director, Child Guidance Clinic, University of Cape Town, Cape Town, South Africa.

Carlos Viesca Treviño, Departamento de Historia de la Medicina, Facultad de Medicina, Universidad Nacional Autonoma de Mexico.

Can Tuncer, Consultant Psychiatrist, Victorian Transcultural Psychiatry Unit, St. Vincent's Hospital, Melbourne, Australia.

Vijoy K. Varma, Department of Psychiatry, Postgraduate Institute of Medical Education and Research, Chandigarh, India.

Mariblanca Ramos de Viesca, Departamento de Historia de la Medicina, Facultad de Medicina, Universidad Nacional Autonoma de Mexico.

William Wedenoja, Professor of Anthropology, Department of Sociology and Anthropology, Southwest Missouri State University, Springfield, Missouri.

Tsoi Wing-Foo, Consultant Psychiatrist, Gleneagles Medical Center, Singapore.

Preface

During the past four decades, transcultural psychiatry has become an important area for both researchers and practitioners and has passed from a previous era of speculation on the exotic behavior of non-Western people, and description of it, to the objective collection of data and the use of sophisticated methodology. Research and general information on the relationship between culture and mental illness have now been published from almost every corner of the globe representing most known cultures and ethnic and religious groups. Although the study of mental illness across cultures had been traditionally conducted by Western researchers, many investigations in non-Western nations are now carried out by native professionals who were trained either in the West or in their own countries. It is the present maturity of the discipline of transcultural psychiatry that inspired me with the idea of this handbook: a publication to provide information on mental illness on a worldwide scale to enable researchers and practitioners to obtain information on sociocultural differences both within and outside the boundaries of their own countries. It is hoped that the handbook will not only highlight international achievements in transcultural psychiatry, but will also demonstrate the biological unity of humankind. Western concepts and theories of mental illness, whether sociocultural or biological, cannot be valid unless they are based on evidence from all humanity, and historical and contemporary psychiatric information within a sociocultural framework from different regions of the world will provide such evidence.

With these ideas in mind, I contacted psychiatrists and other mental health professionals all over the world, either directly or through national psychiatric associations, and asked them to contribute chapters about what they knew and what took place in the relationship between culture and mental illness in their countries. Authors of the chapters are predominantly indigenous to the culture they are writing about or they have intimate knowledge and extensive experience with the ethnic and religious groups they

xiii

discuss. Ideally every region and every ethnic group would be included in a handbook such as this. The limited coverage of countries and ethnic groups may reflect in part difficulties in cross-cultural communication among scientists and researchers.

The material in the chapters is varied and tends to depend on both availability of data in the respective culture, and/or the individual interest of the authors. The methodology (population, setting, diagnostic techniques) used in collecting data reported by the authors is so varied that cross-cultural generalizations are difficult to make about the rates of mental illness and its treatment. However, there are common themes discussed in the chapters illustrating some global research issues and common psychological problems in international psychiatry. Authors provide a brief description of the sociocultural background of the countries, and the ethnic and minority groups with which they deal. There is a global concern with the devastating effects of severe psychopathology and its treatment. Schizophrenia, depression, substance abuse, and suicide are major psychiatric problems. For psychiatrists and psychologists in developing countries, a major problem is how modern psychiatry can accommodate traditional medicine which takes a holistic view of human suffering and does not separate the psyche from the soma. Overall, the handbook will serve as a brief introduction to various countries and cultures and provide a glimpse of the actual and potential achievement of transcultural psychiatry, a microcosm of psychological problems today. It proposes to introduce the reader (whether he or she is a student of psychiatry, psychology, sociology, anthropology, or of any related field in any country) to what can be achieved in understanding abnormal behavior when one steps outside of his or her own culture.

PART I

Introduction

1.

Culture and Mental Illness in an International Perspective

Ihsan Al-Issa

Many definitions have been suggested for the concept of culture (Kroeber and Kluckholm, 1952). Most of these definitions regard culture as those parts of the environment that are human-made, including both its subjective and objective characteristics. The subjective environment consists of beliefs, values, norms, and myths shared by the group and symbolically transmitted to its members from one generation to another. On the other hand, the objective aspect of culture refers to the physical environment which consists of artifacts including roads, bridges, and buildings. The term *culture* is often confused with race, and people who are seen as racially different may be assumed to have a different culture. Race is a socially constructed category which specifies identification of group members. Application of race in a social context is called racism. Ethnic groups are individuals with a sense of belongingness and are thought by themselves and/or by others to share a common origin as well as an important segment of a common culture. The bond that brings members of an ethnic group together may be defined in terms of physical appearance (race) and/or social similarity (culture) (Fernando, 1991).

The term *culture* is originally used by anthropologists in a restricted tribal–traditional sense where mental illness is described in preliterate societies. In its most frequent use in the

3

cross-cultural study of mental illness, *culture* is equated with *nation*. It is assumed that each nation of the world has its own distinct culture and that cultural variations within a nation are less in scope and degree than those that exist between nations. In multicultural nations, the concept of culture is used in the ethnic sense where the nation is divided into "ethnic groups defined on the basis of racial–physical characteristics, shared language, common historic origins, and shared contemporary customs" (Draguns, 1982, p. 56). The inequality of status of various ethnic groups may confound results of research, and differences in mental illness may be a direct result of the stress of inferior status rather than of the ethnic culture itself. This handbook deals with culture on the national and ethnic level. In this introductory chapter, I outline some recent historical events in the study of culture and mental illness, with reference to mental problems that face different nations in the world today as emphasized in the chapters of the handbook, namely acute reactive psychosis, schizophrenia, depression and suicide, culture-specific syndrome, culture and alcoholism, and the mental health of immigrants and ethnic minorities. In conclusion I discuss some major international research problems in the area of culture and mental illness.

HISTORICAL DEVELOPMENTS

Early in this century, Emil Kraepelin traveled to southeast Asia and to other parts of the world and observed that mental illness as known in the West (such as dementia praecox and manic–depressive syndrome) exists in non-Western countries, but differs in incidence and symptomatology from its Western counterpart. Kraepelin also observed culture-specific syndromes (such as *amok* and *latah*) in southeast Asia, but he believed that they are similar to diseases common in the West (hysteria, catatonic episodes, epileptic twilight, for example). Kraepelin also drew attention to the possible differences between different European nations (German, French, Italian, English) in psychiatric morbidity. Kraepelin had a biological orientation, and he concluded that Western disease entities were universal (Lauter, 1965), but his initiative inspired researchers in this century in the area of culture and mental illness. Throughout the major part of this century researchers have posed the same questions that preoccupied Kraepelin himself: Are concepts of mental illness and the Western system of psychiatric diagnosis universal and applicable to other cultures? Are the incidence and symptoms of mental illness the same across cultures? Are there culture-specific syndromes? If culture-specific syndromes do exist, are they the same types of syndromes familiar to Western psychiatrists, but merely expressed differently, or do they represent different psychiatric entities?

One early attempt to study mental illness across cultures was carried out in the 1930s by anthropologists such as Malinowsky and Benedict, guided by the eighteenth-century "nature cult" which attributed the increase of insanity in Europe to a degeneration from "a golden age of natural virtue" (Rosen, 1968). The Freudian conflict model of mental illness also influenced anthropological orientation. In *Civilization and Its Discontents,* Freud (1930) conceptualized neurosis as the result of a conflict between instinctual drives and the repressive processes of civilization. A major cross-cultural hypothesis derived from this approach is that the non-Western style of life may provide immunity against mental illness. An early survey of cross-cultural research by Benedict and Jacks (1954) shows that data in support of this hypothesis are disappointingly negative; the major psychoses occur in all societies.

During the 1930s and 1940s, studies were carried out in the United States and other parts of the world using hospital statistics and surveys to study the epidemiology of mental illness. For example, thousands of cases of first- or second-generation immigrants demonstrated marked differences in morbidity among groups of European cultural origin and native-born Americans (Malzberg, 1940; Ödegaard, 1932). Other epidemiological studies were carried out in the United States (Faris and Dunham, 1939, Chicago; Lemkau, Tietze, and Cooper, 1942, Baltimore), Germany (Brugger, 1931), Japan (Uchimura, Akimoto, Kan, Abe, Takahashi, Inose, Shimazaki, and Ogawa, 1940), Scandinavia (Essen-Moeller, 1956), and Taiwan (Lin, 1953). Many researchers used community data to test a sociocultural hypothesis. Prominent among these studies are those by Leighton and associates to investigate the culture disintegration hypothesis in Nova Scotia, Canada

(Leighton, Harding, Macklin, Macmillan, and Leighton, 1963), Nigeria (Leighton, Lambo, Hughes, Leighton, Murphy, and Macklin, 1963), and Sweden (Leighton, Hagnell, Kellert, Leighton, Harding, and Danley, 1971). Similarly, social disorganization and urbanization hypotheses were suggested by Faris and Dunham (1939), a social class hypothesis by Hollingshead and Redlich (1958), a stress–strain hypothesis by Srole, Langner, Michael, Opler, and Rennie (1962), and a cultural utopia hypothesis by Eaton and Weil (1955). These studies established psychiatric epidemiology as a major research method in psychiatry throughout this century (Robins and Regier, 1991). They also accepted the universality of the Western concept of mental illness suggested earlier by Kraepelin and firmly established the medical model in cross-cultural research. For example, J. M. Murphy (1976) concluded from these epidemiological studies that the rates of mental illness among Canadian villagers in Nova Scotia (18%), the Eskimos (19%), and members of the Yoruba tribe in Nigeria (15%) are similar despite wide differences between these cultures.

Consistent with Kraepelin's observation, researchers accepted similar entities of psychopathology across cultures but recognized variability in their symptoms. This is concisely expressed by Berne (1959) as a result of observing striking similarities among patients in mental hospitals he visited in several tropical African countries, America, and Australia: "Clinically, differences can be affectively treated as mere dialects or accents of a common language; the Italian schizophrenic speaks schizophrenic with an Italian accent; the Siamese manic speaks manic with a Siamese accent" (p. 108). Edgerton (1966) also concluded that the concept of psychosis among four East African tribes was much similar to that in the West. However, he noted differences. "Going naked" was considered an aspect of psychotic behavior by the East African tribes; murder, attempted murder, or serious assault were emphasized more than in the West. Hallucinations, however, which are basic to the diagnosis of psychosis in the West, were seldom mentioned as aspects of psychotic behavior.

Two movements during the 1960s criticized the validity of psychiatric diagnosis: the cultural relativity perspective (social model) and the dimensional approach (psychological model).

Both approaches questioned the concept of mental illness as an absolute entity that is qualitatively different from a state of health. Since normality and abnormality are defined within a social and cultural context, they cannot be considered medical or scientific concepts but rather moral, religious, or political ones. This approach resulted in major changes in public programs for psychiatric care, especially the deinstitutionalization of hospitalized patients to be discussed later in this chapter. The dimensional approach which had been particularly advocated by Eysenck (1960) and Eysenck and Eysenck (1982) used statistical analysis to identify a limited number of dimensions in order to describe patients in terms of their position on dimensions such as psychoticism and neuroticism. These movements brought problems related to diagnosis and institutionalization to the attention of researchers.

THE POLITICS OF PSYCHIATRIC DIAGNOSIS

Kramer (1969) found that age-adjusted first-admission rates to United States mental hospitals for schizophrenia and affective psychoses were 24.7 and 11 per 100,000, respectively, compared with 17.4 and 38.5 in England and Wales. This observation led in part to the U.S.–U.K. Diagnostic Project (Cooper, Kendell, Gurland, Sharpe, Copeland, and Simon, 1972), which demonstrated that much of the differences in rates could be explained by different diagnostic concepts rather than real variations in incidence. The international pilot study of schizophrenia sponsored by the World Health Organization (WHO, 1973, 1979) confirmed this result (broad concepts of schizophrenia in both New York and Moscow). One factor to explain the difference is that Eugen Bleuler's expansion of the Kraepelin concept of schizophrenia has not been as influential in Britain as in the United States. Diagnosis such as psychoneurotic, pseudopsychopathic, simple, borderline, and latent schizophrenia are much less frequently used in the United Kingdom, and a condition such as early childhood autism is differentiated from schizophrenia instead of being incorporated into it. Different hallucinations and delusions are also more differentiated in the United Kingdom than in the

United States. Another factor is that the influence of psychoanalytic theory and its emphasis on intrapsychic processes (projection, primary process) may have been applied to the concept of psychoses in the United States but not in Britain (Wing, 1980).

In reaction to the criticism of psychiatric diagnosis and the results of international research, psychometric diagnosis was consolidated in the 1970s with the development of reliable and valid diagnostic criteria based on clearly defined symptoms involving minimal etiological inferences (Robins and Helzer, 1986; Klerman, 1989). Semistructured interviews were developed to obtain standardized information about a person's history, social functioning, and symptom states such as the Schedule for Affective Disorders and Schizophrenia (SADS, Endicott and Spitzer, 1978), the NIMH Diagnostic Interview Schedule (DIS, Robins, Helzer, Crougham, Williams, and Spitzer, 1981) and the Structured Clinical Interview for DSM-III (SCID). Operational criteria for assigning persons to diagnostic categories were also specified (Feighner, Robins, Guze, Woodruff, Winokur, and Munoz, 1972; Spitzer, Endicott, and Robins, 1978) and this approach was adopted in the DSM-III (APA, 1980).

A broad concept of mental illness in general and schizophrenia in particular in the Soviet Union (WHO, 1973; Report of U.S. Delegation, 1989) clearly demonstrated the political abuse of psychiatry under the communist regime. Some symptoms incorporated into Soviet diagnostic criteria for mild ("sluggish") schizophrenia and, in part, moderate (paranoid) schizophrenia are not acceptable as evidence of psychopathology in the United States or according to an international diagnostic criterion (e.g., "delusion of reformism" or "heightened sense of self-esteem" are used for a diagnosis of schizophrenia). Furthermore, antipsychotic medications were used to treat patients for "delusions of reformism" and "anti-Soviet thoughts" in the absence of psychotic ideation (relatively high doses of neuroleptics are used with some patients who showed no signs of psychotic ideation).

In a review of studies on sluggish schizophrenia, Mersky and Shafran (1986) found that behavior such as being ascetic (quitting smoking, abstaining from alcohol, or sustained energetic productive activity) are considered symptoms of sluggish schizophrenia. In the WHO study (1973), many cases of sluggish schizophrenia were diagnosed as manic-depressive psychosis or most often depressive neurosis. Although international efforts are made to standardize international classification of mental illness, the Soviet experience is a warning against the pitfalls of psychiatric diagnosis.

European nations may not only differ in the broadness of the concept of mental illness (concept of schizophrenia in the former Soviet Union versus Britain), but they may also have their national categories (paraphrenia in Spain and Germany, *bouffées délirantes* in France, and psychogenic psychosis in Scandinavia). Non-Western countries mainly follow DSM-III-R (APA, 1987) and the model of WHO studies in psychiatry. In many Asian and African countries (see parts I and II of this handbook), organic illnesses such as epilepsy are considered mental illnesses and are included in their diagnostic systems. There are also differences in the meaning of concepts used in different nations. One example is *tarjinkyofu* (fear of interpersonal relations) in Korea and Japan (see chapter 9, this handbook), which may be considered a social phobia according to DSM-III-R (Prince, 1991b). North American phobic patients are preoccupied with the disgust or rejection of others while oriental patients tend to be concerned with causing harm or discomfort to others. The concern of oriental patients with their shortcomings may lead Western psychiatrists to give them the diagnosis of delusional disorder rather than phobia.

Attempts are made to make DSM sensitive to cultural and national diversity. The American Psychiatric Association Task Force on DSM-IV (1992) suggested the creation of a subtype of dissociate disorder called "Trance and Possession Disorder," consistent with ICD-10 which contains such a category (WHO, 1992). Most trances and possession states across cultures are normal, and such a psychiatric category may run the risk of misattributing pathology to normal states ignoring the cultural context (Lewis-Fernández, 1992). What is perhaps needed is a classification system with "fluid illness labels" where the meaning of labels or symptoms changes with the social context (see chapter 4, this handbook). The problem facing psychiatry today is how to accommodate patients from different cultural backgrounds.

THE POLITICS OF DEINSTITUTIONALIZATION IN THE UNITED STATES

The 'sixties have seen the beginning of the deinstitutionalization of long-term patients in the United States and other Western countries. The number of patients in the United States declined from 559,000 in 1955 to approximately 110,000 at present (Mechanic and Rochefort, 1990). A major factor for this movement was the introduction of the phenothiazines in the middle 1950s that allow large institutions to change their administrative policies. The new drugs helped control psychotic symptoms and raised hopes for the potential of less coercive restraints and greater predictability of patients' behavior. The new drug therapy was accompanied by the ideology of the deleterious effects of hospitalization on patients' functioning, giving support to the growing community mental health movement (Belknap, 1956; Goffman, 1961). Although studies have documented that alternatives to hospitalization programs attain better outcomes as compared with traditional hospital care (Kiesler and Sibulkin, 1987), they ignored other problematic aspects of deinstitutionalization.

The new system of care following deinstitutionalization resulted in a group of mental patients with psychoses and personality disorders who are difficult to manage outside custodial care. The mentally sick youth and young adults are described as uncooperative with treatment, abuse alcohol and drugs, and generally live an unconventional style of life (Schwartz and Goldfinger, 1981; Pepper and Ryglewicz, 1982; Sheets, Provost, and Reichmank, 1982). This problem is exacerbated by population trends that result in large subgroups in the population at ages of high risk for schizophrenia and drug abuse (Mechanic, 1987).

Problems became more visible and acute with the reduction of public programs during the 1980s in the United States. The large waves of deinstitutionalization in the late 1960s and 1970s occurred with the expansion of social welfare activities, which provided the base for relocation of patients into the community. But this aid was not maintained relative to the growing numbers of seriously mentally ill persons, and in many cases the disabled mentally ill lost their benefits (Osterweis, Kleinman, and Mechanic, 1987). It is estimated that between one quarter to one half of the homeless in the

United States are mentally ill (the number of homeless is estimated between two hundred thousand to more than two million) (Rossie, Wright, Fisher, and Willis, 1987).

European researchers had suggested that the hospital environment may protect patients against stress and thus may reduce diseases such as cardiovascular disorders (Ödegaard, 1936; Masterson, Main, Lever, and Lever, 1975). Masterson and associates found that the blood pressure of long-stay psychiatric inpatients in a Glasgow hospital was significantly below that of normal controls of the same age. This difference was regardless of whether patients were taking drugs or not. It seems that the less restrictive the hospital environment, the higher the blood pressure of the patients. Although deinstitutionalization may be of benefit to some patients, the experience of the last decades in the United States as well as in Britain (Wing, 1980) and Denmark (Licht, Gouliaev, and Lund, 1991) shows that some patients still need the protection of custodial care.

ACUTE REACTIVE PSYCHOSES AND SCHIZOPHRENIA

Acute Reactive Psychoses

Psychotic reactions with short duration and complete recovery are often reported among non-Western patients (see chapters on India, Jamaica, Bali, Tanzania, and Nigeria, this handbook). This reactive psychosis is called *bouffée délirante* in francophone countries (Collomb, 1965a,b), and fear psychosis and anxiety psychosis (Field, 1958), twilight or confusional states (Carothers, 1951), and periodic psychoses (Lambo, 1960) in former British colonies. It is similar to psychogenic or reactive psychosis and schizophreniform psychoses in Anglo-Saxon countries and Scandinavia.

British and German psychiatry tended to attribute acute reactive psychoses to somatic factors such as infection, hormones, or toxins (toxic psychosis). The United States psychiatric thinking is influenced by Bleuler's "group of schizophrenias" which includes acute, transient, and chronic disorders, and thus acute reactive psychosis is included with schizophrenia. There were, however, serious attempts in Scandinavia to distinguish "psychogenic psychoses" from the more chronic ones, but their concepts were different from the French *bouffée délirante*. While the French concept puts emphasis on the presenting clinical picture and a hypothesized constitutional predisposition (Ey, 1954) the Scandinavians drew attention to the involvement of a clear-cut somatic or psychogenic trauma and a favorable prognosis (Faegerman, 1963; Kringlen, 1980).

Acute reactive psychosis may be confused with schizophrenia in international research and may be reflected in the idea of the existence of three types of schizophrenia rather than one (chronic, episodic, and single episode) popularized by the results of the International Pilot Study of Schizophrenia (WHO, 1979). Differences found among nations in the prognosis of schizophrenia may reflect the inclusion of acute reactive psychosis in the study groups. According to Murphy (1982b) acute transient psychoses were more common in the early nineteenth century in Europe than they were at its end. Cooper and Sartorius (1975) attributed this decline to the industrial revolution and suggested that schizophrenia only became recognizable during the 50 years before Kraepelin. Acute reactive psychosis is more common in black Africa (Senegal, Ghana) than in Europe (France, Scandinavia) (Murphy, 1982b). *Bouffée délirante* is also more common among the uneducated than African university students (Lambo, 1956; German and Arya, 1969). It is interesting whether these short-term psychoses are decreasing with westernization in Africa (German, 1972).

Postpartum psychosis may present particular problems for African women and constitute one third of all female psychiatric admissions in Senegal and 10 to 15 percent in North Africa (Ilechukwu, 1991), but only 4 to 5 percent in Western countries. The symptoms of postpartum psychosis are heterogeneous and may reflect mainly affective disorder or organic psychosis (clouding of consciousness) or schizophrenia (hallucinations and delusions). Although Western studies find schizophrenic symptoms only in 2 to 16 percent of patients (Harding, 1989), African studies suggest a predominance of schizophrenialike patterns in between

24 and 53 percent of patients (Ebie, 1972; Swift, 1972). But the picture is changing from high frequency of organic and schizophreniform illness to a more frequent affective disorder (Chkili and El-Khamlichi, 1975; Cox, 1983). This change in the picture of postpartum psychoses in Africa seems to be similar to changes reported in the West (Pothero, 1969).

The behavior involved in *bouffées délirantes* and many other acute reactive psychotic reactions appears to be directed to mobilize the community to take action. It is an attention-getting device which attempts to reintegrate the patient into the social group and which is symbolized, for example, by the rites which take place at the healing shrines in Ghana (Field, 1960) and the Ivory Coast (Piault, 1975). It may be that the extent to which a culture emphasizes individualism determines reaction to conflicts: the more people are brought up to be dependent on the group for social support, the more effective their behavior (symptoms) is likely to be if they depend on the group rather than on themselves. In an individualistic society, the psychological mechanisms used may allow the person to function independently of the group (Murphy, 1982b).

Schizophrenia

Mead (1928) reported that during a nine-month stay in the Manu'a Archipelago, with a population of about 2000, she came across only one case of psychosis, a man of about thirty with a well-systematized delusion of grandeur. That impression was supported by early reports of low hospitalization rates of the Maoris in New Zealand and native Hawaiians. However their rates have later increased to exceed that of caucasians (Schmitt, 1956; see also chapter 23, this handbook). These examples show that sociocultural factors may reduce or increase the risk for schizophrenia. Among the contemporary low-risk groups studied are the Hutterites (active prevalence during one year, 1.9 per 1000), the South Pacific Tongans (1.0 per 1000), and the Taiwan aboriginal tribes (the lowest rate recorded of 0.6 per 1000 in a community study) (Murphy, 1982a,b). These three groups are from contrasting cultural backgrounds with no common genetic or cultural heritage, except that they share a communalistic style of living.

In contrast, the Irish and the Istrians (in Croatia) have a high risk of schizophrenia. These groups also have no common genetic or cultural backgrounds. However, both groups had experienced centuries of resented domination by some neighboring power and extensive overseas emigrations. These massive emigrations may raise the question of whether the high rates of schizophrenia are due to selection, where schizophrenics remain in the home country, while the more healthy grasp the opportunity abroad. Many sociocultural hypotheses have been suggested to explain the high rate of schizophrenia among Irish immigrants, but the selection hypothesis is excluded since Irish immigrants, particularly the Catholics, tend to have higher rates of schizophrenia than other groups in the host countries. There is some evidence for the selection hypothesis in Croatia. When compared with other regions in Croatia with lower rates of schizophrenia, Z. Folnegovic and V. Folnegovic-Smalc (1992) found that high prevalence regions have a population characterized by intensive economic emigration and a greater proportion of autochtonous population, which points to a positive selection of emigrants (the able-bodied leave), or a negative selection of residents is present ("sick" people remaining). Negative selection in the resident population is also increased by mentally ill emigrants returning home. This is in support of the selection hypothesis but against the idea that the schizophrenic-prone tend to emigrate since they are unable to establish satisfactory roots in their native community (Ödegaard, 1932).

The Changing Picture of Schizophrenia: There has been a decrease in the incidence of severe subtypes of schizophrenia, particularly catatonia, with a concomitant increase in the paranoid subtype (see chapter 17 on Germany, this handbook). Morrison (1974) observed this trend in the records of Iowa State Psychopathic Hospital from its opening in 1920 up to 1966. Leff (1988) documented such a change in Britain. For example, in the Bethlem Royal Hospital, catatonic schizophrenia accounted for 6 percent of all admissions in the 1850s, but only 0.5 percent in the 1950s. In the South-East end of London, no case of catatonia was diagnosed among new admissions in 1976. The rates of severe types of schizophrenia is still relatively high in the developing countries. The IPSS data (WHO,

1973) indicates that the catatonic subtype was diagnosed in 22 percent of schizophrenic patients in Agra, 13 percent in Cali, and 8 percent in Ibadan, but in only about 4 percent of patients from the remaining six countries in the study. In another international study (Sartorius, Jablensky, Korten, Ernberg, Anker, Cooper, and Day, 1986), catatonia was diagnosed in 10 percent of schizophrenic cases in the developing nations, but rarely seen in developed countries. Studies in Egypt (Okasha, Kamel, and Hassan, 1968) and Sri Lanka (Chandrasena and Rodrigo, 1979) reveal that the proportion of catatonia among schizophrenic patients is 14.4 percent and 21 percent, respectively (see also chapter 7 on India, this handbook).

Is this a shift from physical expression of distress to a cognitive one as Leff (1988) had suggested (i.e., waxy flexibility, echopraxia, and echolalia are the physical equivalent of delusion of control)? Why is there a change from severe to milder subtypes of schizophrenia? Are the prevalence of subtypes of schizophrenia and their severity related to the standard of living of the population as a Norwegian psychiatrist (Saugstad, 1989) had suggested?

Chronicity and Course of Schizophrenia: It is now accepted that schizophrenia has a variable course that may be influenced by environmental factors and that understanding the stage of the disorder and the cumulative experience with the disorder and dysfunction is important. A followup of patients from different cultures may shed light on the process of chronicity or recovery from the illness.

With some exceptions (Kulhara and Wig, 1978), studies show that in the developed countries, schizophrenia is characterized by poorer prognosis than in the developing countries. The first systematic study, carried out by Murphy and Raman (1971), revealed less chronicity in the island of Mauritius than in Britain. Similarly, the IPSS (WHO, 1979) indicated better prognosis in Nigeria and India than in Britain, Czechoslovakia, Denmark, and the United States. A similar advantageous situation was found in Sri Lanka (Waxler, 1979). Differences in chronicity of schizophrenia among nations may be an artefact of the characteristics of patients studied. Are we, for example, dealing with acute reactive psychosis or are we dealing with true schizophrenia in Asia and Africa? Murphy (1980) pointed out that the IPSS study which had shown that the most technologically developed nations yielded the poorest results also included patients from these nations who had a longer average history of schizophrenia than those patients in the developing countries. However, many sociocultural factors may affect the outcome of schizophrenia such as social rejection, rigidity of role ideals (e.g. sex roles), assignment of responsibility to patients, reality testing, sick role typing (belief that insanity is chronic), acceptance of dependency, and availability of social networks (Murphy, 1982a). Although these factors are not systematically studied, some of them (social rejection, assignment of responsibility, social networks) may involve behavior similar to that in the concept of expressed emotion which is discussed next.

Expressed Emotions and Outcome. Since the pioneering work of Brown, Bone, Dalison, and Wing (1966) on expressed emotion (EE), many studies have confirmed the conclusion that measures of critical comments of relatives and the degree of hostility and emotional involvement are relevant to the relapse of patients. Cultural variations in the level of EE in different households may be related to the degree of Westernization. While the EE level in households is found to be 67 percent in Los Angeles (Vaughn, Snyder, Jones, Freeman, and Falloon, 1984) and 54 percent in Aarhus (Wig, Menon, Bedi, Ghosh, Kuipers, Leff, Korten, Day, Sartorius, Ernberg, and Jablensky, 1987), the Mexican American level was 41 percent (Karno, Jenkins, De La Selva, Santana, Telles, Lopez, and Mintz, 1987) with Indian patients scoring 30 percent and 8 percent in urban and rural areas respectively (Wig et al., 1987).

Cultural variation in EE may be related to the extent to which the patient is held responsible for his symptoms and behavior. Leff and Vaughn (1985) found that most of the critical comments are directed toward negative symptoms such as lack of affect and apathy rather than positive symptoms of hallucinations and delusions. Relatives in non-Western households may be more accepting of these negative symptoms as demonstrated among Mexican Americans by Jenkins, Karno, De La Selva, and Santana (1986). The belief in fate may also affect the reaction to patients in non-Western cultures. There is very little research on attitudes

toward mental illness, but relatives of patients studied reveal tolerance of symptoms and disabilities in the extended family in Sri
Lanka (Waxler, 1979) and in Qatar (El-Islam, 1979, 1982, 1989).
In a thoughtful critique of the study of EE across cultures, Di
Nicola (1988) pointed out that the EE concept focuses on the
negative aspects of family interaction (a reminder of Fromm-
Reichmann's schizophrenogenic mother or Bateson's double-
bind) in contrast to the positive view of the extended family in
non-Western cultures. Objective studies of the characteristics of
families and the sociocultural context in which abnormal behavior is perceived, evaluated, and reacted to may throw light on the
course and outcome of mental illness in general and schizophrenia in particular.

DEPRESSION

In contrast to schizophrenia, the term *depression* may be used to
describe a normal reaction to loss, a symptom of a disorder, or
the disorder itself. In the cross-cultural study of depression researchers have not clearly made such a distinction, and the reader
is not informed whether one is dealing with normal depressive
mood or what Kraepelin called manic-depressive insanity. While
data on schizophrenia are mainly derived from hospital records,
statistics on depression include community studies which make
the distinction between "caseness" and normal depressive mood
more difficult in national and cross-national research. Thus, the
concepts of disease (refers to biological disorder) and illness (social experience with and reaction to the disease) are more applied
to data on depression than on schizophrenia (Kleinman, 1978).
Central issues in the cross-national study of depression are the
low incidence of depression, the lack of guilt feelings, low rates
of suicide and prominence of somatization in non-Western cultures, and the lack of universal validity of the concept of depression (Englesman, 1982).

It is difficult to reach conclusions about the rates of depression in different Western countries because of diagnostic preferences among psychiatrists. The U.S.–U.K. study (Cooper, Kendell,
Gurland, Sharpe, Copeland, and Simon, 1972) demonstrated a

bias toward the diagnosis of affective disorder among British psychiatrists. While American psychiatrists diagnosed 16.6 percent of consecutive admissions as depressed, British psychiatrists gave the same diagnosis to 46.2 percent of a comparable sample of admissions. However, there has been an awareness that the rates of depression have been increasing while those of schizophrenia are decreasing. Studies indicate an increase in the number of manic-depressive patients during this century in Norway (Saugstad, 1989), Denmark (Weeke, Bille, Videech, and Juel-Nielsen, 1975), Sweden (Hagnell, Lanke, Rorsman, and Oyesjo, 1982), and the United States (Klerman, 1978). Hagnell et al. (1982) felt that this increase is so alarming that they entitled their article "Are We Entering an Age of Melancholy?" In contrast, a decrease in the number of hospitalized schizophrenics was reported in Norway (Saugstad, 1989), Denmark (Stromgren, 1987), and Scotland (Eagles and Whalley, 1985).

In non-Western countries and particularly in Africa, early studies reported that true psychotic depression is absent or rare, and when it does occur it is less severe and of short duration (Prince, 1968). However, studies since 1957 revealed higher rates of depression in these countries than in the West. One early example is the study of Leighton et al. (1963) who found depressive symptoms to be four times more frequent among a Nigerian sample than a Canadian one. Orley and Wing (1979) found the rates of depression in Ugandan villages more than double that in London. The reason for the shift in African rates of depression is not clear and the question posed by Prince (1968) ("Is it fact or diagnostic fashion?") remains unanswered.

However, it is agreed that depression is common in non-Western countries but takes a different form from European depression. Non-Western depressive patients show less verbalization of depressive mood, less guilt and more projection, and more somatic symptoms with rare suicidal behavior (Singer, 1975). Reports from Africa reviewed by Singer indicate that depressive patients show paranoid and somatic symptoms in the Senegal, a high frequency of self-accusation of witchcraft in Ghana, and shame rather than guilt in the Sudan. Reports of low guilt feelings in non-Western nations are not consistent (Kim, 1977; Teja, Narang, and Aggrawal, 1971; Rao, 1978). Kim (1977) reported that

Korean patients expressed as much guilt as those in England and the United States and double those manifested by Indian patients. Teja et al. (1971) and Rao (1978) reported regional differences in the expression of guilt in India with some high rates similar to England. Similarly, Kimura (1965) found that guilt is as frequent among Japanese as among German depressives. Is the picture of guilt and self-accusation changing in non-Western countries in a similar fashion to the one described by Murphy (1978) in his history of the symptom in Western countries? Followup and cross-generational study of depressive patients in Asia and Africa is needed to find out changes in symptoms including guilt feelings and self-accusation.

In contrast to the absence of guilt and self-accusation, the prevalence of delusions of persecution in Asian and African patients may reflect "normal" personality trends as opposed to being limited to depression. In many African societies, people are encouraged to attribute misfortune to witchcraft, and therefore patients with different psychopathologies show "paranoid" trends without blaming themselves (see chapter 6, this handbook). Similarly, self-accusation among some Africans may have nothing to do with psychopathology: people with distress including depressives may visit healing shrines to confess and accuse themselves of sins in a stereotyped manner (Field, 1960).

Low rates of suicide are consistently reported in chapters in this handbook on Asia and Africa. They were also reported by Collomb and Collignon (1974), Laubscher (1937), Chaplin (1961), and Asuni (1961). Asuni reported 1 per 100,000 among the Yoruba tribe in Nigeria. Some studies, however, show high rates in Africa, similar to those in Europe (Weinberg, 1965; Rweg-ellera, 1978).

One explanation of low rates of suicide in Asian and African countries is the low feeling of guilt and self-depreciation of depressive patients (see parts II and III of this handbook). Another explanation of low rates in some countries such as the Irish Republic and Moslem countries concerns the condemnation of suicide by Catholicism and the Moslem religion, respectively. However, when suicide is considered as a sin in a culture, this may result in its underreporting. As McCarthy and Walsh (1975) concluded, the actual rates of suicide in Dublin are between two or four times higher than the official figures. One may also wonder about other Christian countries where suicide is considered a sin but the rates of suicide tend to be high.

There is a strong relationship between mental illness, particularly depression, and alcohol and drug abuse on the one hand and suicide on the other. This is clearly evident among aboriginal people of Australia, New Zealand, and North America (see chapters 12, 22 and 23, this handbook). We may be witnessing an increase in suicidal acts on a worldwide level which is concomitant with recent increases in depression, social pathology, and personality disorders (Saugstad, 1989; Paris, 1991).

Finally, a question is raised whether the concept of depression is valid across cultures. It has been suggested by many authors (Kleinman and Good, 1985) that Western psychiatry attempts to medicalize human suffering by considering depression as an illness. For example, Good, Good, and Moradi (1985) consider depressive mood as a normal religious sentiment among Iranians. Similarly, Obeyesekere (1985) pointed out that some of the symptoms of depression such as hopelessness and loss of a sense of pleasure may not be considered abnormal by a Buddhist. Thus depression, according to these authors, should not be studied in another culture without consideration of the cultural context and the meaning of the experience of sadness. These approaches to depression raise the important question of whether sociocultural interpretation and meaning changes the nature of an illness. In other words, when the psychiatrist sees depression, but the Hutterites perceive the hands of the devil tempting the patient (*anfechtung*) (Eaton and Weil, 1955), do these different perceptions change the nature of the physical or emotional suffering of the victim? This question is important in the study of culture-specific syndromes which will be dealt with in another section.

SOMATIZATION

The term *somatization* is part of Western medical terminology and has its roots in psychodynamic theories which suggest that emotions may be repressed and intrapsychic conflicts may be converted into physical symptoms and thus mask the expression of emotions. A "geography of somatization" summarizing major available research in the non-Western world reveals higher levels of somatization than in the Western world (Kirmayer, 1984). In contrast, Western middle-class patients are reported to psychologize. However, a high level of somatization is also found in the West. It is reported that somatization among Western patients constitutes up to three fourths of patients' visits to primary health care physicians, particularly among those patients from low socioeconomic status and educational levels, rural origins, active and traditional religious affiliation, and of certain ethnicity (Harwood, 1981; Katon, Kleinman and Rosen, 1982; Katon, Ries, and Kleinman, 1984; Kleinman and Kleinman, 1985). Krähl (chapter 17, this handbook) reported that a study revealed no difference between somatic symptoms reported by Indonesian and German patients. It may be that somatization attracted more attention among non-Western nations because of its dramatic nature, for example, feeling maggots in the head, crawling feelings, and burning sensations (see chapters on Jamaica and black Africa in this handbook).

Somatization in non-Western cultures was explained in terms of the inability of some people to express emotional distress. The evidence that there is no word equivalent to *depression* in Chinese or Yoruba, a Nigerian language, during the IPSS (WHO, 1973), was used to support such an explanation. Leff (1973, 1988) further reported that the Chinese and Nigerian languages which are not Indo-European do not differentiate between some emotions as compared with other languages (he reported higher correlation between depression, anxiety, and irritability among Chinese and Nigerian subjects as compared with groups from other nations (England, India, Denmark). He suggested that some languages other than the Indo-European have not evolved to a point to differentiate emotional states.

Although language may facilitate the expression of emotions, other sociocultural factors may be involved, since somatization is reported in many cultures with rich emotional vocabulary (e.g., Arabic). One factor emphasized by the authors in this handbook on India, Korea, and the Maoris of New Zealand is that in many traditional theories of medicine, somatopsychic rather than psychological aspects of disease are emphasized. Physical complaints may also have an adaptive social function rather than being a defense against anxiety as conceived by psychodynamic theories. Indeed, they may not "mask" social problems, but serve as devices to draw attention to them. As Koss (1990) pointed out, physical symptoms serve as a key to the social ecology of illness and may form a link between the individual, the social, and the political spheres (Scheper-Hughes and Lock, 1987). For example, Guarnaccia and Farias (1988) have shown that the social meanings of "nervois" among Salvadorian refugees included family and work issues, fears for relatives left in El Salvador, and social commentary on racism and problems of adjustment to life in the United States.

Somatization has been most frequently studied among Asian subjects (Japanese and Chinese). Kawanishi (1992) argued how physical complaints among these peoples have been decontextualized, being studied within a Western frame of reference. The stereotype of Asians as "quiet, shy, deferential and passive" (Sue and Morishima, 1982) may have led to the conclusion that they do not express emotions as overtly as Americans. In many Eastern cultures, open display of emotions in social interactions is undesirable. Somatic symptoms also reduce the stigma of mental illness and legitimize entry into health care (Cheung, 1984). In contrast to mental symptoms, which mean stigmatized mental illness, physical pain is an opportunity to reintegrate the sick person into the social support group and to reaffirm the norms of solidarity and social control in many societies.

Western versus non-Western differences in somatization may be related to cultural differences in causal attribution of distress to somatic or social events by non-Western people rather than to intrapsychic emotional experiences. White (1982) asked Hong Kong Chinese and American students to sort out thirty common illness complaints and psychosocial problems according to their similarity and then proposed a cause for them. There was a tendency among Americans to give emotional causes to physical problems, while the Chinese reported external or situational causes such as "pressures" related to academic concerns. Thus the difference between Western and non-Western groups may reflect differences in causal attribution rather than somatization versus psychologization as claimed by Western researchers.

CULTURE AND ALCOHOL

Alcoholic beverages may serve a wide range of functions across cultures (social organization, recreation, religious and symbolic functions) but its excessive use results in devastating social and physical effects. A major cross-cultural finding is that addiction to alcohol and problem drinking seems to be quite rare outside certain societies of Western civilization (Mandelbaum, 1965; Barry, 1982; Heath, 1986). In many societies where drinking is customary and drunkenness is common, people do not develop withdrawal symptoms or compulsive drinking. The adverse outcomes of the use of alcohol seem to be mediated by sociocultural factors. The occurrence of pathology in a substantial proportion of the people of a society may be related to the presence of each of three conditions: motivation to drink, which causes people to crave severe intoxication; cultural permissiveness and encouragement of alcohol intoxication; and the availability of sufficient alcohol.

The agricultural economic base in Western nations can produce as much alcohol as the population is physiologically capable of consuming. Accordingly, the differences in the drinking customs among these nations seem to be influenced more by variations in social control than availability of alcohol, thus requiring the study of attitudes, values, and behavior associated with drinking. The importance of sociocultural factors in relation to drinking may be illustrated by the contrast between Jews and Irish Americans. Bales (1946) emphasized Orthodox Jewish intrafamilial introduction of children to wine in a sacred ritual context in contrast with the Irish pattern where children are not supposed to drink, but in their adolescence they have to prove their manhood in the secular context of the pub. Since the 1970s, however, a decrease in religious orthodoxy which had weakened the ritual significance of drinking as well as the loosening of family ties, which had undermined parental norms for moderation, had changed the stereotype of Jewish drinking (Blume and Dropkin, 1980; Blume, Dropkin, and Sokolow, 1980). Earlier, Snyder (1958) reported that drinking problems are very rare among Orthodox Jews and progressively more frequent among Conservative, Reform, and Secular Jews. In Israel, it was long reported that problem drinking was rare except among Yemenites (Hes, 1970). Could understanding the Jewish attitude toward drinking and teaching it to the public lead to moderation and prevent problem drinking in Western nations? Moslem countries, where the religion dictates complete abstinence, are known for low rates of alcoholism. However, problems related to drinking are increasing in Moslem countries where strict prohibition is practiced such as in Kuwait (Bilal and El-Islam, 1985; Bilal and Angelo-Khattar, 1989).

Most societies in North America and the Insular Pacific had no alcoholic beverages until the advent of Europeans. Episodes of extreme drunkenness and violence by American Indians resulted in the destruction of individuals and communities, but many people and tribes survived the disruptive effects of liquor and other problems brought about by Europeans (MacAndrew and Edgerton, 1969; Leland, 1976; see chapter 22, this handbook). Although drinking problems are prevalent among American Indians, the majority tend to drink moderately or not at all. The influence of Europeans was less destructive on societies of the Insular Pacific; this is attributed to the more rigid social stratification which might have counteracted the disorganizing effects of alcohol intoxication (Barry, 1982). In Africa, strong spirits were introduced by colonialists and often exchanged for slaves and indigenous merchandise (Tongue, 1976), but their effects varied from one community to another. Alcoholism is more of a problem among Christians and Animists than among Moslems (e.g., the Ivory Coast). There is a high rate of alcoholism among black South Africans (Ben-Arie, Swartz, Teggin, and Elk, 1983; McCabe, 1982) in contrast to West Africans (Leighton, Lambo, Hughes, Leighton, Murphy, and Macklin, 1963). In addition to cultural factors, the "dop" system used in South Africa, whereby part of the wages of a worker are paid as alcohol, also constituted a risk factor (Swartz, 1987). The increase of problem drinking among Moslems in South Africa is due in part to Westernization. Midgley (1971) found that 13 percent of a Moslem community in Cape Town violated religious prohibitions of drinking. Most drinkers lived in a predominantly Christian neighborhood and did not attend the mosque regularly.

Ethnic sensitivity to the short-term physiological effects of ethanol may demonstrate the interaction between biological and cultural factors. Response to alcohol, which is indicated by intense facial flushing, increased heart rate, and the activation of the sympathetic nervous system, is found more among mongoloids than caucasoids. Intense response to alcohol is found among Japanese, Taiwanese, and Koreans (Wolff, 1972), the Eastern Cree tribe of North American Indians (Wolff, 1973), Chinese (Zeiner, Paredes, and Christensen, 1979), and Japanese (Mizoi, Ijiri, Tatsuno, Kijima, Fujiwara, and Adachi, 1979), but this effect is not a universal characteristic of this large racial category. Sensitivity to alcohol may have contributed to the absence of alcohol consumption aboriginally among most North American Indian tribes and rarity of heavy drinking among the Chinese. However, heavy drinking has characterized many mongoloid nations (Japanese, Koreans, American Indians) since the introduction of distilled spirits by Europeans (Yamamoto, Eng-Kug, Chung-Kyoon, and Keh-Ming, 1988).

Differences in drinking patterns among nations may result in different alcohol-related pathology as indicated by the rates of liver cirrhosis. Murphy (1982b) ranked countries in terms of cirrhosis of the liver related to alcohol consumption. He found that nearly all high-ranking countries are wine drinking (Chile, Mexico, France), while the low-ranking ones are not (Iceland, Ireland, England, and Wales). The main difference between wine-drinking and other alcohol-consuming societies is that the former regard wine as part of their daily nourishment to be taken mainly at meals, while the latter tend to regard alcohol as an aid to recreation, mostly consumed outside mealtimes. One result is the quantity consumed per capita tends to be considerably higher in wine-drinking nations than in those that depend on beer and spirits, and mortality rates from cirrhosis and from other aspects of alcoholism are a simple function of the amount of alcohol consumed (a correlation of 0.85 between mortality from cirrhosis and per capita consumption of alcohol among 17 countries was found by Noble [1979]). However, there are some exceptions. Noble found that Austria, which is compared with Italy, has 38 percent less alcohol consumption, but 14 percent more mortality from cirrhosis. Regional variations (16 regions) in an early study in France by Sadoun, Lolli, and Silverman (1965) show an inverse relationship between absolute alcohol consumed and death rates from alcoholism and cirrhosis of the liver ($r = -0.69$). Two areas in the north (Normandy plus Brittany and Alsace) had the highest death rates and the lowest consumption. Four areas in the south had the lowest death rates but an above-average consumption. Southern France is more similar to Italy in its drinking pattern than the northern part of France.

Consumption per capita, however, does not seem to be a valid measure of the tendency of a nation for *excessive* drinking, and it is possible that high consumption per capita is only allowed in countries where controlled drinking without severe intoxication is well established as the social norm. A more valid measure of the tendency for excessive drinking in nations seems to be the frequency of problems associated with alcohol such as hospitalization for alcoholism, arrests for drunkenness, and traffic accidents with alcohol involvements. These problems are limited to a deviant minority of individuals and generally are found more in nations where per capita alcohol consumption is relatively low (Barry, 1982). Thus, the frequency of drinking may be limited more stringently in these nations where many individuals have a stronger desire to experience severe intoxication. For example, in comparison to Italy, the per capita alcohol consumption is much less in Poland, but the frequency of drunkenness (blood alcohol above 0.1%) is more than twice as high (Sulkunen, 1976). Several measures of problems of drunkenness (Nobel, 1979) reveal that the most severe problems occur in countries with low rates of alcohol consumption. Alcohol consumption may be related to more pathology and mental illness in cultures where there are negative attitudes toward or even complete abstinence from alcohol such as in the Moslem countries (Al-Issa, 1990).

CULTURE-SPECIFIC SYNDROMES

Culture-specific syndromes raise the general question whether the Western psychiatric classification is culture-free and could be applied to all nations and cultures and thus could integrate varieties of behavior outside the Western sphere. Although it is now

accepted that the major types of mental illness are found in different nations and cultures, there is certain abnormal behavior that
does not fit within the Western classification of mental illness.
Pfeiffer (1982) suggested that certain syndromes could not be
arranged into a classification system because cultural factors contribute differentially to their etiology (culture-specific areas of
stress), their formation (culture-specific shaping of symptoms),
and their interpretations and treatment. Interpretation and treatment should have nothing to do with designating behavior as
culture-specific because they may vary from one culture to another for the same disorder. Schizophrenia, for example, may be
considered in different cultures as mental exhaustion (treated by
rest), love sickness (treated by marriage), as a bewitched state or
a result of confrontation with a ghost or a curse placed on the
family (treated by exorcism, sacrifice, prayer, and so on), but that
should not change the nature of the illness.

However, the concept of culture-specific syndrome may be
restricted to culturally determined behavior with culture-specific
symptoms (Prince and Tcheng-Laroche, 1987). Many examples
of culturally determined syndromes and symptoms are given in
this volume from Africa, India, and South East Asia. For example,
it is difficult to fit into the DSM-III-R the belief that one is missing
one's genitals after an encounter with a stranger (see chapter 3).
Such a belief is shared by the group who usually lynch the accused, making it difficult to label such a belief as delusional. According to this approach, the application of the concept of
culture-specific syndromes should not be limited to exotic parts
of the world, but could be applied to Western deviant behavior
as a result of Western conditions. Many authors (Swartz, 1985;
Johnson, 1987; Fabrega, 1989) drew attention to the bias in Anglo-American psychiatry where the concept of culture-specific syndrome is applied ethnocentrically to exotic behavior in other
cultures which does not conform to Western classification systems. They suggested that many Anglo-American disorders are
culture-specific. Fabrega (1989) pointed out that Anglo-American
society may produce socially or psychologically deviant behavior
such as Type-A behavior which is "partly an exaggeration of a
time pressured, work driven capitalistic seeking for maximization

of profits'' and eating disorder behaviors which represent "internalized runaway conflicts between biological imperatives and conventional valuations of body physique." Other authors (Swartz, 1985; Littlewood and Lipsedge, 1986; Johnson, 1987) mention many culture-specific syndromes in the West such as premenstrual syndrome and anorexia nervosa, overdose, shoplifting, agoraphobia in women, and domestic siege (cases of child abduction by the father after custody has been awarded to the wife in a divorce settlement), and exhibitionism in men.

Some culture-specific syndromes are clearly related to Western concepts of mental illness (for example, nuptial psychosis, an acute reactive psychosis in women which results from the stress of arranged marriage in North Africa and India [Pfeiffer, 1982], and eating disorders which are now appearing in Africa with a rise in both standard of living and depression [Gregory and Buchan, 1984; Famuyiwa, 1988]). Others may reflect the psychiatric orientation of the observer. Consider, for example, amok in the Malay archipelago. From the sixteenth to the eighteenth centuries amok was traditionally considered as pemeditated behavior with an obvious link between precipitating events and the violent episode, with no signs of mental illness (Murphy, 1973). It is only later, with the introduction of the European criminal law, that a necessity arose for differentiating between acts of violence committed in a state of clear consciousness and those carried out in confusion (Pfeiffer, 1982). Amok as a culture-specific syndrome raises the question whether homicidal manic reaction or panic, which occurs in many parts of the world, should be considered culture-specific syndromes, since mass killing is a social pathology which occurs in different parts of the world (Prince, 1991a) and is not specific to certain countries. Some "syndromes" may represent a myth (Windigo, for example, is a giant man-eating ogre among the Algonquin-speaking Indians of north-eastern Canada [Teicher, 1960]) or an etiological factor to explain illness (Pobough lang, for example, is earth eating among the Serer in the Senegal) (Beiser, Burr, Collomb, and Ravel, 1974) rather than an illness.

IMMIGRANTS AND ETHNIC MINORITIES

With political upheavals, wars, and economic disparity between Western and non-Western nations, our century has witnessed massive population movements that have never been seen in the history of mankind. Immigrants and ethnic minorities have to deal with the stress of adaptations, new language and customs, rejection by the host and dominant group, confusion of one's roles, values and feelings, and the sense of helplessness and ineffectuality in dealing with the new culture (Draguns, 1980). The sense of loss, disruption, and danger may be added to the problems of forced migrants and refugees. However, it has been shown that experiences in the host country during the first years of resettlement seem to have more effect on mental health than past experience before migration (Westermeyer, Vang and Neider, 1983a,b; Beiser, Turner, and Ganesan, 1989).

While early studies of immigrants and refugees used to deal with European populations, the majority of immigrants and refugees in the West now come from Asian, African, and Latin American countries that had been subjected previously to Western colonialism, racism, and discrimination. Historically, Western civilization which is symbolized by industrial supremacy and Christian morality is believed by its proponents to constitute an ultimate stage of human evolution and therefore considered other races and cultures as inferior. Although this traditional belief in hierarchical cultures and civilizations is not officially recognized by Western nations, and race is not overtly mentioned as a factor regarding immigrants, the policies of some countries may be guided by a subtle cultural neoracism in which it is believed that the characteristics and identity of ethnic groups have to be preserved, defended, and developed. For example, white identity could be preserved by separating communities and applying a multicultural policy which is a byproduct of a racial concept of society. This was openly observed in South Africa where such a policy was used as a smokescreen for discrimination (see chapter 4, this handbook).

The degree to which immigrants could assimilate into the dominant culture is related to the reaction of the host society and national differences in racism. This is an area of research that has been neglected by social scientists. In an early study of social distance (the degree of acceptance of various groups) with American subjects whose parents came from different parts of Europe, Triandis and Triandis (1960) found that 77 percent of the variance in the social distance scores was accounted for by race, about 17 percent by occupation, 5 percent by religion, and 15 percent by nationality. Analyses for individuals of various backgrounds showed substantial differences in emphasis on these factors. Subjects whose parents came from Southern and Eastern Europe emphasized occupation and religion more than those subjects whose parents came from Northern and Western Europe; the latter emphasized race more than the former. Could these attitudes determine the acceptance or rejection of immigrants as well as government policies of immigration? Consider the British and French concepts of immigrants. The British concept is based on differentiating between British natives and immigrants in racial terms, while the French differentiation is based on cultural terms such as religion and customs, where the differences between natives and immigrants are less absolute and less permanent than the racial ones. These concepts of the immigrants may facilitate and encourage assimilation (the French) or hinder it (the British) by keeping ethnic groups separate.

It is of interest to compare the mental health of immigrants in countries that follow multicultural policies, such as Britain and Canada, and those that follow an assimilation policy such as France and the United States. Pakistanis in Britain, for example, seem to have relatively low rates of mental illness, and it is interesting to compare them with their North African Moslem counterparts in France. Similarly, Latin Americans who are exposed to the melting pot policy (pressure to lose one's identity) of the United States also tend to have low rates of mental illness. However, blacks in both Britain and the United States tend to have higher rates of mental illness than the general population (Vega and Rumbant, 1991). The low rates of mental illness among Indians and Pakistanis in Britain and Latin Americans in the United States is attributed to the protective features of the extended family (Rack, 1982; Vega and Rumbant, 1991). Whether the high rates of schizophrenia among West Indians in Britain or blacks in the United States are due to true prevalence or an artefact of other factors, such as overdiagnosis of several pathology in blacks, is still an unsettled issue (see chapter 24, this handbook). Indeed, a British author has recently suggested biological factors such as obstetric complications or infectious agents to explain the relationship between schizophrenia and immigration (Eagles, 1991). Race, social class, and stress of immigration may interact in a subtle way to result in the diagnosis of schizophrenia among blacks. There is a tendency to give persons who are black or from a lower class a diagnosis of psychosis rather than neurosis (Baldwin, Floyd, and McSeveny, 1975; Wilkinson, 1975; Littlewood, 1993) or schizophrenia rather than affective disorder (Simon, Fleiss, Gurland, Stiller, and Sharpe, 1973; Bell and Mehta, 1981; Littlewood, 1993). It is possible that police harassment of the black poor and the hostile attitudes of the white population may arouse fear and anger which may be pathologized by the psychiatrists and be designated as paranoia (Fernando, 1991). This may explain the finding in Britain that when the symptoms of West Indians and Africans with schizophrenia were compared with those of natives, the former show an excess of only one psychotic symptom, delusion of persecution (Carpenter and Brockington, 1980). Unless the mental health of immigrants is compared with that in their country of origin, it is difficult to reach conclusions about the relative contribution of psychological stress versus predisposition toward mental illness among immigrants (Ödegaard, 1932). Evidence of the relationship between discrimination against minorities and psychiatric diagnosis is illustrated in many chapters of this book in countries such as Australia, Britain, Israel, South Africa, and the United States.

CONCLUSION

Chapters in this volume illustrate that reaction patterns labeled psychopathological are universal. All over the world, there are people who hallucinate; who express improbable beliefs and delusions, who become fearful, anxious, and depressed, and who reveal excesses or deficits in behavior. The forms of typical symptoms of mental illness seem to be recognizable in different cultural settings. Major mental health problems and concerns all over the world also seem to be quite similar: schizophrenia, depression, suicide, alcoholism, culture-specific syndromes, mental illness among ethnic minorities and immigrants, and so on. Yet, comparative international research involves specific issues and poses several problems which I selectively deal with in this section.

Some useful data in this handbook are concerned with international variation of the rates of mental illness, but these rates may not give a picture of true prevalence or incidence in many countries. The availability of psychiatric services and the degree of tolerance of a given level of dysfunction by the population tend to affect statistics on the rates of mental illness in different nations. This is more so in the developing countries where psychiatric services are limited to a small segment of the population and where alternative native treatment is more available and being frequently used by the population.

Another problem in comparing national data is the transcultural unreliability of psychiatric diagnosis. The professional training of psychiatrists may affect the range of conditions subsumed under a disorder and the threshold of perception of its symptoms. However, serious attempts have been made to make diagnosis more objective in cross-national studies such as those of the U.S.–U.K. project and the WHO studies of schizophrenia and depression. In the WHO projects, psychiatrists from different nations were uniformly trained to interview patients objectively in order to increase the reliability of diagnosis.

Another criticism of diagnosis in international research of mental illness is related to its validity. The WHO studies as well as major research in the developing countries tend to give little consideration to the cultural context by imposing Western diagnostic categories as if they were universal entities, completely ignoring cultural differences between nations. It is not the universality of symptoms of mental illness that is questioned, but it is how they are perceived, evaluated, and reacted to by the patient and his compatriots (Kleinman, 1977; Littlewood, 1990). In Jamaica (chapter 14, this handbook), talking to oneself or believing that someone is out to harm you is a normative behavior. In Mexico (chapter 15, this handbook), psychosis is integrated into religious practice and acquires religious meaning.

How the cultural context influences the meaning of symptoms is expressed by Draguns (1982) as follows:

The proponents of the social learning point of view have reminded us (Higginbotham and Tanaka-Matsumi, 1981; Higginbotham, 1979) that no behavior automatically constitutes a symptom, and that it only becomes an indicator of experienced distress or of perceived disturbance in the course of transaction with the environment. Al-Issa (1977, 1978) demonstrated that hallucinations differ in the social response that they provoke across space and time. Cultural factors facilitate the expression of hallucinations through a sense modality, visual or auditory, and determine their acceptance as normal behavior or even as a supernormal gift, or their rejection as a manifestation of disturbance. It is therefore important to specify where and how the allegedly symptomatic behavior occurs and how it is conceived, labeled, and responded to, both by the person most immediately concerned and by his or her peers. Equally essential is the specification of behaviors and events that have preceded and followed the alleged symptom. Finally, the setting in which the symptomatic behavior occurred must be indicated [p. 52].

Thus, an objective study of symptoms with no consideration of their antecedents or consequences may affect the validity of diagnosis. The WHO study of schizophrenia, indicating better outcome of schizophrenia with no adequate treatment in the developing countries compared with the developed countries, raises the speculation that either schizophrenia is not an illness which is equivalent cross-culturally, or diagnosing schizophrenia as an illness has no predictive validity (Fernando, 1991).

The cultural and ethnic background of the researcher and clinician may influence diagnosis when it is different from that of the subject. The overdiagnosis of severe mental illness and the perception of more impairment in ethnic minorities is an example. Thus differences in the rates of mental illness may be the result of the observer's bias rather than true ethnic differences. Fortunately, the number of psychiatrists from different ethnic groups in Western nations is increasing, and non-Western nations have now their own indigenous psychiatrists. However, psychiatrists in the developing countries obtain their training in specific Western centers (British and American centers dominate the scene), and this may influence international findings. For instance, if the WHO study of schizophrenia had included French psychiatrists where the diagnosis of *bouffée délirante* is recognized, its results and conclusions would have been different. An interdisciplinary approach to mental illness is also needed in order to involve other mental health professionals. The orientation of transnational psychiatric research has been mainly medically oriented, such as the research teams of WHO consisting of only psychiatrists who have influenced the design of its projects and excluded the investigation of psychological, social, and cultural factors.

There is little international research on the effectiveness of psychiatric treatment as compared with native healing practices or on patient-healer relationships in the developing countries. Many authors have discussed similarities between factors involved in Western and non-Western psychotherapies (Frank, 1961; Calestro, 1972; Torrey, 1972; Wittkower and Warnes, 1974; Prince, 1980) (all psychotherapies involve the shared-world view, the warm personal relationship between healer and patient, the expectant hope of the patient, and the high prestige of the healer), but little evaluative outcome research is carried out on native healing. It may be that native healers have advantages over Western trained psychiatrists (see chapter 14, this handbook). With few exceptions of some attempts to integrate native healers into psychiatric settings in Africa and Asia, the emphasis of psychiatric treatment in the developing countries is on organic treatment. Electroconvulsive therapy is still used in the developing countries to treat a variety of psychiatric illnesses and is described by one author (chapter 7, this handbook) as a "safe, cheap and quick" method of treatment. The frequent use of organic treatment in these countries raises the question of whether the tendency of patients to somatize is in part a reaction to the physician who reinforces physical symptoms and helps patients to legitimize their sick role and avoid the stigma of madness. Studies of Chinese patients showing that they report psychological symptoms to friends and relatives but not to physicians suggest that somatization is situation-specific (patient–physician encounters) and could not be generalized to symptoms reported to native healers. It seems that in the developing nations, the majority of patients see a native healer before or simultaneously with a physician (India and Nigeria as examples) and it would be useful to study the report of symptoms to these healers and investigate their consistency with those reported in a psychiatric interview. As in Bali, Indonesia (chapter 13, this handbook), there is a need for "clinical culturation" where a mutual respect may develop between psychiatrists and native healers. In the treatment of Susto in Mexico (chapter 15, this handbook), it was observed that a combination of psychiatric treatment with a symbolic approach to restore the soul is also recognized by psychiatrists.

Problems of acculturation of ethnic groups, minorities, and native people started with colonialism where one powerful ethnic group dominated another. Colonialization brought industrialization, urbanization, and the disruption of stable traditional life patterns and created an environment where hierarchical theories of cultures and civilizations were flourishing (Nazi Germany and apartheid in South Africa were extreme examples of this ideology). The world is now witnessing major population movement of immigrants and refugees as well as a cultural and an ethnic consciousness and pride of minorities within nations. Yet, the striving of these groups to assert themselves or adapt to a new environment may have its costs in terms of mental health. Research is urgently needed to disentangle factors associated with policies of assimilation (e.g., in France) or muticulturalism (e.g., in Britain) that may contribute positively or negatively to the mental health and the adaptation of immigrants and refugees. The study of posttraumatic stress disorder as a result of recent political upheavals and wars (in East Europe and the Middle East) is also urgently needed.

Studies of the influence of culture on normal cognitive, affective, somatic, and motor (behavioral) reaction patterns should form the basis for understanding and differentiating normality from abnormalities across cultures. The study of normal reaction patterns may lead to the understanding of cultural variation in the expression of distress. For example, cultural differences in the expression of cognitive and somatic symptoms may simply reflect a normal cultural bias and the exaggeration of reaction patterns that are common in the normal population (Al-Issa, 1982). In cross-cultural psychiatry, normal coping responses are often confused with symptoms of mental illness. Consider, for example, the description of some West African societies as having a paranoid or persecution complex (see chapter 6, this handbook). This complex may be related to the habit of the population to attribute their problems to witchcraft and consequently blame others, but it has no relationship with psychopathology. If "paranoid" trends do exist in the normal populations of some regions (e.g., in Africa or the Middle East), their study would be as relevant to the understanding of international tension as to mental illness and its treatment. Similarly, in other parts of West Africa, people go to healing shrines to confess their sins, and mental patients, like other clients, may accuse themselves of sins, but these accusations have nothing to do with depression or mental illness (Field, 1960; Piault, 1975).

There is an increasing number of Western psychiatrists, psychologists, and other professionals carrying out research and consultation in the developing countries. Therefore, understanding norms of behavior of various ethnic groups and cultures is necessary to avoid the risk of confusing normality and abnormality (Dubovsky, 1983). Hasty research in the developing countries is often carried out for the benefit of the researcher rather than to meet the expectations of the host professionals and the native population (Beiser, 1977). Publications with limited and superficial information about a culture (after short visits by Western researchers) are unethical.

Finally, with the present increase in international cooperation, the cross-cultural method (Whiting, 1954), which has long been used by anthropologists in the study of preliterate societies, could be usefully applied in international comparison of mental illness. Though this technique is rarely used in international research where each nation could be taken as a single unit, it has many advantages over studies within a nation using single individuals. In the cross-cultural method the index of the rates of mental illness in a nation represents the average among its many individuals and over a span of many years, so that the measure is likely to be more stable and reliable than a tendency of single individuals within a nation. Another advantage in comparing nations is that cultural features that may be related to mental illness show wider variations among nations than within a single nation hence permitting a more comprehensive test of their significance. In comparing nations in one region with similar cultural background (for example Scandinavian countries, Middle East countries, Italy and France), the cross-cultural method also provides an approximation of a natural experiment where all variables are kept constant except the ones under investigation. In this case, researchers from the same region could play a major role in the design and execution of the study. The world is witnessing many sociocultural changes which may result in similar changes in the types and forms of mental illness (e.g., changes in subtypes of schizophrenia and in the symptoms of affective disorders, somatization, and eating disorders), and the cross-cultural method may provide excellent means of tackling many international research problems.

REFERENCES

Al-Issa, I. (1977), Social and cultural aspects of hallucinations. *Psychol. Bull.*, 84:570–587.
——— (1978), Sociocultural factors in hallucinations. *Internat. J. Soc. Psychiat.*, 24:167–176.
——— (1982), Does culture make a difference in psychopathology? In: *Culture and Psychopathology*, ed. I. Al-Issa. Baltimore, MD: University Park Press.
——— (1990), Culture and mental illness in Algeria. *Internat. J. Soc. Psychiat.*, 36:230–246.
American Psychiatric Association (1980), *Diagnostic and Statistical Manual of Mental Disorders*, 3rd ed. Washington, DC: American Psychiatric Association Press.
——— (1987), *Diagnostic and Statistical Manual of Mental Disoders*, 3rd ed., rev. Washington, DC: American Psychiatric Association Press.
American Psychiatric Association Task Force on DSM-IV (1992), DSM-IV options book; Work in progress 9/1/91. Washington, DC: American Psychiatric Association Press.
Asuni, T. (1961), Suicide in Western Nigeria. In: *First Pan African Psychiatric Report*, ed. T. A. Lambo. Ibadan: Government Printers.

Baldwin, B. A., Floyd, H. H., & McSeveny, D. R. (1975), Status inconsistency and psychiatric diagnosis: A structural approach to labeling theory. *J. Health & Soc. Behav.*, 16:257–261.

Bales, R. F. (1946), Cultural differences in rates of alcoholism. *Quart. J. Study Alcohol*, 6:480–499.

Barry, H., III (1982), Cultural variations in alcohol abuse. In: *Culture and Psychopathology*, ed. I. Al-Issa. Baltimore, MD: University Park Press.

Beiser, M. (1977), Ethics in cross-cultural research. In: *Current Perspectives in Cultural Psychiatry*, ed. E. F. Fouks, R. M. Wintrob, J. Westermeyer, & A. R. Favazza. New York: Spectrum.

——— Burr, W. A., Collomb, H., & Ravel, J. L. (1974), Pobough lang in Senegal. *Soc. Psychiat.*, 9:123–129.

——— Turner, R. J., & Ganesan, S. (1989), Catastrophic stress and factors affecting its consequences among Southeast Asian refugees. *Soc. Sci. & Med.*, 28:183–194.

Belknap, I. (1956), *Human Problems of a State Mental Hospital.* New York: McGraw-Hill.

Bell, C. C., & Mehta, H. (1981), Misdiagnosis of black patients with manic-depressive illness: Second in a series. *J. Nat. Med. Assn.*, 73:101–107.

Ben-Arie, O., Swartz, L., Teggin, A. F., & Elk, R. (1983), The colored elderly in Cape Town—A psychosocial, psychiatric, and medical community survey. Part II: Prevalence of psychiatric disorders. *South African Med. J.*, 64:1056–1064.

Benedict, P. K., & Jacks, I. (1954), Mental illness in primitive societies. *Psychiatry*, 17:377–389.

Berne, E. (1959), Difficulties of comparative psychiatry. *Amer. J. Psychiat.*, 116:104–109.

Bilal, A. M., & Angelo-Khattar, M. (1989), Correlates of alcohol-related casualties in Kuwait. *Acta Psychiat. Scand.*, 71:1–4.

——— El-Islam, M. F. (1985), Some clinical and behavioural aspects of patients with alcohol dependence problems in Kuwait psychiatric hospital. *Alcohol & Alcoholism*, 20:57–62.

Blume, S. B., & Dropkin, D. (1980), The Jewish alcoholic: An unrecognized minority? *J. Psychiat. Treat. Eval.*, 2:1–4.

——— ——— Sokolow, L. (1980), The Jewish alcoholic: A descriptive study. *Alcohol, Health & Res. World*, 4:21–26.

Brown, G. W., Bone, M., Dalison, B., & Wing, J. K. (1966), *Schizophrenia and Social Care.* London: Oxford University Press.

Brugger, C. (1931), Versuch einer geistekrankenzahlungin Thuringe. *Z. Gesamte Neurol. Psychiat.*, 1933, pp. 352–390.

Calestro, K. M. (1972), Psychotherapy, faith healing and suggestions. *Internat. J. Psychiat.*, 10:83–113.

Carothers, J. C. (1951), Frontal lobe function and the African. *J. Ment. Sci.*, 97:12–48.

Carpenter, L., & Brockington, I. F. (1980), A study of mental illness in Asians, West Indians and Africans living in Manchester. *Brit. J. Psychiat.*, 137:201–205.

Chandrasena, R., & Rodrigo, A. (1979), Schneider's first rank symptoms: Their prevalence and diagnostic implications in an Asian population. *Brit. J. Psychiat.*, 135:348–351.

Chaplin, J. H. (1961), Suicide in Northern Rhodesia. *African Studies*, 20:145–174.

Cheung, F. (1984), Preferences in help-seeking among Chinese students. *Culture, Med. & Psychiat.*, 8:371–380.

Chkili, T., & El-Khamlichi, A. (1975), Les psychoses puerpérales en milieu morocain. *La Tunisie Méd.*, 53:375–392.

Collomb, H. (1965a), Bouffée délirante en psychiatrie africaine (Abstract). *Transcultural Psychiat. Rev.*, 3:29–34.

——— (1965b), Bouffées délirantes en milieu africain. *Psychopathologie Africaine*, 1:167–239.

——— Collignon, R. (1974), Les conduites suicidaires en Afrique. *Psychopathologie Africaine*, 10:55–114.

Cooper, J. E., & Sartorius, N. (1975), Cultural and Temporal Variations in Schizophrenia: A Speculation on the Importance of Industrialization. Geneva: WHO, Division of Mental Health (Typescript).

Cooper, S., Kendell, R., Gurland, B., Sharpe, L., Copeland, J., & Simon, R. (1972), *Psychiatric Diagnosis in New York and London: A Comparative Study of Mental Hospital Admission*. London: Oxford University Press.

Cox, J. L. (1983), Postnatal depression: A comparison of Scottish and African women. *Soc. Psychiat.*, 18:25–28.

Di Nicola, V. F. (1988), Expressed emotion and schizophrenia in North India. *Transcultural Psychiat. Rev.*, 25:205–216.

Draguns, J. G. (1980), Psychological disorders of clinical severity. In: *Handbook of Cross-Cultural Psychology.* Vol. 6: *Psychopathology*, ed. H. C. Triandis & J. G. Draguns. Boston: Allyn & Bacon.

——— (1982), Methodology in cross-cultural psychopathology. In: *Culture and Psychopathology*, ed. I. Al-Issa. Baltimore, MD: University Park Press.

Dubovsky, S. L. (1983), Psychiatry in Saudi Arabia. *Amer. J. Psychiat.*, 140:1455–1459.

Eagles, J. M. (1991), The relationship between schizophrenia and immigration. Are there alternatives to psychosocial hypotheses? *Brit. J. Psychiat.*, 159:783–789.

———— Whalley, L. J. (1985), Decline in the diagnosis of schizophrenia among first admissions to Scottish mental hospitals from 1969–78. *Brit. J. Psychiat.*, 146:151–154.

Eaton, J., & Weil, R. (1955), *Culture and Mental Disorders*. New York: Free Press.

Ebie, J. C. (1972), Psychiatric illness in the puerperium among Nigerians. *Tropical & Geographic Med.*, 24:253–256.

Edgerton, R. B. (1966), Conception of psychosis in four East African societies. *Amer. Anthropol.*, 68:408–425.

El-Islam, M. F. (1982), Rehabilitation of schizophrenics by the extended family. *Acta Psychiat. Scand.*, 65:112–119.

———— (1979), A better outlook for schizophrenics living in extended families. *Brit. J. Psychiat.*, 135:343–347.

———— (1989), Collaboration with families for the rehabilitation of schizophrenic patients and the concept of expressed emotion. *Acta Psychiat. Scand.*, 65:112–119.

Endicott, J., & Spitzer, R. L. (1978), A diagnostic interview: The schedule for affective disorders and schizophrenia. *Arch. Gen. Psychiat.*, 35:837–844.

Englesman, F. (1982), Culture and depression. In: *Culture and Psychopathology*, ed. I. Al-Issa. Baltimore, MD: University Park Press.

Essen-Moeller, E. (1956), Individual traits and morbidity in a Swedish rural population. *Acta Psychiat. Neurol. Scand.* (Suppl. 100).

Ey, H. (1954), *Etudes Psychiatriques*. Vol. 3: *Structure des Psychoses Aiguës et Destructuration de la Conscience*. Paris: Brounwer.

Eysenck, H. J. (1960), Classification and the problem of diagnosis. In: *Handbook of Abnormal Psychology*, ed. H. J. Eysenck. London: Pitman.

———— Eysenck, S. B. G. (1982), Culture and personality abnormalities. In: *Culture and Psychopathology*, ed. I. Al-Issa. Baltimore, MD: University Park Press.

Fabrega, H., Jr. (1989), An ethnomedical perspective of Anglo-American psychiatry. *Amer. J. Psychiat.*, 146:588–596.

Faegerman, P. M. (1963), *Psychogenic Psychoses*. London: Butterworth.

Famuyiwa, O. O. (1988), Anorexia nervosa in two Nigerians. *Acta Psychiat. Scand.*, 78:550–554.

Faris, R. E. L., & Dunham, H. W. (1939), *Mental Disorders in Urban Areas*. Chicago: University of Chicago Press.

Feighner, J. P., Robins, E., Guze, S., Woodruff, R. A., Winokur, G., & Munoz R., (1972), Diagnostic criteria for use in psychiatric research. *Arch. Gen. Psychiat.*, 26:57–63.

Fernando, S. (1991), *Mental Health, Race and Culture*. New York: St. Martin's Press.

Field, M. J. (1958), Mental disorder in rural Ghana. *J. Ment. Sci.*, 104:1043–1051.

—— (1960), *Search for Security*. London: Faber & Faber.

Folnegović, Z., & Folnegović-Smalc, V. (1992), Schizophrenia in Croatia: Interregional differences in prevalence and a comment upon constant incidence. *J. Epidemiol. Commun. Health*, 46:248–255.

Frank, J. D. (1961), *Persuasion and Healing*. Baltimore, MD: Johns Hopkins University Press.

Freud, S. (1930), *Civilization and Its Discontents*. New York: W. W. Norton, 1961.

German, A. G. (1972), Aspects of clinical psychiatry in sub-Saharan Africa. *Brit. J. Psychiat.*, 121:461–479.

—— Arya, O. P. (1969), Psychiatric morbidity among a Ugandan student population. *Brit. J. Psychiat.*, 115:1323–1329.

Goffman, E. (1961), *Asylums: Essays on the Social Situation of Mental Patients and Other Inmates*. Garden City, NY: Doubleday.

Good, J. B., Good, M. D., & Moradi, R. (1985), The interpretation of Iranian depressive illness and dysphoric affect. In: *Culture and Depression*, ed. A. Kleinman & B. Good. Los Angeles, CA: University of California Press.

Gregory, L. D., & Buchan, T. (1984), Anorexia nervosa in a Black Zimbabwean. *Brit. J. Psychiat.*, 145:326–330.

Guarnaccia, P. J., & Farias, P. (1988), The social meanings of nervios: A case study of the Central American woman. *Soc. Sci. & Med.*, 26:1223–1231.

Hagnell, O., Lanke, J., Rorsman, B., & Oyesjo, L. (1982), Are we entering an age of melancholy? *Psychol. Med.*, 12:279–289.

Harding, J. J. (1989), Post-partum psychiatric disorders: A review. *Comprehen. Psychiat.*, 30:109–112.

Hardwood, A., ed. (1981), *Ethnicity and Medical Care*. Cambridge: Harvard University Press.

Heath, D. B. (1986), Drinking and drunkenness in transcultural perspective. Part I. *Transcult. Psychiat. Res. Rev.*, 23:7–42.

Hes, J. P. (1970), Drinking in a Yemenite rural settlement in Israel. *Brit. J. Addiction*, 65:293–296.

Higginbotham, H. N. (1979), Culture and mental health services in developing countries. In: *Perspectives on Cross-Cultural Psychology*, ed. A. H. Marsella, R. G. Tharp, & T. J. Ciborowski. New York: Academic Press.

—— Tanaka-Matsumi, J. (1981), Social learning theory applied to counseling across cultures. In: *Counseling Across Cultures*, ed. P. B. Pedersen, J. G. Draguns, W. J. Lonner, & I. A. Trimble. Honolulu: University Press of Hawaii.

Hollingshead, A. B., & Redlich, F. C. (1958), *Social Class and Mental Illness: A Community Study*. New York: John Wiley.

Ilechukwu, S. T. C. (1991), Psychiatry in Africa: Special problems and unique features. *Transcult. Psychiat. Res. Rev.*, 28:169–218.

Jenkins, J. H., Karno, M., De La Selva, A., & Santana, F. (1986), Expressed emotion in cross-cultural context: Familial responses to schizophrenic illness among Mexican Americans. In: *Treatment of Schizophrenia: Family Assessment and Intervention*, ed. M. J. Goldstein, I. Hand, & K. Hahlweg. Berlin: Springer-Verlag.

Johnson, T. M. (1987), Premenstrual syndrome as a Western culture-specific disorder. *Culture, Med. & Psychiat.*, 11:337–356.

Karno, M., Jenkins, J. H., De La Selva, A., Santana, F., Telles, C., Lopez, S., & Mintz, J. (1987), Expressed emotion and schizophrenic outcome among Mexican-American families. *J. Nerv. & Ment. Dis.*, 175:143–151.

Katon, W., Kleinman, A., & Rosen, G. (1982), Depression and somatization. *Amer. J. Med.*, 72:127–135; 241–247.

———— Ries, R., & Kleinman, A. (1984), The prevalence of somatization in primary care. *Comprehen. Psychiat.*, 25:208–215.

Kawanishi, Y. (1992), Somatization of Asians: An artifact of Western medicalization? *Transcult. Psychiat. Res. Rev.*, 29:5–36.

Kiesler, C. A., & Sibulkin, A. E. (1987), *Mental Hospitalization, Myths and Facts about a National Crisis*. Newbury Park, CA: Sage.

Kim, K. (1977), Clinical study of primary depressive symptom. Part III: Across cultural comparison. *Neuropsychiat. J. Korean Neuropsychiat. Assn.*, 16:53–60.

Kimura, B. (1965), Vergleichende Undersuchungen über depressive Erkrankungen in Japan ünd in Deutschland. *Fortschr. Neurol. & Psychiat.*, 33:202–215.

Kirmayer, L. J. (1984), Culture, affect and somatization, Part I. *Transcult. Psychiat. Res. Rev.*, 21:159–188.

Kleinman, A. (1977), Depression, somatization and the new cross-cultural psychiatry. *Soc. Sci. & Med.*, 11:3–10.

———— (1978), Culture and depression (editorial). *Culture, Med. & Psychiat.*, 2:295–296.

———— Good, B., eds. (1985), *Culture and Depression*. Los Angeles, CA: University of California Press.

———— Kleinman, J. (1985), Somatization: The interconnections in Chinese society among culture, depressive experiences, and the meaning of pain. In: *Culture and Depression*, ed. A. Kleinman & B. Good. Berkeley: University of California Press.

Klerman, G. L. (1978), Affective disorders. In: *The Harvard Guide to*

Modern Psychiatry, ed. M. Armand & M. D. Nicholi, Jr. Cambridge, MA: Belknap Press, pp. 253–281.

——— (1989), Psychiatric diagnostic categories: Issues of validity and measurement. *J. Health & Soc. Behav.*, 30:26–32.

Koss, J. D. (1990), Somatization and somatic complaint syndromes among hispanics: Overview and ethopsychological perspectives. *Transcult. Psychiat. Res. Rev.*, 27:5–29.

Kramer, M. (1969), Cross-national study of diagnosis of the mental disorder: Origin of the problem. *Amer. J. Psychiat.*, 125 (Suppl. 10).

Kringlen, E. (1980), Schizophrenia: Research in the Nordic countries. *Schizophrenia Bull.*, 6:566–578.

Kroeber, A. L., & Kluckholm, C. (1952), *Culture: A Critical Review of Concepts and Definitions*, 47:1. Cambridge, MA: Peabody Museum.

Kulhara, P., & Wig, N. N. (1978), The chronicity of schizophrenia in North West India: Results of a follow-up study. *Brit. J. Psychiat.*, 132:186–190.

Lambo, T. A. (1956), Neuropsychiatric observations in the Western region of Nigeria. *Brit. Med. J.*, 11:1388–1394.

——— (1960), Further neuropsychiatric observations in Nigeria (with comments on the need for epidemiological study in Africa). *Brit. Med. J.*, 11:1696–1704.

Laubscher, B. J. F. (1937), *Sex, Custom and Psychopathology: A Study of South African Pagan Natives*. London: Routledge & Kegan Paul.

Lauter, H. (1965), Kraepelin's importance for cultural psychiatry. *Transcult. Psychiat. Res. Rev.*, 2:9–12.

Leff, J. (1973), Culture and the differentiation of emotional states. *Brit. J. Psychiat.*, 123:299–306.

——— (1988), *Psychiatry Around the Globe*. London: Gaskell.

——— Vaughn, C. (1985), *Expressed Emotions in Families*. New York: Guilford Press.

Leighton, A. M., Lambo, T. A., Hughes, C. C., Leighton, D. C., Murphy, J. M., & Macklin, D. P. (1963), *Psychiatric Disorder among the Yoruba*. Ithaca: Cornell University Press.

Leighton, D. C., Harding, J. C., Macklin, D. B., Macmillan, A. M., & Leighton, A. H. (1963), *The Character of Danger: Psychiatric Symptoms in Selected Communities*. New York: Basic Books.

——— Hagnell, O., Kellert, S. R., Harding, J. S., & Danley, R. A. (1971), Psychiatric disorder in a Swedish and a Canadian community: An exploratory study. *Soc. Sci. & Med.*, 5:189–209.

Leland, J. (1976), *Firewater Myths: North American Indian Drinking and Alcohol Addiction*, Monograph 11. New Brunswick, NJ: Rutgers Center of Alcohol Studies.

Lemkau, P., Tietze, C., & Cooper, M. (1942), Mental hygiene problems in an urban district. *Mental Hygiene*, 26:100–118.

Lewis-Fernández, R. (1992), The proposed DSM-IV trance and possession disorder category: Potential benefits and risks. *Transcult. Psychiat. Res. Rev.*, 19:301–317.

Licht, R. W., Gouliaev, G., & Lund, J. (1991), Trends in long stay hospitalization in Denmark: A descriptive register study, 1972–1987. *Acta Psychiat. Scand.*, 83:314–318.

Lin, T-Y. (1953), Anthropological study of the incidence of mental disorder in Chinese and other cultures. *Psychiatry*, 16:313–336.

Littlewood, R. (1990), From categories to contexts: A decade of the "new cross-cultural psychiatry." *Brit. J. Psychiat.*, 156:308–327.

——— (1993), Ideology, camouflage or contingency? Racism in British psychiatry. *Transcult. Psychiat. Res. Rev.*, 30:243–290.

——— Lipsedge, M. (1986), The culture-bound syndrome of the dominant culture: Culture, psychopathology and medicine. In: *Transcultural Psychiatry*, ed. J. Cox. London: Croom Helm.

MacAndrew, C., & Edgerton, R. B. (1969), *Drunken Comportment: A Social Explanation*. Chicago: Aldine.

Malzberg, B. (1940), *Social and Biological Aspects of Mental Disease*. Utica, NY: State Hospital Press.

Mandelbaum, D. B. (1965), Alcohol and culture. *Current Anthropol.*, 6:281–293.

Masterson, G., Main, C. J., Lever, A. F., & Lever, R. S. (1975), Low blood pressure in psychiatric inpatients. *Brit. Heart Dis. J.*, 45:442–446.

McCabe, E. M. I. (1982), Life style and disease: Alcoholism—its emergence in the black townships of South Africa. *S. African Med. J.*, 61:881–882.

McCarthy, P. D., & Walsh, D. (1975), Suicide in Dublin: 1—The underreporting of suicide and the consequences for national statistics. *Brit. J. Psychiat.*, 126:301–308.

Mead, M. (1928), *Coming of Age in Samoa*. Morrow: New York.

Mechanic, D., & Rochefort, D. A. (1990), Deinstitutionalization: An appraisal of reform. *Ann. Rev. Sociol.*, Palo Alto, CA, pp. 301–327.

——— (1987), Connecting misconceptions in mental health policy: Strategies for improved care of the seriously mentally ill. *Milbank Memorial Fund Quarterly*, 65:203–230.

Merskey, H., & Shafran, B. (1986), Political hazards in the diagnosis of sluggish schizophrenia. *Brit. J. Psychiat.*, 148:247–256.

Midgley, J. (1971), Drinking and attitudes toward drinking in a Muslim community. *Quart. J. Stud. Alcohol*, 32:148–158.

Mizoi, Y., Ijiri, I., Tatsuno, Y., Kijima, T., Fujiwara, S., & Adachi, J. (1979),

Relationship between facial flushing and blood acetaldehyde levels after alcohol intake. *Pharmacol. Biochem. & Behav.*, 10:303–311.

Morrison, J. R. (1974), Changes in subtype diagnosis of schizophrenia: 1920–1966. *Amer. J. Psychiat.*, 131:674–677.

Murphy, H. B. M. (1973), History and evolution of syndromes: The striking case of latah and amok. In: *Psychopathology*, ed. M. Hammer, K. Salzinger, & S. Sutton. New York: Wiley.

———— (1978), The advent of guilt feelings as a common depressive symptom: A historical comparison on two continents. *Psychiatry*, 41:229–242.

———— (1980), Review of *Schizophrenia: An international follow-up study*. *Transcult. Psychiat. Res. Rev.*, 17:158–161.

———— (1982a), Culture and schizophrenia. In: *Culture and Psychopathology*, ed. I. Al-Issa. Baltimore, MD: University Park Press.

———— (1982b), *Comparative Psychiatry: The International and Intercultural Distribution of Mental Illness*. Berlin: Springer.

———— Raman, A. C. (1971), The chronicity of schizophrenia in indigenous tropical peoples: Results of a twelve-year follow-up survey in Mauritius. *Brit. J. Psychiat.*, 118:489–497.

Murphy, J. M. (1976), Psychiatric labeling in cross-cultural perspective. *Science*, 191:1019–1028.

Noble, E. P., ed. (1979), *Alcohol and Health*. Technical support document. Third special report to the U.S. Congress. (DHEW pubications no. ADM 79-832.) Washington, DC: U.S. Government Printing Office.

Obeyesekere, G. (1985), Depression, Buddhism and the work of culture in Sri Lanka. In: *Culture and Depression*, ed. A. Kleinman & B. Good. Los Angeles, CA: University of California Press.

Ödegaard, Ö. (1932), *Emigration and Insanity*. Copenhagen: Munksgaard.

———— (1936), Mortality in Norwegian mental hospitals from 1916–1933. *Acta Psychiat. Scan.*, 2:323–356.

Okasha, A., Kamel, M., & Hassan, A. H. (1968), Preliminary psychiatric observations in Egypt. *Brit. J. Psychiat.*, 114:949–955.

Orley, J., & Wing, J. K. (1979), Psychiatric disorders in two African villages. *Arch. Gen. Psychiat.*, 36:513–520.

Osterweis, M., Kleinman, A., & Mechanic, D. (1987), *Pain and Disability: Clinical Behavioral and Public Policy Perspectives*. Washington, DC: National Academy Press.

Paris, J. (1991), Personality disorders, parasuicide and culture. *Transcult. Psychiat. Res. Rev.*, 28:25–39.

Pepper, B., & Ryglewicz, H., eds. (1982), The young adult chronic patient. *New Directions for Mental Health Services*, No. 14. San Francisco: Jossey-Bass.

Pfeiffer, W. M. (1982), Culture-bound syndromes. In: *Culture and Psychopathology*, ed. I. Al-Issa. Baltimore, MD: University Park Press.

Piault, C., ed. (1975), *Prophétisme et Therapeutique*. Paris: Hermann.

Pothero, C. (1969), Puerperal psychoses: A long-term study, 1927–1961. *Brit. J. Psychiat.*, 115:9–30.

Prince, R. H. (1968), The changing picture of depressive syndromes in Africa: Is it fact or diagnostic fashion? *Can. J. African Stud.*, 1:177–192.

——— (1980), Variations in psychotherapeutic procedures. In: *Handbook of Cross-Cultural Psychology*. Vol. 6: *Psychopathology*, ed. H. C. Triandis & J. G. Draguns. Boston, MA: Allyn & Bacon.

——— (1991a), Amok, then and now. *Transcult. Psychiat. Res. Rev.*, 28:219–228.

——— (1991b), Transcultural psychiatry's contribution to International Classification Systems: The example of social phobias. *Transcult. Psychiat. Res. Rev.*, 28:124–131.

——— Tcheng-Laroche, F. (1987), Culture-bound syndromes and international disease classifications. *Culture, Med. & Psychiat.*, 11:289–335.

Rack, P. H. (1982), Migration and mental illness: A review of recent research in Britain. *Transcult. Psychiat. Res. Rev.*, 19:151–172.

Rao, A. V. (1978), Some aspects of psychiatry in India. *Transcult. Psychiat. Res. Rev.*, 15:7–27.

Report of the US Delegation to Assess Recent Changes in Soviet Psychiatry (1989), *Schizophrenia Bull.* (Suppl. 15):1–78.

Robins, L. N., & Helzer, J. E. (1986), Diagnosis and clinical assessment: The current state of psychiatric diagnosis. *Ann. Rev. Psychol.*, 37:409–432.

——— ——— Crougham, J. L., Williams, S. B., & Spitzer, R. (1981), *The N.I.M.H. Diagnostic Interview Schedule, Version III*. Washington, DC: Public Health Service (HSS) ADM-1-423 (5/81, 8/81).

——— Regier, D. (1991), *Psychiatric Disorders in America: The Epidemiological Catchment Area Study*. New York: Free Press.

Rosen, G. (1968), *Madness in Society*. Chicago: University of Chicago Press.

Rossie, P., Wright, J. D., Fisher, G. A., & Willis, G. (1987), The urban homeless: Estimating composition and size. *Science*, 235:1336–1341.

Rwegellera, G. G. G. (1978), Suicide rates in Lusaka, Zambia: Preliminary observations. *Psychol. Med.*, 8:423–432.

Sadoun, R., Lolli, G., & Silverman, M. (1965), *Drinking in French Culture.* New Brunswick, NJ: Rutgers Center of Alcohol Studies.

Sartorius, N., Jablensky, A., Korten, G., Ernberg, G., Anker, M., Cooper, J. E., & Day, R. (1986), Early manifestations and first contact incidence of schizophrenia in different cultures. *Psychol. Med.,* 16:909–928.

Saugstad, L. F. (1989), Social class, marriage, and fertility in schizophrenia. *Schizophrenia Bull.,* 15:9–43.

Scheper-Hughes, N., & Lock, M. M. (1987), The mindful body: A prolegomenon to future work in medical anthropology. *Med. Anthropol. Quart.,* 1:6–41.

Schmitt, R. C. (1956), Psychosis and race in Hawaii. *Hawaii Med. J.,* 16:144–146.

Schwartz, S., & Goldfinger, S. (1981), The new chronic patient: Clinical characteristics of an emerging subgroup. *Hosp. & Commun. Psychiat.,* 32:470–474.

Sheets, J., Provost, J., & Reihmank, J. (1982), Young adult chronic patients: Three hypothesized subgroups. *Hosp. & Commun. Psychiat.,* 33:197–202.

Simon, R., Fleiss, J. L., Gurland, B. J., Stiller, P. R., & Sharpe, L. (1973), Depression and schizophrenia in hospitalized black and white mental patients. *Arch. Gen. Psychiat.,* 28:509–512.

Singer, K. (1975), Depression disorders from a transcultural perspective. *Soc. Sci. & Med.,* 9:289–301.

Snyder, C. R. (1958), *Alcohol and Jews.* Glencoe, IL: Free Press.

Spitzer, R. L., Endicott, J., & Robins, E. (1978), Research diagnostic criteria: Rationale and reliability. *Arch. Gen. Psychiat.,* 35:773–782.

Srole, L., Langner, T. S., Michael, S. T., Opler, M. K., & Rennie, T. A. C. (1962), *Mental Health in the Metropolis.* New York: McGraw-Hill.

Stromgren, E. (1987), Changes in the incidence of schizophrenia? *Brit. J. Psychiat.,* 150:1–7.

Sue, S., & Morishima, J. K. (1982), *Mental Health of Asian Americans.* San Francisco: Jossey-Bass.

Sulkunen, P. (1976), Drinking patterns and the level of alcohol consumption: An international overview. In: *Research Advances in Alcohol and Drug Problems,* Vol. 3, ed. R. J. Gibbins, Y. Israel, H. Kalant, R. E. Popham, W. Schmidt, & R. G. Smart. New York: John Wiley.

Swartz, L. (1985), Anorexia nervosa as a culture-bound syndrome. *Soc. Sci. & Med.,* 20:725–730.

——— (1987), Transcultural psychiatry in South Africa. II. *Transcult. Psychiat. Res. Rev.,* 24:5–30.

Swift, C. R. (1972), Psychosis during the puerperium among Tanzanians. *East African Med. J.,* 9:651–657.

Teicher, M. I. (1960), *Windigo Psychosis. A Study of the Relationship between Belief and Behavior among the Indians of North-Eastern Canada.* Seattle: American Ethnological Society.

Teja, J. S., Narang, R. L., & Aggrawal, A. K. (1971), Depression across cultures. *Brit. J. Psychiat.*, 119:253–260.

Tongue, E. (1976), Alcohol related problems in some African countries. *African J. Psychiat.*, 3:351–363.

Torrey, E. F. (1972), *The Mind Game: Witchdoctors and Psychiatrists.* New York: Emerson Hall.

Triandis, H. C., & Triandis, L. M. (1960), Race, social class, religion and nationality as determinants of social distance. *J. Abnorm. & Soc. Psychol.*, 61:110–118.

Uchimura, Y., Akimoto, H., Kan, O., Abe, Y., Takahashi, K., Inose, Y., Shimazaki, T., & Ogawa, N. (1940), Uber die vergleichende psychiatrische und erbpathologische untersuchung auf einer Japanischen isel. *Psychiat. & Neurol. Japonica*, 44:745–782.

Vaughn, C., Snyder, K. S., Jones, S., Freeman, W. B., & Falloon, I. R. H. (1984), Family factors in schizophrenic relapse: A California replication of the British research on expressed emotion. *Arch. Gen. Psychiat.*, 41:1169–1177.

Vega, W. A., & Rumbant, R. G. (1991), Ethnic minorities and mental health. *Ann. Rev. Sociol.*, Palo Alto, CA, pp. 351–384.

Waxler, N. E. (1979), Is outcome for schizophrenia better in nonindustrial societies? The case of Sri Lanka. *J. Nerv. & Ment. Dis.*, 167:144–158.

Weeke, A., Bille, M., Videech, T., Juel-Nielsen, N. (1975), Incidence of depressive symptoms in a Danish county. *Acta Psychiat. Scand.*, 51:28–41.

Weinberg, S. K. (1965), Cultural aspects of manic-depression in West Africa. *J. Health & Human Behav.*, 6:247–253.

Westermeyer, J., Vang, T. F., & Neider, J. (1983a), Migration and mental health among refugees: Association of pre- and post-migration factors with self-rating scales. *J. Nerv. & Ment. Dis.*, 171:92–96.

———————— (1983b), Refugees who do and do not seek psychiatric care: An analysis of pre-migratory and post-migratory characteristics. *J. Nerv. & Ment. Dis.*, 171:86–91.

White, J. M. (1982), The role of cultural explanations in "somatization" and "psychologization." *Soc. Sci. & Med.*, 16:1519–1930.

Whiting, J. W. M. (1954), The cross-cultural method. In: *Handbook of Social Psychology.* Vol. 1: *Theory and Method*, ed. G. Lindzey. Reading, MA: Addison-Wesley.

Wig, N. N., Menon, D. K., Bedi, H., Ghosh, A., Kuipers, L., Leff, J.,

Korten, A., Day, R., Sartorius, N., Ernberg, G., & Jablensky, A. (1987), Expressed emotion and schizophrenia in North India. 1. Cross-cultural transfer of ratings of relatives' expressed emotion. *Brit. J. Psychiat.*, 151:156–173.

Wilkinson, G. S. (1975), Patient-audience social status and the social construction of psychiatric disorders: Toward a differential frame of reference hypothesis. *J. Health & Soc. Behav.*, 16:28–38.

Wing, J. K. (1980), Social psychiatry in the United Kingdom: The approach to schizophrenia. *Schizophrenia Bull.*, 6:556–565.

Wittkower, E. D., & Warnes, H. (1974), Cultural aspects of psychotherapy. *Amer. J. Psychother.*, 28:566–573.

Wolff, P. H. (1972), Ethnic differences in alcohol sensitivity. *Science,* 175:449–450.

———— (1973), Vasomotor sensitivity to alcohol in diverse Mongoloid population. *Amer. J. Human Gen.*, 25:193–199.

World Health Organization (1973), *The International Pilot Study of Schizophrenia*, Vol. 1. Geneva: WHO.

———— (1979), *Schizophrenia: An International Follow-Up Study.* New York: Wiley.

———— (1992), *The ICD-10 Classification of Mental and Behavioral Disorders.* Geneva: WHO.

Yamamoto, J., Eng-Kung, Y., Chung-Kyoon, L., & Keh-Ming, L. (1988), Alcohol abuse among Koreans and Taiwanese. In: *Cultural Influences and Drinking Patterns: A Focus on Hispanic and Japanese Populations*, ed. L. H. Towle & T. C. Harford. Washington: National Institute of Alcohol Abuse & Alcoholism.

Zeiner, A. R., Paredes, A., & Christensen, H. D. (1979), The role of acetaldehyde in mediating reactivity to an acute dose of ethanol among different racial groups. *Alcoholism*, 3:11–18.

PART II

Africa

2.

Transcultural Psychiatry in Egypt

Mahmoud Sami Abd El-Gawad

Ancient Egyptian papyri record mental disorders including many descriptions of depression, but apart from Cleopatra's suicide, this problem was not a major issue in ancient Egyptian medical literature (Ghaliongi, 1963).[1] In Pharaonic Egypt the concept of hysterical disorders was known and ascribed to the movement of the uterus, long before Hippocrates described it under the term *hysteria*. The therapeutic approach to this disorder was physical rather than spiritual and involved fumigating the vagina. Dementia, retardation, negativism, subacute delirious states, and thought disorders similar to schizophrenia were described in detail in the book of the heart in Eber's papyrus (1600 B.C.). The heart and the mind were regarded as synonymous, and the etiology of all these states was ascribed to vascular problems, purulence, fecal matter, a mysterious poison, and only in two conditions was spiritual etiology alleged (Okasha, 1978). These two conditions are

---

[1]There was no particular period under the pharaohs when medical matters were recorded; this went on over the centuries as could be detected from the small available number of medical papyri: (1) **Kahun Papyrus (1900 B.C.)**—a rather incomplete and fragmentary record dealing with the morbid states attributed to the displacement of the uterus; (2) **Eber Papyrus (1600 B.C.)**—the greatest Egyptian medical document (translated by B. Ebbell [Copenhagen: Lexin and Munskgaard, 1937]); (3) **Edwin Smith Papyrus (1600 B.C.)**—deals mainly with surgery; (4) **Hearst Papyrus**—similar to that of the Eber Papyrus; (5) **Berlin Medical Papyrus (1250 B.C.)**—deals with prescriptions in an unsystematic arrangement; (6) **London Medical Papyrus (1350 B.C.)**—composed mainly of incantations against a variety of diseases and few prescriptions.

"perishing of the mind" and "forgetfulness" ("It is the breath of the activity of the priest that does it; it enters into the lungs several times and the mind becomes confused . . ." [Ebbell, 1926, p. 14]). Kalawoon General Hospital was built in Cairo early in the fourteenth century; it had four main departments: surgery, ophthalmology, internal medicine, and mental diseases. Thus in Egypt, mental patients were treated in a general hospital before many Western countries did so. The first mental hospital, Abbassia, was established in the nineteenth century and patients in Kalawoon hospital were transferred to it.

In the early 1960s, a decentralization of health care was implemented in Egypt. Psychiatric services were provided in small hospitals in various governorates, in the inpatient units of district hospitals, and in outpatient clinics. Mental hospital beds vary from 50 to 2500, and inpatient units in general hospitals vary from 4 to 30. There is approximately one psychiatric bed for every 6000 people. Free service is provided throughout the country by 52 outpatient clinics, 31 inpatient psychiatric units, and eight mental hospitals. Private practice is permitted, and there are six private psychiatric institutes.

SOCIOCULTURAL BACKGROUND

Psychiatric practice in Egypt generally follows the British school. Most textbooks on psychiatry in Egypt are British. The majority of Egyptian psychiatrists do their psychiatric residencies in Britain. Almost all groups of psychoactive drugs—major and minor tranquilizers, antidepressants, anticonvulsants, and anxiolytics—are used, and controlled studies on the effectiveness of such drugs are carried out in university hospitals before any imported drug can be marketed. Advances in pharmacotherapy together with the development of psychiatric wards in general hospitals have reduced the use of electroconvulsive therapy (ECT). Psychoanalytically oriented psychotherapy is practiced in private centers and in a few public ones such as the Kasr Al-Aini School of Medicine; orthodox psychoanalysis is employed sporadically by a few trained psychoanalysts. The Ain-Shams school tends to emphasize the organic basis of mental disease. The Al-Azhar School is humanistic and analytically oriented. Sponsored by the World Health Organization, Bashaar, El-Hakim, Galal, and Habashy (1979) developed a plan to extend mental health to the primary care level.

In our culture, nonmedical healers are assuming an active role in the management of dissociative and conversion disorders. Religious healers encourage people to visit a sheikh or a priest, to read the hegab (any sacred writing), and attend El-Zar ceremonies.[2] Relatives of psychiatric patients resort to nonmedical methods and folk prescriptions due to their inability to relate the behavioral changes to symptoms of mental illness. Rather, they assume the illness is due to magic, the rage of God, spirits, envy, supernatural forces, and demons. Some folk prescriptions used involve putting papers written by witches in water for a specific number of days and bathing the patient with this water or spreading it in front of the patient's door. In other instances the patient drinks this water in the morning for seven days. Some birds are used, but with special characteristics such as color, number of claws, and type, according to the witch's instructions: pigeons, hens, ducks, geese, and roosters are examples. A family member will cut the throat of the bird over the patient's head and body until its blood covers him. After these trials, when the patient's condition has deteriorated and the family can no longer tolerate the situation, the relatives seek medical help.

KNOWLEDGE AND ATTITUDES OF RELATIVES LIVING WITH A PSYCHIATRIC PATIENT

Relatives perceive a certain event or stressful situation which the patient has faced prior to the onset of the illness as being the

---

[2]El-Zar is one of the traditional healing cults in Egypt, and is neither inspired by nor practiced with religious motives; it is, in fact, antireligious. With the advent of modern therapies it has lost much of its former popularity. It is only uneducated, highly suggestible women of the lower and middle classes who resort to the cult. El-Zar seems to have been introduced into Egypt from Sudan through Ethiopia. The word *Zar* in Amharic means the *devil* or *spirit*. Literally, the word implies the intermittent visit of a wicked spirit. In practice, it generally connotes the gathering of some women, headed by a woman called "Kodia," with the purpose of exorcizing evil spirits. When some patients become ill and cannot find a cause for their illness, they attribute it to a "djenne." They therefore seek treatment from Zar healers, who are usually well known among the people. A simple form of psychotherapy is then conducted in a festive atmosphere, usually at the home of the "Kodia" or at a private residence (Okasha, 1966).

main cause for his trouble (mainly an emotional crisis due to loss of a loved person, financial problems, overwork, or failure in school). They lay the blame on some particular reason, and this helps them maintain their self-esteem and relieves their guilt feelings about their responsibility for the patient's illness. Hereditary factors are mentioned only by those who have a positive family history. Relatives associate mental illness with meaningless speech, the patient talking to himself, violence, excitement, bizarre behavior, hallucinations, aimless walking, strange body movements, and overall appearance.

Relatives reject the idea of having a mentally ill patient in the family. They tend to deny that the illness is mental and try to get the patient not to exhibit signs of illness. They try to keep the patient's illness as a secret. Those who are unable to do so, express sorrow and despair at their failure to protect the patient and hide his illness. One of the reasons for keeping the patient's illness a secret is to avoid humorous comments, especially from neighbors, and adverse effects on the patient's reputation and his social status in school or work, which might make his condition worse (Gawad, Loutfi, and Rahman, 1989).

PSYCHIATRIC SERVICES FOR CHILDREN AND THE ELDERLY

In Egypt, children from birth to 6 make up approximately 40 percent of the population. The presidential decree of January 24, 1988, established the National Council for Childhood and Motherhood. The main objective of this council is to formulate proposals for a comprehensive general national plan which would aim at the protection of mothers and children, especially with regard to social and family welfare, health, education, culture, information, and social security.

A study of the psychological effects of hospitalization on children revealed that children hospitalized with rheumatic heart disease showed an increase in anxiety scores. The most common manifestations of anxiety were fear of injections, irrational fear of ghosts, anorexia, reduced activity, sleep disturbances, and poor relationships with others.

The elderly in Egypt are traditionally cared for at home. This is dictated by custom and religion and is a part of the extended family system prevalent in most parts of the country. A verse in the Holy Koran states: "The Lord has commanded: Worship none but Him, and show Kindness to parents. If one of them or both of them attain old age with you at your home, never say to them any word expressive of disgust, nor reproach them, but address them with excellent speech. And lower to them the wing of humility out of tenderness. And say: My Lord, have mercy on them even as they nourished me in my childhood."

Yet, in the last decade, hostels for the elderly started to erupt in modern sections of Egyptian cities and particularly in the metropolitan areas. Currently we have sixteen such hostels in Cairo, eleven in Alexandria, and six in other governorates (Ashour, Okasha, Sadek, Hambali, Lotaif, and Bishry, 1982). In 1981, the population above 60 years was 5.3 percent of the total Egyptian population, i.e. about 2 million. (M.P.H., 1981).

TRANSCULTURAL STUDIES

Schizophrenia

A cross-national comparison of the symptomatology of schizophrenia, considering the rank order of symptom importance in the diagnosis, was carried out between a British study (Willis and Bannister, 1965), and American study (Edwards, 1972), and an Egyptian study (Gawad, Rakhawy, Mahfouz, and Howaidy, 1981): thirty-one symptoms were tabulated in descending order according to their rank in the diagnosis of schizophrenia by the three studies. Rank correlation coefficients between Egypt and Britain, and Egypt and the United States were 0.829 and 0.625 respectively. The top ten symptoms in this hierarchy are shown in Table 2.1. Results showed that incongruity of affect ranked first in Egypt, second in Britain, and fourth in the United States. Apathy ranked eighth in the Egyptian results, sixteenth in the American, and twenty-third in the British results. Thought disorder (formal) ranked second in Egypt, and first in both Britain and the United States. Incoherence ranked fifth in Egypt, eleventh in

TABLE 2.1
The "Top Ten" Symptoms in the United States, United Kingdom, and Egypt

Rank Order of Importance	United States	United Kingdom	Egypt
1.	Thought Disorder (formal)	Thought Disorder (formal)	Incongruity of Affect
2.	Delusions	Incongruity of Affect	Thought Disorder (formal)
3.	Paranoid Delusions	Neologisms	Thought Block
4.	Incongruity of Affect	Thought Block	Thought Withdrawal
5.	Hallucinations	Passivity Feelings	Incoherence
6.	Ideas of Reference	Paranoid Delusions	Passivity Feelings
7.	Neologisms	Stereotype	Neologisms
8.	Depersonalization	Delusions	Apathy
9.	Mannerisms	Thought Withdrawal	Hallucinations
10.	Thought Block	Ideas of Reference	Delusions

the United States, and sixteenth in Britain. The differences between the Egyptian hierarchy and the British hierarchy are less than those differences between the Egyptian and the American hierarchies. This might be explained by the fact that textbooks and training in psychiatry in Egyptian medical schools are predominately British.

Depression

A sample of 100 Egyptian depressed patients diagnosed according to the *Egyptian Diagnostic Manual of Psychiatric Disorders* (Diagnostic Manual of Psychiatric Disorders [DMP-I]) was selected randomly from the Kasr El-Aini outpatient psychiatric clinic. The presence or absence of a particular symptom was rated on Hamilton's rating scale for depression (Hamilton, 1960). The symptoms exhibited by the Egyptian patients were then compared with those reported in three other studies: one Indian study by Teja, Narang, and Aggarwal (1971), and two British studies by Kiloh and Garside (1963) and Carney, Roth, and Garside (1965) (Table 2.2). The

TABLE 2.2

Frequency Distribution in Percentages of Various Symptoms in the Four Studies

Symptoms	Egyptian	Indian (Teja et al., 1971)	British (Carney et al., 1965)	British (Kiloh & Garside, 1963)
1. Depressed Mood	100	100	60	63
2. Guilt Feelings	23	48	59	31
3. Suicidal Ideations	93	80	48	60
4. Insomnia, Initial	55	84	75	61
5. Insomnia, Late	23	92	67	37
6. Retardation	40	77	50	36
7. Agitation	8	68	NA[+]	41
8. Anxiety	99	80	61	48
9. Somatic Symptoms	87	76	13	INA
10. Hypochondriasis	31	73	51	57
11. Diurnal Variation	31	58	41	41
12. Paranoid Symptoms	25	14	28	19
13. Obsessional Symptoms	18	3	INA[+]	29

NA = Information not available

comparison between the symptomatological pattern of depression in the three cultures showed the following features:

1. Somatic symptoms and anxiety were present in a significantly higher percentage of Egyptian and Indian depressed patients as compared to the British patients. Increased somatic symptoms can be explained in terms of lower differentiation of emotional states or, in other words, as incapacity to verbalize feelings in developing societies and thus stressing the somatic concomitants of emotions. The same applies to people of lower social classes and lesser education. Another explanation might be related to the concept of "sick people" in that physicians expect physical symptoms in their practice. Third, it can be a defense mechanism against the experiencing of the painful background affect (Gawad and Arafa, 1980). In a study, "Alexithymia and Upper Gastrointestinal Disorders" (Gawad, 1989), 230 peptic ulcer patients and 167 patients with upper gastrointestinal tract symptoms were compared, but proved to be endoscopically free (somatizers). A control group not suffering from gastrointestinal troubles was included. The study revealed that personality characteristics of the duodenal ulcer and somatizers groups were nearly the same, but they both

differed from the control group. On the other hand, peptic ulcer patients tend to have a higher educational level, more were married, they smoked more, and complained less of depression and anxiety, with a higher number of previous endoscopies than somatizers (Gawad, 1989).

2. Suicidal ideations in our Egyptian depressives are relatively high compared with the low rates of suicide and attempted suicide. This can be explained by the fact that the suicidal act has two components: an emotional one which is part of the disease, and an ideational one which causes the execution of the act. So suicidal feelings may be prevalent, but family cohesion, lack of social alienation, religious condemnation of the act, and its lack of social acceptance, can explain the discrepancy between ideation and the attempt or act.

   A survey of the Ain-Shams University psychiatric outpatient clinic revealed affective disorders in 24 percent with neurotic depression 10.4 percent, manic-depression 8.6 percent, and involutional melancholia 5.2 percent (Okasha, 1977). Suicidal attempts and suicide were most common among depressives especially in the young age groups. Another study in Cairo by Okasha and Lotaif (1979) gave a rough estimate of suicide at 4/100,000 and attempted suicide at 38/100,000.

3. Guilt feelings in our Egyptian sample were low. This may be explained by the fact that Egyptians viewed their life roles more as part of a social system and thus their guilt feelings take a rather impersonal attitude externally directed, while in the West, guilt is internalized, personal, and self-centered owing to a greater degree of individual self-responsibility and independent role playing. The Christian religious concept of original sin may also contribute to feelings of self-guilt in Western depressed patients (Gawad and Arafa, 1980).

THE EGYPTIAN DIAGNOSTIC MANUAL OF PSYCHIATRIC DISORDERS (DMP-I)

The Egyptian Psychiatric Association was founded in 1971 as an independent society of the World Psychiatric Association. The

Egyptian Journal of Psychiatry has been published semiannually since 1978. This Manual was first published in 1975 in English. In 1979 an Arabic version of the same manual was published (both English and Arabic versions are included in the same volume). This classification is mainly derived from the ICD-8 (1968). Other sources are the French classification (Ey, Bernadr, and Bresset, 1967), DSM-I (1952) and II (1968), traditional British textbooks, and Egyptian works. International nomenclature is preserved whenever possible, and the coding system is independent with the corresponding international code cited, modifications are referred to and explained. Drug dependence was included with alcoholism and alcoholic psychoses as one category. Alcoholism does not represent a major psychiatric problem in our culture. The Scientific Committee of the Egyptian Psychiatric Association is now revising the manual and preparing the DMP-II, guided by both the ICD-10 (WHO, 1992) and the DSM-III-R (APA, 1987).

REFERENCES

American Psychiatric Association (1952), *Diagnostic and Statistical Manual of Mental Disorders (DSM-I)*. Washington, DC: American Psychiatric Association.

—— (1968), *Diagnostic and Statistical Manual of Mental Disorders (DSM-II)*. Washington, DC: American Psychiatric Association.

—— (1987), *Diagnostic and Statistical Manual of Mental Disorders (DSM-III-R)*. Washington, DC: American Psychiatric Association.

Ashour, A., Okasha, A., Sadek, A., Hambali, M., Lotaif, F., & Bishry, Z. (1982), Portrait of old people in Cairo hostels: A morbidity prevalence survey and some empirical correlations. *Egyptian J. Psychiatry*, 5:75–94.

Bashaar, T., El-Hakim, A., Galal, A., & Habashy, E. (1979), Rural psychiatry: The Fayoum experiment. *Egyptian J. Psychiatry*, 2:77–87.

Carney, M. W., Roth, M., & Garside, R. F. (1965), The diagnosis of depressive syndromes and the prediction of E.C.T. response. *Brit. J. Psychiat.*, 31:659–674.

Ebbell, B. (1926), *Eber Papyrus*. Copenhagen: Lexin and Munskgaard, 1937.

Edwards, G. (1972), Diagnosis of schizophrenia: An Anglo-American comparison. *Brit. J. Psychiat.*, 120:385–390.

Egyptian Psychiatric Association (1975), *Diagnostic Manual of Psychiatric Disorders*. Cairo: Egyptian Psychiatric Association.

El-Hamid, H. A., El-Geneidy, M., Banna, S. M., Kamal, S. A., & Gawad, M. S. A. (1984), Psychological effects of hospitalization on children. *Egyptian J. Psychiatry*, 7:121–130.

Ey, H., Bernadr, P., & Bresset, C. (1967), *Manuel de Psychiatrie*. Paris: Masson.

Gawad, M. S. A. (1989), Alexithymia and upper gastrointestinal disorders. Paper presented to the 4th Pan Arab Congress of Psychiatry, SANA'A, Yemen Arab Republic.

——— Arafa, M. (1980), Trans-cultural study of depressive symptomatology. *Egyptian J. Psychiatry*, 3:163–181.

——— Loutfi, Z., & Rahman, A. A. (1989), Knowledge of relatives of psychiatric patients about mental illness. *Arab J. Psychiatry*, 1:22–29.

——— Rakhawy, Y. T., Mahfouz, R., & Howaidy, M. (1981), Relative symptom importance in the diagnosis of schizophrenia. *Egyptian J. Psychiatry*, 4:39–56.

Ghaliongi, P. (1963), *Magic and Medical Science in Ancient Egypt*. New York: Hodder & Stoughton.

Hamilton, M. (1960), A rating scale for depression. *J. Neurosurg. Psychiat.*, 23:56–62.

Kiloh, L. G., & Garside, R. F. (1963), The independence of neurotic depression and endogenous depression. *British J. Psychiat.*, 109:451–463.

Kunzman, L. (1972), Some factors influencing a young child's mastery of hospitalization. *Nurs. Clin. North Amer.*, 7:13–26.

M.P.H. (1981), Demographic data. Report of the Ministry of Health, Cairo, Egypt. Typescript.

Okasha, A. (1966), A cultural psychiatric study of El-Zar Cult in U.A.R. *Brit. J. Psychiat.*, 112:1217–1221.

——— (1977), Psychiatric symptomatology in Egypt. *Mental Health & Soc.*, 4:121–125.

——— (1978), Mental disorders in Pharaonic Egypt. *Egyptian J. Psychiatry*, 1:3–12.

——— (1984), Depression and suicide in Egypt. *Egyptian J. Psychiatry*, 7:33–45.

——— Lotaif, F. (1979), Attempted suicide: An Egyptian investigation. *Acta Psychiat. Scand.*, 60:69–75.

Teja, J. S., Narang, R. L., & Aggarwal, A. K. (1971), Depression across cultures. *Brit. J. Psychiat.*, 119:253–260.

Willis, J. H., & Bannister, D. (1965), The diagnosis and treatment of schizophrenia: A questionnaire study of psychiatric opinion. *Brit. J. Psychiat.*, 111:1165–1171.

World Health Organization (1968), *Manual of the International Classification of Diseases (ICD-8)*. Geneva: World Health Organization.

―――― (1977), *Manual of the International Statistical Classification of Diseases (ICD-9)*. Geneva: World Health Organization.

―――― (1992), *The ICD-10 Classification of Mental and Behavioural Disorders*. Geneva: World Health Organization.

3.

Culture, Religion, and Mental Illness in Nigeria

O. A. Sijuwola

Nigeria, in West Africa, with an estimated population of 80 million, is the most populous country in Africa. It spans a wide climatic range, from the arid semidesert in the north to the green, tropical forests of the south. It is a multiethnic society with over 200 linguistic groups. There are three main ethnic groups, which overshadow the other ethnic groups: Hausa predominates in the north, the Igbos in the southeast, and the Yorubas in the southwest. Most people live in the rural areas and are farmers with a good admixture of animal husbandry, particularly in the savannah lands of the north. The overall literacy rate is still low and estimated at about 40 percent of the total population. An estimated 60 percent of the population is under the age of 20 years, however, and they have benefited from the free universal primary education first introduced in the Western Region of the country in 1955 and later made available nationwide in the early 1970s. This has led to a higher literacy rate amongst those under 20, whilst the rate for those over 20 remains low.

THE CULTURAL BACKGROUND OF MENTAL HEALTH

Prior to the advent of the colonialists, mental illness was the exclusive preserve of the traditional healers. They still command a large following. The indigenous concept of the etiology of mental illness is governed to a large extent by the traditional belief system. While the role of natural causes in the etiology of mental illness is not denied, the traditional healers more often than not attribute it to curses and the work of evil spirits. When traditional healers in the city of Ibadan, Nigeria were asked about their concept of the etiology of mental disorders, 76 percent cited curses, 67 percent epidemic infections, and 47.2 percent attributed them to spirits. The contribution of genetic factors to mental illness is recognized. This forms one aspect of the family investigations which are usually carried out prior to giving family consent to a proposed marriage. Any history of mental illness in a family almost invariably leads to opposition to the marriage.

Consistent with the traditional belief system, a substantial proportion of patients seek traditional treatment first before considering hospital care. In a study of 160 consecutive new cases seen at the outpatient psychiatric clinic of University College Hospital, Ibadan, Nigeria, 40 percent of the patients were found to have been treated earlier by traditional or religious healers or both for the current illness (Jegede, 1981).

The traditional methods of treatment are derived from indigenous theories of causation. Demonology and possession by evil spirits call for treatment with flogging and rituals involving offering of sacrifices to gods to win divine favor. Offenses against the gods required penitence and appeasement of the offended deity by the offering of sacrifices.

Whether the etiology is viewed as organic or spiritual, drugs are still given to the patient. Drugs obtained from mineral, vegetable, or animal sources are administered and the route of administration may be oral or parenteral. The parenteral administration takes the form of multiple incisions onto which the drug, usually in powdered form, is applied.

Physical restraint is used to control the restless, aggressive, or violent patient. Ropes are at times used to tie both hands and legs together in order to restrain the patient. Equipment such as handcuffs and leg chains is also used by the traditional healers. Severe injuries, infections, and necrosis as a result of ischemia from the patient being tied too tightly and for too long may occur, and may lead to amputation of a hand or a leg to save the patient's life. Terrible pressure sores on the buttocks have also been seen in patients who have been treated by traditional healers. The mortality rate can be very high among the patients treated in these facilities. In a study of pueperal psychosis, the morality among those who have been to such facilities was found to be 19.7 percent as against 10.9 percent among controls.

Chronically ill patients are subjected to long periods of treatment within the traditional healer's compound, which is often used to house the patients. In effect, there is prolonged "hospitalization" of the patient, and, as the patient improves, rehabilitation is initiated. The patient gradually takes on part of the domestic chores and as the mental state improves may be sent out to work on the farm. It is not unusual for the traditional male healer to marry a female patient after recovery.

The Islamic and Christian religions coexist with the traditional religions, and they appear to command more official recognition as major Islamic and Christian festivals are observed as public holidays unlike the festivals of the indigenous deities. In times of stress, however, the adherents of these two newer religions still find solace in the traditional gods. The Islamic religion is predominately the religion of the Hausas in the north, and the Christian religion that of the Yorubas and Igbos in the south. Both religions have inputs into the treatment of psychiatric disorders.

Management of mental disorders under the Islamic religion involves prayers repeated several times, and the oral administration of the ink solution obtained by washing off passages from the Koran inscribed on slates. Passages from the Koran are also made into charms or amulets which the individual wears on his person or carries about in his pocket. These are designed to drive out the evil spirits, fortify the individual against further violation, or surround him or her with benevolent spirits.

Christian churches, particularly the syncretic religious groups which have incorporated a substantial proportion of local culture into their practices, command a strong following in times of stress, illness, and other misfortunes. A lot of psychiatric patients are treated in these facilities, particularly neurotic patients. Treatment involves fasting, prayers, and the application of "holy water." Prayers and night vigils accompanied by drumming and *or be*

make better

emotional release

singing often produce cathartic effects, and this may lead to amelioration of symptoms. In some cases, a trance state is induced and this may last from a few minutes to two or three days. In this state, the individual speaks "in tongues" and the behavior undergoes radical changes. The language spoken in such a state is usually not comprehensible, and an initiate has to interpret what is said to the congregation. Recovery from the trance state is often associated with disappearance of symptoms. The "holy water," which in most cases is potable water subjected to hours of prayers, is usually drunk and also used for bathing. In recent times patients have been presented with extrapyramidal signs after drinking the "holy water." This suggests the possibility that neuroleptics may have been added to the "holy water."

MENTAL HEALTH SERVICES

Current psychiatric practice in Nigeria presents an interesting mixture of traditional practices, which have fallen into disuse in the developed countries, religious healing practices, and orthodox Western psychiatric practices. There is a constant flow of patients between the different systems and in many cases the patient appears in a hospital only when the other systems have been tried and failed. This has implications as regards early therapeutic intervention in the major psychoses, as it delays hospital care. The acute features of the illnesses in most cases will have disappeared by the time the patient finally arrives in a hospital.

The Western type of services for the mentally ill was introduced in 1907 with the establishment of the Yaba asylum. Just like Western countries at that time, treatment consisted only of custodial care in the isolated asylum. The asylum had no doctor on its staff until 1927 when a general duty medical officer was employed. Treatment consisted of sedation with paraldehyde and maintenance of order in the institution.

The first modern psychiatric hospital was opened in 1954 and modern treatment of psychiatric disorders began. Therapies such as insulin coma, electroconvulsive treatment (ECT), and barbiturates were introduced into the care of the patients.

At the primary care level, heavy recourse is made by the

patient to the traditional and religious systems of care. The secondary care level involves treatment by a general practitioner. At present, the country has a total of sixty-seven psychiatrists serving a population of about 80 million. Over 80 percent of these psychiatrists are based in tertiary institutions, that is, psychiatric institutions, with a sprinkling at the secondary, and none at the primary care level. This lopsided deployment of the few experts available has contributed greatly to ensuring the continued strength of alternate modes of psychiatric care.

THE EFFECT OF CULTURE ON MENTAL HEALTH

An analysis by ethnic group of the admissions into the Jos University Teaching Hospital revealed that the nomadic Fulanis have the highest rate of hospitalization for psychiatric disorders. Though they form only 4 percent of the population, they contribute 25.1 percent of the admissions. The nomadic Fulanis are further subclassified according to the degree of stability of domicile, into (1) "Settled Fulani" (i.e., has fixed residence and does not move outside his area in search of pasture; some have given up cattle rearing); (2) semisettled (i.e., a person who has a permanent residence where some members of the family have taken up agriculture and only the young people move with the cattle in dry season); and (3) nomadic (i.e., a person with no fixed residence and moving with the entire family and livestock). The rate of psychiatric disorders as evidenced in the admission rate increased in the descending order. The commonest psychiatric disorder among the Fulanis was found to be schizophrenia, 41.2 percent, followed by affective disorders, 29.9 percent (Ikwuagwu, 1991). The author explained the high rate of psychiatric disorders on the basis of the stress of being constantly on the move and the difficulties associated with locating grazing areas without coming into conflict with farmers, and indiscriminate burning of forests and farm lands after harvesting the crops.

DEPRESSIVE DISORDERS

The controversy as to the rarity of depressive disorders among Africans has now been laid to rest. The consensus is that Africans do indeed suffer from depressive disorder, and that the prevalence is not much different from the prevalence among Europeans and Americans. Lambo (1960) revised his earlier position that depression may have distinct features such as asthenia, multiple hypochondriacal symptoms, and general mental inertia in Africans. He also wrote that a profound sense of sorrow, self-accusation, or ruin may be lacking. Rwegellera (1981) pointed out that phenomenologically, depressions may be experienced as a sense of personal decay, decline, or retardation, along with the cessation of body functions. The individual describes the changes using myths and symbols acceptable to his culture. Among Yoruba Nigerians, claims of being a witch, a crawling sensation in the body, and a feeling of bodily heat, often referred to as "central heat syndrome," are frequent manifestations of depressive illness. The nonrecognition of these symptoms as such will tend to create the erroneous impression that depressive disorders are rare in the population.

Guilt feelings are rare among Nigerian depressives. Lambo (1960) reported that "Ideas of self accusation or ruin, fear for the future and a profound sense of sorrow are often completely lacking or may feature in terminal stages." Binitie (1971) in his study of ninety-eight cases with affective disorders reported 17 percent of patients had ideas of guilt, self-blame, or feeling of unworthiness. Hallucinations, particularly auditory hallucinations, are common among the depressed population. Binitie reported auditory hallucinations in 39 percent of the patients he studied and the hallucinatory experience was usually centered around death and killings. Persecutory delusions were found to be common and were reported by 29 percent of the depressed patients he studied. He reported that the persecutory delusions were similar to the beliefs held by members of the community. This has been linked with the tendency to externalize misfortune, thus minimizing personal responsibility such that self-reproach or a feeling of guilt is absent. Studies suggest that suicide is rare and was estimated at less than one per 100,000 in Western Nigeria.

CULTURE-SPECIFIC SYNDROMES

In the last year or so, there have been frequent reports of cases of "missing genitals." The subject, almost invariably a man, exchanges greetings with another person, usually another man or at times a woman, and the greetings usually involve a handshake. The exchanges are usually between total strangers, and are followed by fear that the genitals of one of the parties have disappeared. It is usually claimed that the alleged offending party had invoked supernatural forces to make the genitals disappear. In the rare cases involving women, it is claimed that the breasts have been "stolen or changed." Objective examination of the genitals or breasts reveal they are intact but pointing this out to the complainant usually does not convince him or her, and often the person responds that the parts are now different from what they had been prior to the exchange of greetings.

Some psychiatric disorders have never been reported by workers in this country; for example anorexia nervosa. The reason for this is surely that in a country where food is often difficult to come by and where the little available has to be competed for by family members, the nutritional needs of the individual are likely to be just barely met.

PSYCHIATRIC SERVICE AND TRADITIONAL HEALING

As mentioned earlier, there is constant flow of patients between the modern and traditional psychiatric facilities. In the rural areas, psychiatric services are offered almost entirely by the traditional healers. Given this state of affairs, recognition of the traditional healers will be an important step in effectively monitoring their practices and also in raising the standard of such practices. Attempts have been made in the recent past to integrate the traditional and modern healers into a unified health care delivery system for the country, but this has not met with success. The move has proved to be unpopular with those professionals trained in the West while the traditional healers hailed it as a

welcome development. Because of the popularity traditional healers continue to enjoy among the people, they may have something
to offer the health care system.

REFERENCES

Binitie, A. (1971), *A Study of Depression in Benin Nigeria.* Unpublished
    doctoral dissertation. University of London.
Ikwuagwu, P. (1991), A prospective study of the social and clinical char-
    acteristics of patients admitted at Jos University Teaching Hospital.
    Unpublished FMCPsych. dissertation. Jos University, Nigeria.
Jegede, R. O. (1981), A study of the role of socio-cultural factors in the
    treatment of mental illness in Nigeria. *Soc. Sci. & Med.,* 15A, 49.
Lambo, T. A. (1960), Further neuropsychiatric observations in Nigeria.
    Brit. Med. J., 2:1696–1704.
Rwegellara, G. G. C. (1981), Cultural aspects of depressive illness. *Psycho-
    pathologie Africaine,* 17:41–63.

4.

The Politics of Culture and Mental Illness: The Case of South Africa

Leslie Swartz

South Africa is a heterogeneous country. Over three-quarters of South Africans are considered to be of African origin, and smaller proportions of European origin ("whites"), and of Asian origin ("Indians"). According to the Population Registration Act of 1950 (repealed in 1991) the remaining South Africans are "coloureds"—a ragbag category made up of all people who do not fit into any of the other categories, and including people of mixed origin and Malay descent. South Africa is also a polylingual country, and under the apartheid system African native speakers of different languages have been viewed as coming from different cultural groups, whereas white native speakers of different languages—such as English and Afrikaans—have not. The problems with South African race classification have been extensively documented (Swartz, 1985; Boonzaier, 1988). Research on culture and mental illness in South Africa has focused almost exclusively on Africans, and this bias, though recognized as highly problematic, will necessarily be reflected in the material reviewed in this chapter. Clearly, even the issue of how cultural groups are defined in South Africa is political, and this chapter will begin with a brief consideration of the politics of culture and mental illness. Indigenous illness concepts and healing approaches will then be examined before turning to epidemiological data on mental illness.

The practice of psychiatry in South Africa's multicultural context will then be considered, along with a discussion of the possibilities for integrating biomedical and non-Western approaches. In the final section, key issues for further research and practice will be suggested.

THE POLITICS OF CULTURE AND MENTAL ILLNESS IN SOUTH AFRICA

The apartheid system, now at last crumbled, depended for its ideological justification on the notion of "cultural" differences. Gross discrimination and disparities in service provision were explained away by reference to the need to protect ethnic identities. In the health field, this has led, for example, to the extravagance of fourteen separate departments of health, each supposedly catering to a culturally "separate" group (De Beer, 1984, 1986).

Muticulturalism and cultural relativism, therefore, while often associated with liberal political views elsewhere in the world (Shweder and Bourne, 1982), are often seen in South Africa simply as smokescreens for discrimination (Boonzaier and Sharp, 1988; Swartz, in press a). The political environment has had a profound effect on the nature of knowledge produced on culture and mental health, with a number of key texts on cultural difference quite clearly racist in their orientation, and with a hesitance on the part of politically progressive authors to assert anything other than an overarching universalist position, for fear of reproducing racist views (Ngubane, 1988; Kottler, 1990; Swartz, in press a,b).

INDIGENOUS ILLNESSES AND HEALING

The better-known work in this area has been conducted on speakers of the Nguni family of languages (Zulu and Xhosa). Ngubane (1977), in her influential study of Zulu healing, distinguishes between *ukufa kwabantu* (diseases of the African people) and universal illnesses which are not specifically African. Indigenous illnesses such as *amafufunyane* are typically forms of negative spirit possession caused either by bewitchment (*ubuthakathi*) or by a negative relationship with one's ancestors, or both. A positive relationship with the ancestors, by contrast, may lead to one's experiencing a socially sanctioned form of spirit possession, *ukuthwasa*, through which illness one is "called" by the ancestors to become a traditional healer (Bührmann, 1983).

Not all mental illness, though, is interpreted in terms of the social and spiritual network of the sufferer. *Phambana* is a form of madness which is of no known origin and "just happens" (Schweitzer, 1977). Some debate exists as to the precise nature of the illness categories. In its narrow sense, for example, *amafufunyane* is reported to have a set of fairly standard possible manifestations which may include, in the case of a Xhosa-speaking woman, talking in Zulu in a male voice. A recent study of relatives of psychiatric patients, though, indicates that a substantial proportion of them label a wide range of symptoms as *amafufunyane* (Spiro, 1991). Some authors have drawn up taxonomies of African mental illnesses largely along lines which mimic the construction of Western systems in that they use symptom profiles rather than notions of etiology; for example, as defining the boundaries of disorder (Edwards, Cheetham, Majozi, and Lasisch, 1982). Others, though, have demonstrated a fluidity in the way that illness labels are used: different labels may be used for the same symptoms in different contexts, and the same label for different symptoms, depending on the interpretive network surrounding the illness (Mills, 1985). Even the African/non-African illness distinction cannot be taken as rigid.

Theories concerning the etiology of spirit possession states, positive and negative, tend to focus on social stressors ranging from industrialization and the migrant labor system to more general aspects of gender relationships (Ngubane, 1977; O'Connell, 1980, 1982). Some forms of spirit possession, such as *indiki* and *amafufunyane*, seem to be of fairly recent origin—occurring for the first time this century (Ngubane, 1977)—and a complete history of spirit possession in South Africa remains to be undertaken.

Similar to elsewhere in Africa, indigenous treatment tends to be undertaken by two forms of healer, the herbalist/doctor (*inyanga* in Zulu), and the diviner (*isangoma* in Zulu). Herbalists train by means of apprenticeships, usually lasting at least a year

(Ngubane, 1977). In order to become a diviner one has to go through a state of spirit possession as described above. Another major treatment resource lies in faith healers of the African independent churches, of which there are a large and apparently increasing number in this country (West, 1975a,b; Farrand, 1980; Edwards, 1983a,b). These churches vary considerably in orientation but some, such as the Zionist churches, combine the American Pentacostal tradition with elements of local healing traditions. The work of both diviners and faith healers tends to rely on music and dance, with a strong emphasis on clan and community participation and often on dream interpretation (Ngubane, 1977, 1981; van der Hoofdt, 1979, 1980; Bürhmann, 1978, 1980, 1981, 1984a,b). The issue of the integration between indigenous and Western medicine will be discussed later in the chapter.

EPIDEMIOLOGY OF MENTAL ILLNESS

The few hospital archive studies available yield a remarkably uniform picture for patterns of diagnosis of psychiatric illness. Most common disorders seen by a clinical psychologist at a hospital catering for Xhosa-speaking people in the Transkei were schizophrenia, depression, epilepsy, and anxiety states (Gijana and Louw, 1981). Of 261 African patients seen at a psychiatric clinic in Soweto, 40 percent were diagnosed schizophrenic, 14 percent epileptic, and 13 percent toxic psychosis (Luiz, 1981). Of 1889 patients seen in the psychiatry section of a general hospital in Soweto, 38 percent were diagnosed organic brain syndrome with alcohol playing a major part, 35 percent were schizophrenic, and 15 percent had affective disorder (Freed and Bishop, 1980). The issue of disorders induced by substances such as alcohol, cannabis, and methaqualone is a prominent one in South Africa (Rottanburg, Robins, Ben-Arie, Teggin, and Elk, 1982; Teggin, Elk, Ben-Arie, and Gillis, 1985; Oberholzer, 1986; Farrand, 1988). Of 52 Black adolescent patients admitted to Valkenberg Hospital, Cape Town, during the first six months of 1988, almost half (25) were diagnosed with "toxic psychosis" (Schoeman, Robertson, Lasisch, Bicha, and Westaway, 1989). The authors are at pains to point out, however, that like the diagnosis "traditional illness," the label of "toxic psychosis" refers to an "uncertain" diagnostic category (Schoeman et al., 1989, p. 2). There are concerns that attributions concerning toxic psychoses may to some extent reflect underlying racial prejudice, as has been suggested in Britain (Littlewood, 1988; Littlewood and Lipsedge, 1989; Swartz, 1989).

Hypertension rates for African, coloured, white, and Indian South Africans respectively have been estimated to be 12.9, 14.9, 21.6, and 31.8 per 100,000, and various hypotheses concerning stress in Indian South Africans have been put forward (van Rensburg and Mans, 1987). The rates in India itself are far lower than amongst Indian South Africans. Duodenal ulceration and gastrointestinal problems are thought to be increasing rapidly in prevalence among African migrant workers; stressful factors have once again been implicated (see Swartz [1987] for a review). Coronary heart disease is far higher in white and Indian South Africans than in Africans, but the prevalence is increasing amongst Africans (Swartz, 1987). It is tempting to assign this increase simply to urbanization and an increasingly "Western" life-style, but it has been argued that coronary heart disease in Africans tends to be associated with malnutrition and high rates of alcohol consumption (van Rensburg and Mans, 1987).

THE PRACTICE OF PSYCHIATRY IN SOUTH AFRICA

By Western standards, South Africa is poorly served in terms of health personnel. It is estimated that there is one psychiatrist and three clinical psychologists per 100,000 population in South Africa, compared to Western countries where there are five to fifteen psychiatrists and fifteen to thirty-five clinical psychologists per 100,000 population (Centre for the Study of Health Policy, 1990), with disparities of provision by race (Ben-Arie and Nash, 1986). Fragmentation of services by race has serious consequences for patient care (Freeman, 1989a,b). The ratio of number of psychiatric beds to population in Johannesburg in 1989 was approximately 1:6300 for Blacks, and 1:2500 for whites (calculated from Freeman [1989a, pp. 11–12]), with a range of sophisticated services available to whites which are not available to Blacks. Access to resources in rural areas is probably even more difficult for poor people (Freeman, 1989a; Miller and Swartz, 1990). Although it has recently become policy for all facilities to be open to all races, linguistic and financial barriers still operate.

Given the political history of South Africa it is not surprising that the literature on culture and mental illness has tended to focus more on differences between groups than on the question of how Western medicine can learn to accommodate a range of patients. The implicit theme that runs through much of the literature is that African people choose indigenous healing over Western medicine because it is in keeping with their cosmology (Cheetham and Griffiths, 1982a,b; Bührmann, 1984a; Schoeman, 1989). It is, of course, spurious to speak of a choice when basic Western-style mental health facilities are simply not available or accessible to large numbers of people. Africans, like people everywhere in the world, make use of the range of healing resources available to them (Farrand, 1980; Boonzaier, 1985; Spiro, 1991).

Recent work has begun to explore the ways in which the concept of cultural difference actually affects practice within the environment of the psychiatric institution (Swartz, 1989, in press a,b). It is clear that considerable conflict surrounds the notion, much of it related to more general conflicts concerning the politics of culture in South Africa as discussed above.

There have been many calls for a greater collaboration between psychiatry and traditional healing, and reports of successful collaboration (Oberholzer, 1985; Psychological Association of South Africa, 1989). The question of the politics of collaboration with regard to such issues as who makes final decisions about patient care has been less adequately addressed. An important recent development has been the interest on the question of traditional healing on the part of authors concerned with policy issues in a democratic South Africa (Freeman and Motsei, 1990; Korber, 1990). Given the limited financial resources in South Africa, this will be a central concern for a future democratic government.

The desegregation of psychiatric facilities by race, long called for by anti-apartheid mental health workers, has been occurring largely over the past year. The ways in which this change has affected everyday life in psychiatric hospitals has not yet been studied formally. There is, however, considerable interest in the practice of psychiatry in this time of change, and no doubt interesting analyses will be forthcoming.

THE FUTURE

South Africa is currently in a time of social change, accompanied by a high degree of turmoil and political violence. This fact in itself has been the subject of much work on the part of mental health practitioners (Foster, Davis, and Sandler, 1987; Dawes, Tredoux, and Feinstein, 1989; Swartz and Levett, 1989; Swartz, Gibson, and Swartz, 1990). Predictions about the future in such a climate are difficult, if not foolhardy, to make, but responsible planning in the mental health care sector does require some prognostication.

From a financial point of view, providing Western-style individually oriented, and specialized psychiatric and psychological services for the entire population is simply not feasible. Community-based care, better integrated into primary health care in general, seems to be a more realistic option. Training of primary health care practitioners in identification, basic management, and referral skills in the mental health field should be useful (Seedat and Nell, 1990). The increasing number of community health worker projects in South Africa also need development in the mental health area.

As far as research and formal training developments in the culture and mental illness field are concerned, there is probably one salient factor which bears consideration. It is to be hoped that South Africans will be able in the not too distant future to explore the area of culture and mental illness in an environment in which to speak of multiculturalism is not necessarily to raise the specter of apartheid. Only then will we be in a position to give adequate attention to both the strengths and weaknesses of the approach.

REFERENCES

Ben-Arie, O., & Nash, E. (1986), Deficiencies and inequalities in psychiatric services (letter). *SA Med. J.*, 69:343–344.

Boonzaier, E. (1985), Choice of healer: An important area of interest for general practitioners. *SA Fam. Pract.*, 6:235–240.

—— (1988), "Race" and the race paradigm. In: *South African Keywords: The Use and Abuse of Political Concepts*, ed. E. Boonzaier & J. Sharp. Cape Town: David Philip, pp. 58–67.

—— Sharp, J., eds. (1988), *South African Keywords: The Use and Abuse of Political Concepts*. Cape Town: David Philip.

Bührmann, M. V. (1978), Tentative views on dream therapy by Xhosa diviners. *J. Anal. Psychol.*, 23:105–121.

—— (1980), Why are certain procedures of the indigenous healer effective? In: *Economics of Health in South Africa*, Vol. 2, ed. F. Wilson & G. Westcott. Johannesburg: Ravan, pp. 338–342.

—— (1981), The Xhosa healers of Southern Africa. 1. Intlombe and xhentsa: A Xhosa healing ritual. *J. Anal. Psychol.*, 26:187–201.

—— (1983), Training of Xhosa medicine-men and analytical psychologists: A comparative study. In: *Money, Food, Drink and Fashion and Analytical Training: Depth Dimensions of Physical Existence*, ed. J. Beebe. (Papers of the 8th International Congress of Analytical Psychology.) Fellbach-Oeffingen, Germany: Bonz, pp. 237–245.

—— (1984a), *Living in Two Worlds: Communication Between a White Healer and Her Black Counterparts*. Cape Town: Human & Rousseau.

—— (1984b), The health care of an *iggira* (indigenous healer). In: *Jung in Modern Perspective*, ed. R. K. Papadopolous & G. S. Saayman. London: Wildwood House.

Centre for the Study of Health Policy (1990), *The Need for Improved Mental Health Care in South Africa*. Briefing document, Centre for the Study of Health Policy, University of the Witwatersrand, South Africa.

Cheetham, R. W. S., & Griffiths, J. A. (1982a), Sickness and medicine—An African paradigm. *SA Med. J.*, 62:954–956.

—— —— (1982b), The traditional healer/diviner as psychotherapist. *SA Med. J.*, 62:957–958.

Dawes, A. R. L., Tredoux, C., & Feinstein, A. (1989), Political violence in South Africa: Some effects on children of the violent destruction of their community. *Internat. J. Ment. Health*, 18:16–43.

De Beer, C. (1984), *The South African Disease: Apartheid Health and Health Services*. Johannesburg: South African Research Service.

—— (1986), Apartheid, health and health services in South Africa. In: *Proceedings of the Organization for Appropriate Social Services "Apartheid and Mental Health" Conference*. Johannesburg: OASSSA, pp. 13–20.

Edwards, F. S. (1983a), Amafufunyana spirit possession: A report on some current developments. Paper presented at the Fifth Annual Congress for the Study of Religion. University of Durban-Westville.

———— (1983b), Healing and transculturation in Xhosa Zionist practice. *Cult., Med. & Psychiatry,* 7:177–198.

Edwards, S. D., Cheetham, R. W. S., Majozi, E., & Lasisch, A. (1982), Zulu culture-bound psychiatric syndromes. *SA J. Hosp. Med.,* 8:82–86.

Farrand, D. (1980), *An Analysis of Indigenous Healing in Suburban Johannesburg.* Unpublished master's dissertation, University of the Witwatersrand, Johannesburg.

———— (1988), *Idliso: A Phenomenological and Psychiatric Comparison.* Unpublished doctoral dissertation, University of the Witwatersrand.

Foster, D., Davis, D., & Sandler, D. (1987), *Detention and Torture in South Africa.* Cape Town: David Philip.

Freed, E. D., & Bishop, E. (1980), Major psychiatric disability in open ward patients referred by medical and surgical units at Baragwanath Hospital: A study of 1889 patients. *The Leech,* 50:56–62.

Freeman, M., & Motsei, M. (1990), *Is There a Role for Traditional Healers in Health Care in South Africa?* Paper No. 20. University of the Witwatersrand, Johannesburg: Centre for the Study of Health Policy.

Freeman, M. C. (1989a), *Mental Health Care in Crisis in South Africa.* Paper No. 16. University of the Witwatersrand, Johannesburg: Centre for Health Policy.

———— (1989b), The structure of mental health care services in South Africa. Paper presented at the Conference of the Organisation for Appropriate Social Services in South Africa, University of the Witwatersrand, Johannesburg.

Gijana, E. W. M., & Louw, J. (1981), Psychiatric disorders in a developing community as reflected by archival material. *SA Med. J.,* 59:988–991.

Korber, I. (1990), Indigenous healers in a future mental health system: A case for cooperation. *Psychol. in Soc.,* 14:47–62.

Kottler, A. (1990), South Africa: Psychology's dilemma of multiple discourses. *Psychol. in Soc.,* 13:27–36.

Littlewood, R. (1988), Community initiated research: A study in psychiatrists' conceptualisations of "cannabis psychosis." *Bull. Roy. Coll. Psychiatrists,* 12:486–488.

———— Lipsedge, M. (1989), *Aliens and Alienists: Ethnic Minorities and Psychiatry,* 2nd ed. London: Unwin Hyman.

Luiz, H. A. (1981), Profile of a psychiatric clinic in Soweto. *Transactions Coll. Med. SA,* 25, (Suppl.):187–190.

Miller, T., & Swartz, L. (1990), Access to psychiatric resources: The case of Mamre. Presented at the Association for Sociology in Southern Africa Conference, Stellenbosch, July.

Mills, J. (1985), The possession state *intwaso*: An anthropological re-appraisal. *SA J. Sociol.*, 16:9–13.

Ngubane, H. (1977), *Body and Mind in Zulu Medicine: An Ethnography of Health and Disease in Nyuswa-Zulu Thought and Practice.* London: Academic Press.

———— (1981), Aspects of clinical practice and traditional organization of traditional healers in South Africa. *Soc. Sci. & Med.*, 15B: 361–365.

———— (1988), Reshaping social anthropology. Paper presented at the University of Durban-Westville, August.

Oberholzer, D. (1986), Depression in the eighties: Black population. *Psychotherapeia*, 43:9–11.

———— (1985), Co-operative venture with traditional healers in providing a community mental health service in the Odi I district, Bophuthatswana: A preliminary review. *Psychother. & Psychiatry in Pract.*, 36:36–42.

O'Connell, M. C. (1980), The aetiology of thwasa. *Psychotherapeia*, 6:18–23.

———— (1982), Spirit possession and role stress among the Xesibe of Eastern Transkei. *Ethnology*, 21:21–37.

Psychological Association of South Africa (1989), *Mental Health in South Africa.* Pretoria: Psychological Association of South Africa.

Rottanburg, D., Robins, A. H., Ben-Arie, O., Teggin, A. F., & Elk, R. (1982), Cannabis-associated psychosis with hypomanic features. *Lancet*, 2:1364–1366.

Schoeman, J. B. (1989), Psigopatologie by tradisionele swart Suid-Afrikaners. In: *Suid-Afrikaanse Handboek van Abnormale Gedrag*, ed. D. A. Louw. Johannesburg: Southern, pp. 448–470.

———— Robertson, B., Lasisch, A. J., Bicha, E., & Westaway, J. (1989), Children and adolescents consulted at four psychiatric units in the Transvaal, and the Cape Province. *SA J. Child & Adol. Psychiatry*, 1:1–15.

Schweitzer, R. D. (1977), *Categories of Experience Amongst the Xhosa: A Psychological Study.* Unpublished master's dissertation, Rhodes University, Grahamstown.

Seedat, M., & Nell, V. (1990), Third world or one world: Mysticism, pragmatism, and pain in family therapy in South Africa. *SA J. Psychol.*, 20:141–149.

Shweder, R. A., & Bourne, E. (1982), Does the concept of the person vary cross-culturally? In: *Cultural Conceptions of Mental Health and Therapy*, ed. A. Marsella & G. M. White. Dordrecht: Reidel, pp. 97–137.

Spiro, M. (1991), *Illness Models of Relatives in African Psychiatric Patients: Implications for a Family-Based Service.* Unpublished MA dissertation. University of Cape Town.

Swartz, L. (1985), Issues for cross-cultural psychiatric research in South Africa. *Cult., Med. & Psychiatry,* 9:59–74.

———— (1987), Transcultural psychiatry in South Africa. Part II. *Transcult. Psychiatric Res. Rev.,* 24:5–30.

———— (1989), *Aspects of Culture in South African Psychiatry.* Unpublished doctoral dissertation, University of Cape Town.

———— (in press, a), Professional ethnopsychiatry in South Africa: The question of relativism. In: *Ethnopsychiatry: The Cultural Construction of Professional and Folk Psychiatries,* ed. A. D. Gaines. New York: State University of New York Press.

———— (in press, b), The politics of Black patients' identity: Ward-rounds on the "Black" side of a South African psychiatric hospital. *Cult., Med. & Psychiatry.*

———— Gibson, K., & Swartz, S. (1990), State violence in South Africa and the development of a progressive psychology. In: *Political Violence and the Struggle of South Africa,* ed. N. C. Manganyi & A. du Toit. London: Macmillan.

———— Levett, A. (1989), Political repression and children in South Africa: The social construction of damaging effects. *Soc. Sci. & Med.,* 28:741–750.

Teggin, A. F., Elk, R., Ben-Arie, O., & Gillis, L. S. (1985), A comparison of PSE CATEGO "S" Schizophrenia in three population groups: Psychiatric manifestations. *Brit. J. Psychiatry,* 147:683–687.

van der Hoofdt, G. A. (1979), *De Malopodans: een transcultureel-psychiatrische studie.* Doctoral dissertation, Rijksuniversiteit of Leiden. Leiden: Rodopi.

———— (1980), Some possibly paranormal aspects of Malopo dancing. *Parapsychol. J. SA,* 1:32–43.

van Rensburg, H. C. J., & Mans, A. (1987), *Profile of Disease and Health Care in South Africa,* 2nd ed. Pretoria: Academica.

West, M. E. (1975a), *Bishops and Prophets in a Black City: African Independent Churches in Soweto, Johannesburg.* Cape Town: David Philip. London: Rex Collings.

———— (1975b), The shades come to town: Ancestors and urban independent churches. In: *Religion and Social Change in South Africa,* ed. M. G. Whisson & M. West. Cape Town: David Philip. London: Rex Collings, pp. 185–206.

5.

Mental Disorders in Tanzania: A Cultural Perspective

N. K. Ndosi

The current population of Tanzania is 27.4 million people. For every 100 females there are 96 males. The annual population growth rate is 2.8 percent. A household contains 5.3 persons on the average. Nearly half of Tanzanians are less than 15 years old. There are about 8000 registered villages in Tanzania which contain 75 percent of the rural population, and Tanzania is thus one of the least urbanized African countries. These villages facilitate the provision of social services. The agricultural sector employs more than 80 percent of the work force and accounts for more than half the Gross National Product. Tanzanian society is predominantly one of agricultural peasant communities.

More than 40 percent of the people are Christians, half of the remaining 60 percent are Muslims, and the rest belong to other religions. The majority of Tanzanians follow religions which emphasize the unity of their world. Members of the indigenous religions travel to sacred groves to make sacrifices to ensure the well-being of their clans. Despite the impact of changes brought about by technology and religion, most Tanzanians do not draw a clear distinction between the animate and inanimate, natural and supernatural, physical and psychic. This world of the living forms a continuum with an invisible world occupied by similar

groups of ancestral spirits. Dead ancestors protect the social affairs of the community. The elderly are not only guardians of
tradition but also function as an important link between the living
and their dead ancestors.

Despite two generations of colonization of Tanzania and
thirty years of rapid postindependent sociocultural changes, most
Tanzanians still believe in the supernatural causes of disease, irrespective of their educational levels. Traditional views on causes
of mental disorders vary widely. A mental disorder is considered
a misfortune like a physical illness, a bad harvest, or floods. Sometimes it is taken as a penalty for misdeeds of the affected person
or of their family members, or as a manifestation of an ill-omen
or even as a curse from an ancestor (Neki, Joinet, Hogan, Hauli,
and Kilonzo, 1985).

PREVALENCE OF MENTAL DISORDERS IN TANZANIA

The World Health Organization (WHO) estimates the prevalence
of severe mental retardation in Tanzanian adults at 100,000 (1%)
and severe mental retardation in children and cerebral palsy at
37,500 (0.5%). Research into the logistics of mental health disorders carried out by the Ministry of Health in 1984 in two pilot
regions (Morogoro and Kilimanjaro) established that 7 percent of
patients attending rural health facilities complained of psychiatric
symptoms and 2 percent got psychiatric diagnoses. Other diagnoses were: epilepsy 0.5, alcohol 0.2, cannabis abuse 0.1, social problems 0.1, schizophrenia 0.3, depression 0.1, and neurosis 1.2
percent.

The above figures represent an estimation from only about
10 percent of the population of Tanzania. They could portray an
underestimation of the mentally ill because of fears of stigmatization or inadequate diagnostic criteria. Little is known concerning
the number of mental patients in rural areas who do not seek
help from health centers.

Schizophrenia and psychotic states carry the social stigma of
kichaa or wazimu. These psychotic conditions occur with a welter of
symptoms including aggression, confusion, paranoid symptoms,
inappropriate behavior, social withdrawal, self-neglect, auditory

and visual hallucinations, mutism, negativism, feelings of being controlled by external forces, and religious delusions. Schizophrenia in African patients has been reported to be fundamentally similar to that in European patients (German, 1987). However, a psychotic presentation colored by delusions of being bewitched, ancestral requisites, religious ideation, and somatization is stronger and more frequent among Tanzanian psychotic patients.

Acute episodes of brief or transient psychoses tend to be classified under the rubric of schizophrenia when, in fact, organic causative factors such as encephalopathy, toxic agents, falciparum malaria, sleeping sickness, or psychomotor epilepsy are responsible. Such inadequacy of diagnosing schizophrenia has in the past led to the notion that schizophrenia in developing countries carries a better prognosis than in industrialized nations (Stevens, 1987).

Though rare, severe depressive stupor with muteness, malnourishment, and encopresis and enuresis does occur (Ndosi, 1990). In most Tanzanian patients, depression is predominated by somatic complaints, which are culturally more acceptable than the expression of emotional complaints. Anxiety, nihilistic views of self with suicidal ideas may also be featured. Furthermore, hypochondriacal delusions may feature with bodily changes, gastrointestinal and cardiorespiratory.

In his study of puerperal psychiatric disturbances in Tanzania, Harris (1981) found that 38 percent of puerperal Tanzanian women showed similar "maternal blues" to other cultures.

Irarata is a malignant form of depression observed in the Meru tribe of Northern Tanzania. It is a severe reactive form of depression which characteristically affects menopausal women. When a healthy elderly woman loses her spouse through death, she becomes so severely depressed that the will to live on is affected. Anhedonic, she loses appetite and body weight. As if to escort her dead spouse, she dies within weeks or months of his death.

The typical neurotic patient usually gives a polysymptomatic history often dating back for several months or years. Vague physical complaints like things crawling under the skin, heat on the head, coldness and numbness in the limbs, choking, heaviness of head or chest, blurred vision, tremulousness, and shifting headaches of varying intensity may be present.

Common psychological complaints include excessive worries, nervousness, labile mood, irritability, inadequate intellectual concentration, apprehension, fearfulness, deficient self-assertiveness, and sexual inadequacy (Swift and Asuni, 1975). Neurotic symptoms may result from identifiable stressful experiences like divorce, loss of property, illness, or the death of a cherished person. Holmes and Speight (1975) found that 48 percent of patients attending general outpatient services in urban Dar es Salaam accounted for neurosis. The main complaints were abdominal pain, palpitations, chest pain, general body weakness, and genital complaints. Other less common symptoms were dizziness, headache, skin rash, musculoskeletal and limb weakness. In that study, anxiety was not only the most common and crippling disorder, as found in other African studies, but also the central core of other neurotic reactions (Lambo, 1962; Swift and Asuni, 1975).

The chief symptoms seen in conversion consist of laughing mania, weeping, overtalkativeness, stripping off clothes, fainting, and paralysis. Tremor, aphonia, blindness, and deafness are less frequent.

"Brain-fag" syndrome is a reactive disorder in adolescence described by Prince (1960) in Nigeria. This syndrome of anxiety depression commonly affects secondary school pupils under an academically competitive atmosphere. The sufferer tends to be rather anxious, complains of headache, burning, a crawling feeling, visual difficulties, poor comprehension, poor memory, general physical tiredness, and insomnia.

Phobia occurs predominantly in women since men are not expected culturally to show fear. Fear of heights, thunderstorms, darkness, animals, snakes, ghosts, or insects (Dudu-phobia) are not rare.

Malignant anxiety as described by Lambo (1960) occurs rarely. In this condition, the ego is subdued by severe psychic stress to the extent of social incapacitation and may sometimes lead to violence or even to a sudden death.

Mori is a frequent morbid rage experienced by Masai warriors. The affected warrior experiences a heightened state of aggressiveness which leads to irrational acts. The warrior progressively gets into a state of psychomotoric excitement as he growls with rage, hyperventilates, trembles with wide open eyes until he froths at the mouth. When he misses his target, he is usually physically restrained lest he turn homicidal.

Kupandisha mashetani (literally meaning to raise demons in oneself) is a form of spirit-possession which more frequently occurs amongst coastal women in Tanzania. The affected woman, who is usually a highly suggestible individual, becomes increasingly anxious until the anxiety reaches levels of ego disorganization and depersonalization. Dramatic bizarre behavior, including shouting, inappropriate acts, and hyperventilation, follow. *Jazba* is another dissociation state which occurs in a religious context. This condition occurs ordinarily in Muslims when reciting prayers. The praying person loses memory and mental coherence during an emotionally touching religious session and utters unintelligible speech.

ORGANIC BRAIN DISORDERS AND DRUG ABUSE

Acute organic reaction commonly referred to as confusional state is a temporary, usually reversible feature whose cardinal symptom is disturbance of consciousness. Other important symptoms include loss of memory, disorientation, especially to place, labile mood, insomnia, and visual hallucinations.

Major causes of organic brain disorders in Tanzania include infections such as severe falciparum malaria, meningitis, typhoid, H.I.V., pneumonia, trauma to the head, cerebral degenerative diseases, tumors, hepatic failure, diabetes mellitus, vitamin deficiencies, endocrine disorders, anemia, and malnutrition.

Alcohol and cannabis are at present the most widely abused drugs in Tanzania (Kilonzo and Maselle, 1986). Other less abused drugs include tobacco, Khat, cocaine, heroin, mandrax, benzodiazepines, analgesics, and solvents. The drug abusers are mostly young, unemployed males.

The majority of people in Tanzania who take alcoholic beverages do so to promote social intercommunication. In the precolonial area, brewing of alcohol was mainly for festivities and religious rites and the drinking of alcoholic beverages was mainly confined to adults. Rapid sociocultural and economic changes have altered the traditional drinking patterns and the production of alcoholic beverages in the last three decades has shifted more to the commercial area.

Our experience with cannabis is markedly at variance with previous reports from the West, where it is considered to be relatively harmless. Acute psychosis occurs in those who abuse cannabis, and it also tends to exacerbate psychotic processes like schizophrenia. The acute psychosis is characterized by auditory and visual hallucinations. Patients are irritable and aggressive, hyperactive and impulsive in their behavior. Formal thought disorders, delusions, anxiety, impairment of memory, and panic reaction do occur.

MANAGEMENT OF MENTAL DISTURBANCES

Traditional healers had been treating mental illness for hundreds of years before the dawn of modern medicine. The Tanzanian traditional healer, *mganga*, has always adopted a holistic view of the illness affecting the client. Some traditional healers are not only capable of effective care of psychotic patients by using tranquilizing herbs, but have considerable insight into the patient's circumstances, problems, and anxieties. Since large portions of rural populations have no access to medical practitioners, they consult the *mganga*. Even in cities, where Western medicine is accessible, patients consult traditional healers, often postponing medical treatment.

Drug therapy with appropriate doses of psychotropic drugs are increasingly becoming popular in treating psychiatric disorders. Antidepressants are effective in treating psychotic depression. Electroconvulsive treatment combined with antidepressants effectively treats long-term depression or postpartum depression. Low doses of 75 to 150 mg of Amitriptylene are better tolerated than higher doses because of the warm climate and small body weight of most patients. Communal response in providing support in times of bereavement or illness has an important cushioning psychotherapeutic effect. Treatment with minor tranquilizers over a week or two may alleviate anxiety and enable the patient to sleep better. Currently, psychiatric villages are tenable alternative means of rehabilitating chronic mental patients.

REFERENCES

German, A. G. (1987), Mental health in Africa. II The nature of mental disorder in Africa today. Some clinical observations. *Brit. J. Psychiat.*, 151:440–446.

Harris, B. (1981), Maternity blues in East African clinic attenders. *Arch. Gen. Psychiat.*, 38:1293–1295.

Holmes, J. A., & Speight, A. N. (1975), The problem of non-organic illness in Tanzanian urban medical practice. *E. African Med. J.*, 52:225–236.

Kilonzo, G. P., & Maselle, A. Y. (1986), Substance misuse in Tanzania. *Tanzania Med. J.*, 3:21–22.

Lambo, T. A. (1962), Malignant anxiety in the African. *J. Ment. Sci.*, 108:256–264.

Ndosi, N. K. (1990), Primary affective disorders. *Med. Digest*, 16:3–8.

Neki, J. S., Joinet, B., Hogan, M., Hauli, J. G., & Kilonzo, G. (1985), Therapeutic perspective of cultural relationship. *Acta Psychiat. Scand.*, 71:543–550.

Prince, R. (1960), The "brain-fag" syndrome in Nigerian students. *J. Ment. Sci.*, 106:559–570.

Stevens, J. (1987), Brief psychoses: Do they contribute to the good prognosis and equal prevalence of schizophrenia in developing countries? *Brit. J. Psychiat.*, 151:393–396.

Swift, C. R., & Asuni, T. (1975), *Mental Health and Disease in Africa.* New York: Churchill, Livingstone.

6.

The Interface Between Culture and Mental Illness in French Speaking West Africa

René Collignon and Momar Gueye

Institutions for psychiatric care are of recent origin in French-speaking West Africa. They have been increasing in number in recent years, and are still undergoing development. The history of psychiatry in this region has been deeply influenced by the work, teachings, and publications of Henri Collomb[1] who directed the psychiatric clinic of the Centre Hospitalier Universitaire de Fann-Dakar (Senegal) from 1959 to 1978.

At its creation in 1956, the neuropsychiatric service at Fann was designed to fit the classic model of custodial care; it replaced the locked cells and isolation wards of the existing overcrowded general hospitals during the colonial period. After Senegal was declared a Republic in 1958, the neuropsychiatric clinic of Fann lost its federal status[2] and became an open service. The development of certain institutional practices and various fields of research introduced by Collomb and his team attested to the growing awareness of the inadequacies of both psychiatric structures and the applicability of imported models of psychiatric care.

Acknowledgments. The authors wish to express their gratitude to Dr. Robert R. Franklin for his kind assistance in reviewing the English translation of this article.

[1]Of whom the present authors were a collaborator and a student respectively.

[2]The former Federation of French West Africa (AOF: Afrique Occidentale française).

PSYCHIATRIC RESEARCH IN THE WEST AFRICAN CONTEXT

Confronted with the problem of trying to communicate with patients from different cultures, in 1962 the psychiatrists (who were almost exclusively Europeans during that time) developed a multidisciplinary team (clinical psychologists, psychosociologists, and sociologists and one psychoanalyst) which devoted itself to research. This team worked closely with the psychiatrists; yet, was not directly concerned with delivering psychiatric care.

An outpatient clinic in the field of clinical psychology was established for children and adolescents with learning difficulties (but was also open for adults). The opening of that clinic turned attention to the special difficulties to be encountered with such an enterprise in a cross-cultural setting: methods of operation, clinical setting, language barriers, cultural landmarks, speech patterns, dynamics of relationships, interviews with the child and the family, attitudes of adults toward children (Ortigues, 1963). Simultaneously, studies were initiated on the psychomotor development of Senegalese children (Valantin, 1970) and forms of socialization from the weaning period to integration into their age group (Zempléni-Rabain, 1966, 1968; Rabain, 1979). Research was also conducted on questions surrounding education, viewing it as an indicator of the transition between two cultures; the questions of entrance into the educational system, the relation between the family and the school (Colot, 1965), the authority of the parent over the children (Le Guérinel, Ndiaye, Ortigues, Berne, and Delbard, 1969), and juvenile delinquency (Hugot, 1969; Ortigues, Colot, and Montagnier, 1965) were important subjects for reflection and study.

On the side of ethnological research, Andràs Zempléni (1966, 1968) studied the interpretations and traditional methods of treatment of mental disorders among the Wolof and Lebou ethnic groups. These populations had developed few nosological concepts,[3] but instead emphasized etiological interpretations conceiving of mental illness as the byproduct or final result of some

---

[3]They recognize the prevalence of nosology over the etiology in only two cases: epilepsy and mental retardation which are considered incurable.

outside intervention by forces experienced as persecutory. As the underlying principle for explaining such problems, these beliefs also serve the major criteria for their classification, the instruments for their interpretation, and the operating principles for their therapy (Zempléni, 1968, pp. 90–92). The belief system identifies four types of aggression: (1) that involving ancestral spirits (*rab, tuur*); (2) that involving Islamic spirits (*jinn, seytanne*), and those originating from aggressive relationships among human beings; (3) attacks by witches (*dëmm*); (4) interpersonal magic or sorcery (*liggéey*). A remarkable characteristic of these beliefs is that they are shared by everyone and provide a common language which helps the patient to overcome the alienating effects of his experience by means of the mediations of the therapist and the ritualized therapeutic procedures that integrate the disturbed person into his social environment and reestablish him in his place in society. The successive steps in this therapeutic process include the interpretation of the pathological experience, the reorganization and manipulation of it around collective beliefs (persecutory figures). The distressing experience of the individual is shared by the immediate group and then mediated by the consulting therapist. Thus, the individual experience is transformed into a group experience and with group responsibility for the illness, which then allows for a cure through symbolic approaches (Zempléni, 1968). Several publications by this author analyze and describe in detail certain ritual procedures (Zempléni, 1966) and illustrate through life histories, particularly that of a Wolof priestess (officiant) of the *ndëpp* ritual (Zempléni, 1974), how the articulation of cultural meanings permits the formulation and resolution of conflicts by reinstating the person into his system of filiation and descent.

Still taking an anthropological perspective which adopts an emic point of view, Andràs Zempléni and Jacqueline Rabain have shown in the description of a traditional psychopathological picture of the child among the Wolof, "how a culture constructs and describes, utilizes and explains a pathological entity by using its own meanings" (Zempléni and Rabain, 1965, p. 331). The child who is labeled *nit ku bon* (literally means "the person who is bad") is characterized by refusal to respond, extreme sensitivity, frequent crises, and violent reactions to everything he or she considers hostile. He is thought to be either an ancestral spirit that desires to visit humans, or a reincarnated ancestor, or a *doom u yaradal* (a child of a mother whose children successively die) in which case the later children are considered to be reappearances of the original one who do nothing but return again and again.[4] Such a child is an alien, and his behavior refers only to his personal subjectivity (he acts, does not react). In the group's ambivalence (promised a great future, threatened with death), he is considered to be able to leave again on his own initiative at the least annoyance from his group. This is because of his closeness with ancestors or *rab*. The beliefs surrounding the *nit ku bon* are very much related to questions about identity which neither entirely correspond to a social identity nor to a cultural one; they also show what behavior is expected from children and how deviations from the norms are interpreted.

NOSOLOGICAL DATA

At the same time more and more important information was being collected in the clinical field. Information gathered from the hospital allowed better understanding of the semiological and nosological characteristics of psychopathology in an African environment (Collomb, 1965a, 1967). Concerning neuroses, there was found to be a high frequency of anxiety states and reactions, often accompanied by agitated motor or verbal symptoms and various somatic complaints (unpleasant sensations, particularly on the skin), vegetative and metabolic disorders. Acute anxiety states were found to be experienced as attacks on the body with a threat of imminent death (attacks by witches). It seems that these reactive symptoms rarely corresponded to an organized neurotic structure. If hysteria was frequent, many of its somatic manifestations were associated with a more general synchretic expression shown in bodily complaints as well as in speech and

---

[4]Similar representations related to children born after a series of deaths exist throughout West Africa; *o kin a paxeer* among the Serer (Senegal), the *burdo* of Peul, the *kinkirga* child of Mossi (Birkina Faso), the *abiku* of the Yoruba (Nigeria, Benin) the *Ogbanji* of Igbo (Nigeria), etc.

behavior. Other frequently seen forms of neurosis close to hysteria are: enuresis, impotency, physical or intellectual inhibitions (the "brain fag" syndrome of Anglo-Saxon authors), fear of competing. Phobic behavior was found to be part of daily life, imposed from outside and experienced collectively in a socialized expression of the prohibitions and rituals which seemed to help the individual to avoid obsessional neuroses. It is often difficult to separate psychoses from neuroses; and the boundaries between delusions and hallucinations are often imprecise. Dreams, fantasies, vivid images, and hallucinations are often confused and it is sometimes difficult to separate delusional interpretations from collective beliefs which are the basis of sociocultural organization.

What seems to emerge from hospital data is that the rates of psychoses are lower than those encountered in France and in the West. This is often thought to be related to the educational and cultural methods in Africa which might protect against schizophrenic dissociation. On the other hand, the high level of tolerance present avoids or delays permanent alienation. Some peculiarities worth mentioning are: the rarity of catatonic states, the frequency of somatization and hysterical symptoms, and the difficulty of the differential diagnosis with chronic depressive states when characterized by social withdrawal and autistic behavior. The *bouffée délirante* (Collomb, 1965b), with its high frequency and clinical symptoms, constitutes a noticeable feature of psychiatric pathology in Africa. It occurs everywhere and is the expression of a specific personality structure and the prevailing type of sociocultural organization. As an indicator of some weakness in the personality, *bouffée délirante* also constitutes a regulatory system at both the personal and social levels. The persecutory attitudes and values of an individual and his persona within the makeup of the African personality allow us to better understand the high frequency and wide variety of forms of this common syndrome. Although the clinical picture is sometimes similar to schizophrenia, the *bouffée délirante* maintains an open dialogue with his community since the group shares the same beliefs; its prognosis is also quite good due to its potential reversibility.[5] Manic-depressive

---

[5]Murphy writes the following about *bouffées delirantes* in the West Indies: "still more appear to have become psychotic at a moment of crisis in some internal conflict, a conflict which in Europeans would be expected to give rise to a neurosis rather than a psychosis." And later: "In West Africa the same can be said of some of the delusional cases described

psychosis is rare with clear predominance of the manic over the depressive form. Rarely if ever are there delusions of a self-accusatory nature; the feeling of self-deprecation is not externalized the same way among Africans as in the West; suicidal behavior is also less often observed (Collomb and Collignon, 1974). Beliefs in possession and persecution, or hypchondriacal preoccupations, which are more evident, can mask the underlying depression. One must emphasize the particular difficulty of a differential diagnosis between confusional states in psychosis (frequent in tropical environments) and stuporous states in depression. It is also worth noting the relatively high frequency of hospitalization for puerperal psychosis, which many authors associate with sociocultural factors such as: the importance of motherhood and producing descendants, the early age of marriage for young women, taboos surrounding procreation, traditional beliefs concerning the dangers of pregnancy and childbirth (Gueye, 1976; Durand-Comiot, 1977).

This brief summary of the psychopathology found in the hospital environment in Senegal is intended to give only a glimpse of the field of psychiatry there. The efforts to interpret the findings dealt mostly with recognizing the specific role played by sociocultural factors in influencing the elements that intervene in the etiology, symptomatology, and evolution of mental illness.[6]

In comparing anthropological data gathered in the field and clinical data recorded during consultation, psychiatrists have quickly learned to recognize how much the theme of persecution

---

in the book *Oedipe africain*, and we have an admirably clear picture of the transition from what we would call psychotic to neurotic mechanisms of defense in an Ivory Coast patient described by Zempléni (1975)" (Murphy, 1982, pp. 104–105).

[6]The epidemiological approach in terms of the number and distribution of mental disturbances in the population and the factors influencing this distribution was undoubtedly the aspect least developed by the Fann team. In comparison with the general demands of this branch of medicine, the epidemiological approach is concerned with characteristic difficulties in practicing psychiatry in the region: scarcity of personnel and specialized institutions; the multitude of beliefs and traditional interpretations of illness; turning to unfamiliar means of care, and intercultural practice. However, clinicians have noticed the importance of epidemiology which aims beyond the descriptive statistics at the knowledge of favorable factors and consequently establishes methods of care and prevention. Collomb (1965a, p. 50; 1967, p. 241) attempts to clarify the comment on the nosological distribution of 2000 hospitalized patients in the neuropsychiatric clinic of Fann from 1959 to 1965 (Table 6.1) and compares them with the then current standard French classification system (Table 6.2), and with the standard international classification (Table 6.3).

TABLE 6.1
Senegalese Data

C	M	D	BD	DC	Sch	N
5%	5%	15%	30%	5%	5%	5%

PO = 20%

TABLE 6.2
Standard French Classification (Ey, 1958)

C	MD	BD	Sch	N
5%	20%	5%	20%	5%

PO = 20%

TABLE 6.3
Standard International Classification (Ey, 1958)

C	MD	Sch	N
5%	20%	35%	20%

PO = 20%

C	= *états confusionnels* [confusional disorders]
MD	= *états maniaques, états dépressifs, psychoses périodiques* [manic disorders, depressive disorders, periodic disorders]
BD	= *bouffeés délirantes* [acute psychosis, paranoid reactions . . .]
DC	= *délires chroniques* [chronic delusions]
SCH	= *schizophrénie* [schizophrenia]
N	= *névroses* [neuroses]
PO	= *psychoses organiques* [organic psychosis]

In another context, the study which was carried out between 1976 and 1979 in a rural region in the Serer country of Senegal (Diop, Collignon, Gueye, and Harding, 1982) has considered the frequency and the nature of psychological symptoms and mental disturbances in the primary health care services and their detection by officials of the services. Among 545 children examined, the frequency of mental disturbance was 16.9 percent. Among 897 adult medical records, 8.8 percent showed mental health disturbance. There have been other statistical studies conducted at Fann as well as in other psychiatric services. The lack of rigor in these works, their use of different methodologies, and their sectarian character does not allow one to make a comparison. We will cite as an illustration the thesis of Adam Andrade (1979) who studied 1742 files of patients seen in the outpatient consultation ward of CHU of Fann during a year (September 1, 1977–August 31, 1978).

The following was the distribution of patients.

C	M	D	BD	DC	Sch	N
2%	6.4%	8.2%	10.5%	5.5%	15%	5%

The rest that are included together are drug addiction, other unspecified behavior disturbances, and epilepsy.

colors all psychopathology in Africa: Whether "Experienced through a delusion or interpretation, or cultural belief, [persecution] becomes an explanation of everything that disturbs the general social order, destroys personal relationships and affects the individual's physical and mental, or spiritual being. It is first experienced by the individual, then proposed by the family or group, and finally given form by the healer or marabout" (Diop, Zempléni, Martino, and Collomb, 1964). In many publications[7] with a psychodynamic perspective based on psychoanalytical concepts and approaches, clinicians advanced hypotheses to correlate models of traditional beliefs with the individualization of oedipean positions (Ortigues and Martino, 1965; Ortigues, Diop, and Collomb, 1964; Ortigues, Martino, and Collomb, 1966). These hypotheses rely on clear similarities between traditional persecutory beliefs and certain stages of personality organization. As much from the point of view (1) of the form of the relationship and (2) its imaginary content, as (3) from that of the body-image which underlies it, the dynamics of *witchcraft* correspond to a pregenital oral level. On the other hand the interpretation of *sorcery* is considered to be at the level of the dynamic phallic stage in light of its analogous functioning at the same three levels. The structural similarity is clear enough from these three points of view that the beliefs used by the patients take on a psychological significance and thus become manageable to the therapist. In contrast to witchcraft and sorcery, the interpretations involving the *rab* do not correspond to a particular stage of organization but rather to a mode of resolution of conflicts. Where the interpretations of witchcraft and magic allow a personal formulation of aggressivity—you should fight against the witch which devours you and protect yourself against a *liggéey* by a more powerful *liggéey*—the relation with the *rab* implies a total submission to their will (Ortigues and Ortigues, 1966, chap. 5, chap. 4).

AFRICAN DEPRESSION

We will now deal briefly with a group of studies carried out in Dakar on the long-debated question of depression in Africa, before reconsidering some criticisms directed toward the hypotheses of the Fann team concerning the place of persecutory

---

[7]The most complete theoretical and clinical elaboration is found in the work of Marie-Cécile and Edmond Ortigues (*Oedipe africain* [1966] of which there were three editions).

interpretations and the importance of somatic expression of mental problems.

From the early 1960s, psychiatric hospital statistics from Dakar have noted the frequency of depressive states, finding an approximate rate of 15 percent (Collomb and Zwingelstein, 1962; Diop, 1961; Collomb, 1965a).[8] Among the general characteristics found in these studies, are the importance of somatic signs and symptoms, the almost constant presence of delusional ideas of persecution, and the rarity of ideas of worthlessness, self-accusation,[9] and suicidal behavior. The frequency of somatic complaints hinders a more in-depth investigation of depression at the conflict level; on the other hand, the traditional persecutory beliefs provide a common and convenient screen for projections. During the following years, we witnessed an evolution in depressive symptomatology. René Ahyi (1977), confirming the previous observations, drew attention to the difference in symptomatology occurring in the same hospital service among the most acculturated subjects, and which approached the classical picture of depression observed in Europe and the West. In a retrospective study of a period of twenty years (1961–1980), Michel M'Boussou (1981) traces trends in the evolution of depression in Senegal from hospitalized cases with a diagnosis of the depressive syndrome at Fann. He clarifies three "types" of syndromes; which helps to clarify the evolution of symptoms of depression. Type I corresponds to the form of African depression described earlier. Type II corresponds to a symptomatology that could be superimposed upon the classic syndrome in the West and in which one

---

This work suggests profound methodological reflection on the relations between ethnology and psychoanalysis. It tackles on a theoretical level the problem of the universality of the Oedipus complex by presenting clinical data which allows one to clarify the particular modalities of organization of oedipal positions in the Senegal; these data were examined from a psychoanalytical point of view which was activated from inside the categories of African traditions.

[8]It will be remembered that Prince (1968), in a review of the literature on depression in Africa, emphasized that all reports during the colonial period recorded the absence or the rarity of depression in Africa. He points out that only from the fifties were quite frequent rates of depression noted: attention was given to more specific manifestations of depression and it was consequently recognized more often behind the masks of physical complaints.

[9]One cannot reach any conclusion about the absence of feelings of depreciation. These feelings are not expressed in the same way, but rather as impotence, fatigue, and so on.

observes a tendency for the localization of somatic complaints; the presence of verbalized feelings of guilt, self-accusation, and worthlessness; lack of delusions of persecution; and an increased frequency of suicidal behavior. Type III produces a mixture of type I and II in which anxiety and suicidal behavior are dominant. We witness during these two decades an evolution of somatic complaints in which they tended to be reduced in intensity, became more fixed on a specific organ, and lost the diffused character more frequent in the past. This transformation of "somatic symptoms" was encountered more often among subjects imbued with Western culture. Women more than men presented the rich body symptomatology often described in Africa. An evolution also took place in the interpretation of persecution: systematized delusions of persecution, formed in accordance with various interpretations involving the supernatural world, began to lose their mysterious and magical character, ending up as more "rational" systems. Although always present, the systematizing of delusions gave way to complex and diffused feelings of persecution which could no longer succeed in channeling anxiety. Current economic changes facing African states because of the world situation, and their devastating effects on traditional family organization as well as other solidarity enhancing groups such as those of the same age, forced the individual into meeting the demands of competition and all that it implies, such as the management of aggressiveness. Traditional interests are losing their relevance in the new and changing situation and the development of clinical material over a twenty-year period seems to emphasize the progressive appearance of guilt in association with increasing modernity.

DISCUSSION

The importance of persecutory beliefs as well as somatic symptoms as put forward by clinicians and researchers at Fann, has been the object of criticism by some authors. In an article proposing a program to restore the individual dimension of African psychology, Corin (1980) proceeds to criticize the widespread notion that the African personality is essentially communal, a notion she considers to represent a vision too homogenizing and exclusively socializing. She shows in a convincing manner from material gathered first hand in a matrilineal clan in Zaire that "the hierarchical, collectivizing structure of traditional societies often described, whose impact on personality has been stated, constitutes only the most manifest level of functioning of the social structure" (1980, p. 146). She continues: "it is important to understand that the society itself has established mechanisms to permit the person to individualize his position and to protect himself against the homogeneous and collective character of his relationship to the clan" (1980, p. 146). Next, examining the relationship to the notion of evil and to the notion of conflict within the traditional beliefs, she observes that anthropologists and psychiatrists are mainly interested in a level of interpretation of causality which is profound, unnatural, or mystical, and lies at the heart of cultural studies. Starting from the diagnoses made by healers themselves in the context of illness, Corin thinks that it is the notion of "persecutory themes" themselves that should be criticized. An analysis of her material from Zaire shows that the cultural explanation has most often been put into effect by what she calls a "primary cause" (Corin and Bibeau, 1975). It is at this primary level that the person participates in the etiological dynamics of his illness; the second level of causality, the evoked cultural explanations (the etiological agents) are only mobilized afterwards. It appears to Corin to be important therefore to distinguish between two aspects in the matter of the traditional etiological interpretations: that of the dynamics at the origin of the conflict and that of the manner of action of the conflict on the person. On the other hand, she considers that one should try to understand the organization of the person at two different levels in his relation to the community in African societies, "that of the *diktat* of the society which emphasizes the importance of the communal dimension, and that of the experience of the individual for whom this dimension is shown in conflict with a more individual orientation" (Corin, 1980, p. 151). These remarks are welcome for their help in clarifying the levels of analysis and because of their appeal for rigorous reflection on the conceptions of the person in black Africa.[10] They seem, however, to be more relevant to some of the general articles containing ideas which are sometimes a little hastily prepared and reductionist concerning the effects of forms of education and socialization on individuals in Africa, than to clinical articles (particularly case studies), or to anthropological works on etiological beliefs and ritualistic or therapeutic procedures associated with them. "The story of Khady Fall," a presentation and interpretation of the autobiography of a Wolof priestess–therapist (*ndëppkat*) which was presented by Zempléni (1974), is undoubtedly one of the most successful attempts in anthropology for "defining a *method* which makes individual cases expressed through and in the language of socio-religious meanings of traditional cultures" accessible to the clinical perspective. A number of case studies illustrate the frequent use of themes of persecution (Diop and Collomb, 1965a,b; Martino, Zempléni, and Collomb, 1965; Ortigues and Ortigues, 1966; Ortigues et al., 1966, 1967). These, however, do not exclude the use of other themes. They show great flexibility in using the traditional beliefs, which were in turn found to be dependent upon the needs and abilities of the individual and his group in a context of religious syncretism. There is a place here for the consideration of professional ethics. As was emphasized by M. C. Ortigues et al. (1967, p. 145), the physician, clinician, and therapist would be as open to criticism if they did not recognize traditions and their organizing power as to discharge the patient who will have, if that is the case, no choice. What is important in an authentic psychoanalytical approach is to try to understand the place of the person in what he says. The cultural decoding of his discourse is not the aim in itself. Even in so-called traditional societies, personal searching manifests itself and new elaborations search themselves by questioning social data or by more personalizing cultural references. The role of the therapist is to accompany the patient in his own questioning of himself and in following his destiny, while respecting his choice of means of expression. With this approach, some patients go a bit far in taking complete control as subjects of their own lives. This takes place in the context

---

[10]In this regard, the late Paul Riesman has carried out an extensive review of the literature on the notion of the person in black Africa (Riesman, 1986).

of a changing society where people are confronted more and more by being between two worlds where the subjects' reference systems are confused and searching for themselves. In this respect, the case of the therapeutic community of Bregbo in the lower part of the Ivory Coast, built around the charismatic figure of Albert Atcho who invoked the Harriste prophetic religious movement, seems to suggest a sort of intermediate situation between the persecutory model and that of internalized guilt, between sociocollective beliefs of evil and the internalization of the idea of evil and illness. Zempléni is able to conclude from cases of confession in Bregbo that:

> In substituting the ideology of the diabolical offense for the former persecutory schema, it (the prophetic movement) sanctions for some (the confessors) and denies for others (their families) the decline of a sociopsychological mechanism which has in any case already turned against the individual. In instituting an intersubjective structure characterized (yet) by the stated external division of a subject who speaks and his projected, evil double about whom he speaks . . . , he brings about the process of internalization of guilt. In making the prophet not only the witness of the person's evil double but also a charismatic master who focuses the hostile wishes thus projected, he establishes a protective structure which mediates the effects of taking care of his own aggressiveness [Zempléni, 1975, pp. 215–216].

The apparent evolution of symptomatology over time and the relatively personalized positions of patients in their recourse to different ways of interpreting their misfortunes, such as those emerging from studies on depression, and case studies mentioned earlier, as well as traditional and prophetic therapies, underline the importance of putting these basic questions into a historical and comparative perspective. In our view, one of the most interesting attempts in this regard is that of the late Henry B. M. Murphy (1978, 1979) who points out a striking similarity between the symptoms of depression in England in the sixteenth century and the situation described by the first psychiatrists in Africa in the twentieth century. He explains that if melancholy has existed in all periods of known history, up until the sixteenth century the number of documented cases presenting exaggerated feelings of guilt and self-accusation was so small that physicians did not even take them into account in their descriptions of the phenomenon. The feelings of guilt, therefore, appeared as a common symptom of depression secondarily between 1620 and 1670 giving English melancholia its modern form. To account for the emergence of these symptoms, Murphy suggests a relationship between the development of economic, social, and cultural processes in the sense of the promotion of the dimension of individuality in the culture with the effects of internalization of the intrapsychic superego in association with changes in the modification of the parent–child relationship and in conceptions of educational systems.

The data emerging from clinical, psychosocial, and ethnological research encouraged the Fann-Dakar team to make institutional improvements at the hospital to make psychiatry more open to a social mission: emphasis was put on the integration of patients into society. A therapeutic community was established in the hospital: the *pénc* (meeting of the hospital ward modeled after a village palaver) was initiated and organized with an open door policy and the admission of patients' companions who came to stay on the wards with the patients while they were hospitalized. Limited attempts to integrate the healer within the hospital demonstrated the difficulties, ambiguities, and misunderstandings of such an approach. Inspired by traditional African therapeutic communities and the Nigerian experience of professor T. A. Lambo (Aro village program), attempts were also made to establish village psychiatric communities for mental patients.[11]

The establishment of these innovations was in part due to the sustained effort of Collomb's team to develop training in neuropsychiatry. About ten candidates received a *certificat d'Etudes Spéciales* (CES) in neuropsychiatry between 1965 and 1971. After 1968, following a transitional period, the separation between neurology and psychiatry was completed; a four-year CES program was organized. In 1972, the ''Internat en Psychiatrie des hopitaux

---

[11]For these different experiences, the reader should refer to the indexed works in the annotated bibliography of Collomb's team (Collignon, 1978) as well as to the files on the ''psychiatric villages'' (Collignon, 1983).

de Dakar (a more intensive training program in psychiatry) was created. About thirty young African physicians (from Senegal, Burkina Faso, Cameroon, Bénin, Gabon, Guinea, Mali, Niger, and Togo) were trained. Many of these physicians have since returned to their countries to establish structures more responsive to patient needs. For further information, we point out some of the following publications on psychiatry and mental health in Bénin (Tall and Ahyi, 1988–1989); in Burkina Faso (Mitelberg, Sanou, and Ouedraogo, 1986–1987); in Mali (Coulibaly, Koumare, and Coudray, 1983; Koumare, Coudray, and Miquel Garcia, 1989; Uchoa, 1988; Coppo and Keita, 1990). The near future heralds quite promising developments in psychiatric research: we particularly note the appearance (1992) of a special issue of the journal, *Psychopathologie Africaine*, which was devoted entirely to mental health in Mali, edited by professor Baba Koumaré and his colleagues; and finally the participation of some colleagues from the Ivory Coast and Mali in a comparative study dealing with "the systems of signs, meanings, and actions" coordinated by Ellen Corin and Gilles Bibeau, a study that should be taking place simultaneously in selected areas of Mali, the Ivory coast, Brazil, Peru, and India.

REFERENCES

Ahyi, R. G. (1977), Les états dépressifs au Sénégal (à propos de 246 observations). Unpublished doctoral dissertation, Faculty of Medicine, University of Dakar.

Andrade, A. (1979), *La demande d'assistance psychiatrique au Sénégal. Approche statistique* (The demand for psychiatric treatment in Senegal. A statistical approach). Unpublished doctoral dissertation, Dakar University, Faculty of Medicine, Dakar, Senegal.

Bibeau, G. (1981), Préalables à une épidémiologie anthropologique de la dépression (Preliminary studies for a epidemiological-anthropological study of depression). *Psychopathologie Africaine*, 17:96–112.

Collignon, R. (1978), Vingt ans de travaux à la clinique psychiatrique de Fann-Dakar (Twenty years of work at a psychiatric clinic in Fann-Dakar). *Psychopathologie Africaine*, 19:287–328.

——— (1983), À propos de psychiatrie communautaire en Afrique noire. Les dispositifs villageois d'assistance. Eléments pour un dossier (On community psychiatry in black Africa. The apparatus of village aid. Notes for a study). *Psychopathologie Africaine,* 19:287–328.

Collomb, H. (1965a), Assistance psychiatrique en Afrique (expérience sénégalaise) (Psychiatric help in Africa [Experience in Senegal]). *Psychopathologie Africaine,* 1:11–84.

—— (1965b), Les bouffées délirantes en psychiatrie africaine (Acute psychosis in African psychiatry). *Psychopathologie Africaine,* 1:167–239.

—— (1967), Aspects de la psychiatrie dans l'ouest africain (Sénégal) (Aspects of psychiatry in West Africa [Senegal]). In: *Contributions to Comparative Psychiatry,* ed. N. Petrowitsch. Basel/New York: Karger, pp. 229–253.

—— (1977), La mort en tant qu'organisateur de syndromes psychosomatiques en Afrique (Death as an organizer of psychosomatic syndromes in Africa). *Psychopathologie Africaine,* 13:137–147.

—— Collignon, R. (1974), Les conduites suicidaires en Afrique (Pathways to suicide in Africa). *Psychopathologie Africaine,* 10:55–113.

——Zwingelstein, J. (1962), Depressive states in an African community. *First Pan-African Psychiatric Conference* (Abeokuta, 1961). Conference Report, ed. T. A. Lambo. Ibadan, Government Printer, pp. 227–234.

Colot, A. (1965), Note sur l'entrée à l'école dans l'agglomeration dakaroise (Entrance into school in the Dakar region). *Psychopathologie Africaine,* 1:130–150.

Coppo, P., & Keita, A., eds. (1990), *Médecine traditionnelle. Acteurs, itinéraires thérapeutiques* (Traditional medicine. Therapeutic personnel and delivery systems). Trieste: Edizioni E.

Corin, E. (1980), Vers une réappropriation de la dimension individuelle en psychologie africaine (Towards reestablishing the individual dimension in African psychology). *Revue canadienne des études africaines (Can. J. African Studies),* 14:135–156.

—— Bibeau, G. (1975), De la forme culturelle au vécu des troubles psychiques en Afrique: propositions méthodologiques pour une étude interculturelle du champ des maladies mentales (On the cultural element in psychiatric disorders in Africa: Proposed methodology for an intercultural field study on mental illnesses). *Africa,* 45:280–315.

Coulibaly, B., Koumare, B., & Coudray, J.-P. (1983), La demande de soins psychiatriques au Mali: données d'épidémiologie hospitalière (The demand for psychiatric care in Mali: Data on the epidemiology of hospitalization). *Psychopathologie Africaine,* 19:261–286.

Diop, B., Collignon, R., Gueye, M., & Harding, T. W. (1982), Diagnosis and symptoms of mental disorder in a rural area of Senegal. *African J. Med. & Med. Sci.*, 11:95–103.

Diop, M. (1961), La dépression chez le Noir Africain (Depression in the black African). *Psychopathologie Africaine*, 3:183–184, 1967.

———— Collomb, H. (1965a), Pratiques mystiques et psychopathologie: à propos d'un cas (Mystical practices and psychopathology: A case study). *Psychopathologie Africaine*, 1:304–322.

———— ———— (1965b), A propos d'un cas d'impuissance (On a case of impotence). *Psychopathologie Africaine*, 1:487–511.

———— Zempléni, A., Martino, P., & Collomb, H. (1964), Signification et valeur de la persécution dans les cultures africaines (The meaning and import of paranoia in African cultures). In: *Congrès de Psychiatrie et de la Neurologie de langue française*, Vol. 1. Paris: Masson, pp. 333–343.

Durand-Comiot, M.-L. (1977), La psychose puerpérale? Etude en milieu sénégalais (Puerperal psychosis? A study in the Senegalese context). *Psychopathologie Africaine*, 13:169–335.

Ey, H. (1958), Les problèmes cliniques des schizophrénies (Clinical problems of schizophrenics). *L'Evolution psychiatrique*, 11:149–212.

Gueye, M. (1976), *Les psychoses puerpérales en milieu sénégalais (a propos de 92 observations)* (Puerperal psychoses in Senegal (92 cases)). Unpublished doctoral dissertation, Faculty of Medicine, Dakar University, Dakar, Senegal.

Hugot, S. (1969), Le problème de la délinquance juvénile a Dakar (The problem of juvenile delinquency in Dakar). *Psychopathologie Africaine*, 5:75–99.

Koumaré, B. (1992), Sauté mentale au Mali (numéro spécial sans la direction de). *Psychopathologie Africaine*, 24:133–287.

————Coudray, J.-P., & Miquel Garcia, E. (1989), Der psychiatrische Dienst in Mali. Überlegungen zur Unterbringung von chronischen Psychiatrischen Patienten bei traditionellen Heilkundigen (Psychiatric services in Mali. Reflections on treating chronic psychiatric patients with traditional healing methods). *Curare*, 12:145–152.

Le Guérinel, N., Ndiaye, M., Ortigues, M. C., Berne, C., & Delbard, B. (1969), L'autorité et son évolution dans les relations parents–enfants à Dakar (The evolution of authority in parent–child relations in Dakar). *Psychopathologie Africaine*, 5:11–73.

Martino, P., Zempléni, A., & Collomb, H. (1965), Delire et représentations culturelles. A propos du meurtre d'un sorcier (Delirium and cultural representations. On the murder of a sorcerer). *Psychopathologie Africaine*, 1:151–157.

M'Boussou, M. (1981), Contribution à l'étude des états dépressifs au Sénégal (A propos de 417 observations à la clinique psychiatrique du CHU de Fann-Dakar). Unpublished doctoral dissertation, Faculty of Medicine, University of Dakar.

Mitelberg, G., ed. (Conceived and developed collectively by Sanou, Z., Ouedraogo, A., & Mitelberg, G.) (1986–1987), Projet de développement de la santé mentale au Burkina-Faso. Ministère de la Santé et de l'Action Sociale de Burkina Faso (Project to develop mental health in Burkina-Faso. Ministry of Health and Action Sociale, Burkina Faso). *Psychopathologie Africaine*, 21:19–65.

Murphy, H. B. M. (1978), The advent of guilt feelings as a common depressive symptom: A historical comparison on two continents. *Psychiatry*, 41:229–242.

———— (1979), Depression, witchcraft beliefs and super-ego development in preliterate societies. *Can. J. Psychiatry*, 24:437–449.

———— (1982), *Comparative Psychiatry: The International and Intercultural Distribution of Mental Illness*. New York: Springer Verlag.

Ortigues, M.-C. (with Colot, A., Pierre, E., Rabain, J., & Valantin, S. (1963), Problèmes de psychologie clinique concernant les enfants sénégalais. La situation d'examen (An examination of the problem of clinical psychology in regard to Senegalese children). *Bull. et Mémoire de la Fac. mixte de Médecine et de Pharmacie de Dakar*, 11:160–174.

———— Colot, A., & Montagnier, M.-T. (1965), La délinquance juvénile à Dakar. Etude psychologique de 14 cas (Juvenile delinquency in Dakar. A psychological study of 14 cases). *Psychopathologie Africaine*, 1:85–129.

———— Diop, M., & Collomb, H. (1964), Syndromes de possession, niveaux d'organisation de la personnalité et structures sociales (Possession syndromes, standards of personality organization and social structures). In: *Congrès de Psychiatrie et de Neurologie de langue française*, Vol. 1. Paris: Masson.

———— Martino, P. (1965), Psychologie clinique et psychiatrie en milieu africain (Clinical psychology and psychiatry in an African milieu). *Psychopathologie Africaine*, 1:240–253.

———— ———— Collomb, H. (1966), Intégration des données culturelles africaines à la psychiatrie de l'enfant dans la pratique clinique au Sénégal (Integration of African cultural givens in the psychiatric treatment of a child in a clinic in Senegal). *Psychopathologie Africaine*, 2:441–450.

———— ———— ———— (1967), L'utilisation des données culturelles dans un cas de bouffée delirante (The use of cultural givens in a case of acute psychosis). *Psychopathologie Africaine*, 3:121–147.

———— Ortigues, E. (1966), *Oedipe africain* (African Oedipus), 3rd ed. Paris: L'Harmattan, 1984.

Prince, R. (1960), The "brain fag" syndrome in Nigerian students. *J. Ment. Sci.*, 106:559–570.

———— (1968), The changing picture of depressive syndromes in Africa. *Can. J. African Studies*, 1:177–192.

Rabain, J. (1979), *L'enfant du lignage. Du sevrage à la classe d'âge chez les Wolof du Senegal* (The child of lineage. From weaning to entrance into the age group amongst the Wolofs of Senegal). Paris: Payot.

Riesman, P. (1986), The person and the life cycle in African social life and thought. *African Studies Rev.*, 29:71–138.

Tall, E. K., & Ahyi, R. G. (1988–1989), Le centre de neuro-psychiatrie de Jacquot: un itinéraire, ou les difficultés de la mise en place des structures de la psychiatrie en Afrique (l'exemple du Bénin) (The Jacquot center for neuro-psychiatry: A guide to the difficulties of setting up psychiatric structures in Africa [An example from Benin]). *Psychopathologie Africaine*, 22:5–20.

Uchoa, M. E. (1988), *Les femmes de Bamako (Muli) et la santé mentale. Une étude anthropo-psychiatrique* (The women of Bamako [Mali] and their mental health. An anthropological–psychiatric study). Unpublished doctoral dissertation, University of Montreal, Montreal.

Valantin, S. (1970), *Le développement de la fonction manipulatoire chez l'enfant sénégalais au cours des deux premières années de sa vie* (The development of the manipulative function in a Senegalese child during the first two years of her life). Unpublished doctoral dissertation, Faculty of Letters and Human Sciences, University of Paris.

Zempléni, A. (1966), La dimension thérapeutique du culte des Rab, Ndop, Tuuru, et Samp, rites de possession chez les Lebou et les Wolof (The therapeutic element in the cult of Rab, Ndop, Tuuru, and Samp, possession rites amongst the Lebou and Wolof). *Psychopathologie Africaine*, 2:295–439.

———— (1968), *L'interprétation et la thérapie traditionelle du désordre mental chez les Wolof et les Lebou (Sénégal)* (Interpretation and traditional therapy for mental disorders with the Wolof and Lebou). Unpublished doctoral dissertation. Faculty of Letters and Human Sciences, University of Paris.

———— (1974), From symptom to sacrifice: The story of Khady Fall. In: *Case Studies in Spirit Possession*, ed. V. Crapazano & V. Garrison. New York: John Wiley, pp. 87–239.

———— (1975), De la persécution à la culpabilité. In: *Prophétisme et thérapeutique*, Albert Atcho et la communauté de Bregbo, ed. C. Piault. Paris: Hermann, pp. 153–218.

──── Rabain, J. (1965), L'enfant Nit-Ku-Bon. Un tableau psychopatho-
logique traditionnel chez les Wolof and les Lebou du Sénégal (The
child Nit-Ku-Bon. A description of traditional psychopathology
amongst the Wolof and Lebou of Senegal). *Psychopathologie Africaine*, 1:329–441.
Zempléni-Rabain, J. (1966), Modes fondamentaux de relations chez
l'enfant wolof, du sevrage à l'intégration dans la classe d'âge. I. Les
relations de contact physique et de corps à corps (Basic patterns of
relations with Wolof children from weaning to integration into the
tribe. I. The relationship between physical and bodily contact).
Psychopathologie Africaine, 2:143–177.
──── (1968), L'aliment et la stratégie de l'apprentissage de l'échange
avec les frères chez l'enfant wolof (Food and strategies for appren-
ticeship in exchanges with siblings amongst Wolof children). *Psychopathologie Africaine*, 4:297–311.

PART III

Asia

7.

Social Correlates and Cultural Dynamics of Mental Illness in Traditional Society: India

Vijoy K. Varma and Subho Chakrabarti

India is the ideal ground for the cross-cultural psychiatrist. A population of over 890 million with numerous languages, dialects, religions, and faiths gives rise to an amazing diversity. An array of ancient texts and epics, myths and legends, customs and traditions, and a rich folklore provide a bewilderingly rich cultural input. Despite modernization, the influence of these cultural factors has hardly waned. This reliance on the past is both the strength and weakness of Indian culture, a characteristic this country shares with other traditional societies.

Mental illness has been known in India since pre-Vedic times. Psychiatry as a separate discipline, however, emerged around the fifth century B.C. with the advent of *Ayurveda*, a formal system of medicine. Ayurvedic physicians conceptualized the mind as a sense organ, the finest state in the hierarchy of the evolution of matter. Mental illness was explained on the basis of endogenous factors such as a disturbance in the three humors: *Vayu* (wind), *Pitta* (bile), and "*Kapha*" (phlegm). Apart from this, psychological factors and exogenous factors (such as visitations by evil spirits) could cause mental problems. Graphic descriptions of various

categories of mental illnesses, of bodily constitutions, and personality configurations were given in ancient texts. The treatment
through rituals, chanting of mantras, psychological techniques
such as hypnotism, or through herbal medicines was prescribed
(Dube, Dube and Kumar, 1982). Some of these concepts have
filtered down and influenced popular notions regarding mental
afflictions. Thus, as latter day Indian psychiatrists are finding out,
a knowledge of these ancient texts is an essential ingredient of
modern psychiatric practice.

MENTAL MORBIDITY

Studies on mental morbidity have been conducted in almost all
parts of India. Community surveys in rural and urban population
and hospital statistics constitute the major sources of information.
Prevalence rates from some major surveys are shown in Tables
7.1 and 7.2.

TABLE 7.1
Psychiatric Field Surveys in India

Year	Region	Population Size	Urban–Rural	Prevalence of Mental Morbidity (Rates Per 1000)
1964	South	2,731	Urban	9.5
1967	North	1,733	Urban	72.7
1970	North	29,468	Mixed	17.99
1971	East	1,383	Rural	27.
1972	North	2,691	Rural	39.4
1973	South	1,887	Urban	66.5
1975	North	2,696	Urban	82.
1975	East	1,060	Rural	102.8
1980	East	647	Urban	207.1
		1,225	Rural	88.8
1980	West	2,712	Urban	47.
1982	South	1,658	Rural	184.

Source = NMHP—Progress Report, 1988

A marked variation of rates is seen across different surveys.
Much of the variance stems from differences in methodology. A
few facts can, however, be derived from the available data. Mental

TABLE 7.2
Prevalence Rates of Common Psychiatric Illnesses in India

Mental Illness	Prevalence Rates/ 1000.
Schizophrenia	0.9–5.3
Depression	1.5–32.9
Neurosis	1.4–2000
Epilepsy	2.2–10.4
Mental Retardation	1.4–25.3
Organic Psychosis	0.6–1.7

morbidity rates are considerably higher in the urban population. Mental retardation, epilepsy, and depression are the commonest disorders seen in the community. The average prevalence rate of schizophrenia compares well with the West. Depression is less prevalent, whereas the prevalence rates for neurosis are similar to the West. Studies from mental hospitals and the general hospital psychiatric units have shown that a higher proportion of psychotics, as compared to neurotics, attend these facilities (Khanna, Wig, and Varma, 1974).

SOCIOCULTURAL CORRELATES OF MENTAL ILLNESS

The uniqueness of Indian socioeconomic and cultural processes merits a detailed consideration of these factors and their impact on mental illness. A summary of the findings from various Indian studies is given in Table 7.3.

Most studies have shown the highest rate of mental illness to be amongst those of 20 to 45 years with a sharp decline after 50 years (Mehta, Joseph, and Verghese, 1985). The reasons advanced for the difference are a shorter life span, and considerably more care and concern for the aged among Indians. Mental morbidity is higher amongst married people and more so for married women who do not work outside the home (Nandi, Ajmany, Ganguli, Banerjee, Boral, Ghosh, and Sarkar, 1975).

For generations, life in India has revolved around the extended family. The extended family provides succor for the weak, the aged, the unemployed, and the ill. It acts as a buffer against

TABLE 7.3
Sociocultural Correlates of Mental Morbidity

Sociocultural Correlate	Association with Prevalence Mental Disorders	Explanation Given
Age	Decrease in prevalence after 50 years	Short life span, better care, and concern for the aged
Sex	Increased prevalence in females	Lack of education, neglect, superstition, early marriage, etc.
Marital Status	Increased prevalence in married, more so in housewives	Marriage, source of stress especially for housewives with added responsibilities
Domicile	Increased prevalence in urban areas	Living conditions, increasing competition, etc.
Birth Order	Increased in the eldest, early born children	Premature responsibilities cause additional stress
Migration	Increased prevalence in migrants	Unclear, probably stress of migration
Family	Increased in nuclear families (controversial), hysteria more in extended families, increased in transitional families	Extended family a buffer against various stresses
Social Class	Increased prevalence in middle class (inconsistent data)	Unclear, lack of facilities for lower classes
Caste	No consistent data	—

stress, and is suited to the agrarian pattern of Indian society (Sethi and Sharma, 1982). With rapid urbanization and industrialization, however, extended families are breaking up into smaller units. Nuclear families, especially in urban areas, are subject to a number of new stressors. Does this lead to increased psychiatric morbidity? Opinions differ, with some insisting that such is not the case (Carstairs and Kapur, 1976).

Most studies have shown higher morbidity in the middle class (Dutta Ray, 1962; Thacore, Gupta and Suraiya, 1971). Indian Hindus were once rigidly categorized according to the caste system, with Brahmins at the top and Shudras (untouchables) at the bottom of the hierarchy. Studies dealing with caste and mental illness have shown both high (Nandi, Das, Chaudhari, Banerjee, Datta, Ghosh, and Boral, 1980) and low rates of prevalence (Carstairs and Kapur, 1976) in Brahmins.

Since India is a developing country, it has witnessed more emigration than immigration. There have been two large scale shifts, however, the first involving 90 million people from Pakistan in 1947. The second was relatively smaller (10 million people) and was a transient shift from Bangladesh in 1971. A study of migrants from Pakistan showed higher frequency of mental disorders even three decades after migration (Sethi, Gupta, Mahendru, and Kumari, 1972). There was more illness in the aged, depression and neurosis were common, though schizophrenia was rare. Similar findings have been replicated by other authors (Dube, 1970).

CULTURE-BOUND SYNDROMES

Hysterical psychosis is an acute psychosis developing in young patients especially females following a stressor (Venkoba Rao, 1986). The illness is short lasting, the picture is polymorphic with a predominance of conversion symptoms and possession states. Possession states are common in all parts of India and all languages have a name for it. These are dissociative states where verbal and motor behavior is governed by the possessing agent (god, devil, ancestral spirit, etc.). It is common among rural women of low socioeconomic status and is fostered in certain environs, such as temples. Epidemics are known to occur.

Sexual neuroses are culture-bound syndromes distinct from other neuroses, such as anxiety or hysteria. Semen, according to Ayurveda, is one of the seven essential elements of the body. It imparts physical and mental vigor, and longevity. Loss through masturbation or nocturnal emission is believed to lead to weakness (Venkoba Rao, 1986). The "Dhat" syndrome is seen in young males and is characterized by a whitish discharge in urine, impotence, premature ejaculation, hypochondriasis, anxiety, and weakness (Singh, 1985). The "ascetic" syndrome (Neki, 1973) involves a morbid concern over control of sexual impulses in young adolescent males. The patient typically becomes withdrawn, abstinent, and loses weight.

Koro, a complaint of the penis shrinking in size, was first reported from China. An attenuated form of Koro characterized by fear of retraction of the penis into the abdomen has been reported from many parts of India (Venkoba Rao, 1986). Additional features include fears about size and shape of penis, quality and quantity of semen, and impotence. In females shrinking of the breast has been reported (Dutta, Phookan, and Das, 1982). The symptoms are usually attributed to masturbation.

Certain syndromes are rare in India, a prime example being anorexia nervosa. The fact that Indians attach more value to obesity than to excessively low weight could be the likely explanation.

CULTURE-SPECIFIC SYMPTOMS

Several studies have shown that depression is not uncommon in India as was once believed (Venkoba Rao, 1984). Indian depressives tend to somatize more often (Kulhara and Varma, 1985). The prevalence of guilt feelings has been reported to be less in Indian patients (Venkoba Rao, 1973; Sethi, Prakash, and Arora, 1980). Some authors, however, feel that the frequency of guilt feelings is the same, though the content differs (Teja, Narang, and Aggarwal, 1971). The classical elated and frankly grandiose picture of mania seen in the West is less common in India. Irritability, hostility, and some sort of dysphoria is usually seen instead (Varma, 1986). The rates of completed suicide are much less in India though suicidal ideas and attempts are quite frequent. Catatonic forms are more common in schizophrenia; confusion and perplexity predominate in the early stages (Bhaskaran and Saxena, 1970). Delusions are less systematized and the contents reflect cultural beliefs and religious preoccupation (Kala and Wig, 1978). Hysteria, neurotic depression, and anxiety states are the common neurotic disorders in India. Obsessive compulsive disorders are rare probably due to the social sanction accorded to certain compulsive practices. A culturally sanctioned form of this disorder has also been reported (Chakraborty and Banerji, 1975). Some forms, for example, multiple personality disorders, are virtually unknown (Varma, Bouri, and Wig, 1981). Mental retardation, neurosis, behavior disorders, and hyperkinesis are the common problems encountered in childhood. Childhood psychosis and infantile autism are rare.

CULTURAL PSYCHODYNAMICS IN HEALTH AND ILLNESS

Varma (1986) has pleaded for the need to correlate the differences across cultures in mental illness so as to arrive at a dynamic model of transcultural psychiatry. The cultural factors influencing mental illness identified by him are: (1) basic/ethnic/social/"modal" personality, particularly on a dependence-autonomy continuum; (2) linguistic competence; (3) cognitive style; (4) social support system; (5) material culture and (6) psychological sophistication.

Autonomy-Dependence and Mental Illness

Drawing on the concept of basic/social/ethnic/"modal" personality in the transcultural perspective, Varma (1986) has elucidated the variability across cultures in one important dimension, namely autonomy vs. dependence. Whereas dependence characterizes the social inter-relationship in the traditional, agrarian societies of the East, autonomy is more a hallmark of the developed, technologically advanced Western cultures. It is argued that on account of the emphasis on self-reliance, an autonomous individual may resist mental breakdown to a larger extent. However, such a breakdown when it occurs will represent a greater psychopathology in him and as such spell a less favorable course and outcome.

Linguistic Competence and Mental Illness

Drawing attention to the differences across societies in language parameters, Varma (1982a) hypothesized a relationship between linguistic competence (intrinsic ability) and mental illness. It was argued that linguistic competence may importantly determine the typology, course and outcome of mental illness. To illustrate, in an incipient schizophrenic, high linguistic competence may take over from the psychotic anxiety and lead to the development, systematization and ramification of delusions, making them more entrenched and thus less amenable to therapeutic change. Similarly, in neuroses, high competence may cause the transformation of anxiety into obsessions (rather than somatization). Subsequent research by Varma and his colleagues (Varma, Das, and Jiloha, 1985) has substantiated the above hypothesis relating high linguistic competence to paranoid and positive schizophrenia, anxiety and obsessional neuroses and low competence with catatonic and undifferentiated schizophrenia and hysterical and hypochondriacal neuroses.

Characterizing the *cognitive style* of traditional, developing societies as synthetic in contrast to the analytic style of the West, Varma (1986) has pointed out that the synthetic style fits in well with the sense of dependence and loose ego boundaries. The nature of the *material culture* will influence the thought content of delusions (e.g., perceiving a malevolent force as a ghost or spirit as opposed to gamma rays, Martians, etc.). Defining *psychological sophistication* as the ability to see conflicts in intrapsychic terms rather than externally, he has pointed out its relationship to coping mechanisms and to certain illnesses, e.g., hysteria.

Culture and Positive Mental Health

As opposed to pejorative connotation to "culture" given by some as regards mental health, Varma (1982b) has pointed out the health-sustaining and health-promoting aspects of culture. In addition to the role of social institutions, norms and mores, he has pointed out the contribution of customs, rituals, traditions, folkways and symbolisms in protecting and promoting mental health. He has developed the concept of "cultural defenses" meaning thereby the above which serve the functions of alleviation of anxiety and gratification of drives and are available for the use of all members of the society in a readymade form. Rituals associated with life events such as birth, puberty, marriage, illness, and death exemplify such cultural defenses through denial, repression, sublimation, projection, identification, introjection, incorporation, and undoing.

TREATMENT AND PROGNOSIS—CULTURAL ASPECTS

Doubts have been expressed time and again about the suitability of the Western model of psychotherapy for Indian patients. Western concepts of intrapsychic integration, of separation and individuation are wholly different from the Indian concepts of integration into the family and society. Indians are more dependent on their therapist which prompts a more active and directive kind of psychotherapy. Indian patients believe more in the physical and metaphysical rather than the psychological. Explanations have to place proper emphasis on religion and faith. Lesser use of dynamic interpretation and greater use of suggestion and reassurance prove more helpful (Varma, 1988). The confidentiality and the one-to-one relationship between patient and therapist is of little importance in India, where the family is routinely involved in the psychotherapeutic relationship.

In general, psychotherapy should be briefer, crisis oriented, supportive, flexible and eclectic, and tuned to cultural and social conditions (Varma, 1988). Alternative paradigms of psychotherapy such as the *Guru–Chela* (literally teacher-disciple) relationship have also been suggested (Neki, 1973). The principles enshrined in religious texts like the Gita form the backbone of many a psychotherapeutic intervention (Venkoba Rao, 1986). Psychotherapy for the illiterate and less privileged also needs to be culturally tailored and made more medically oriented. Involvement of paramedical personnel and emphasis on group therapy has been recommended (Varma, 1988).

Other indigenous forms of psychotherapy have been used in treatment of psychiatric disorders. Among them yoga has definitely found to be useful in neurotic and psychosomatic disorders. Recent reports of the usefulness of Ayurvedic rituals in substance abuse prove that these forms have as much potential as any other kind of therapy.

Most Indians especially villagers prefer to visit a faith healer before going to a psychiatrist. Various studies have estimated that about 30 to 60 percent of the patients in psychiatric facilities have also taken treatment from these healers (Venkoba Rao, 1986). Cultural beliefs in the supernatural causes of illness also hinder acceptance of treatment at a psychiatric hospital, because, according to common belief, a hospital is the place to treat physical illnesses.

The majority of the cases treated by faith healers or priests are neurotics, mainly hysterics. Illiterate villagers, especially women with low socioeconomic status, form the bulk of those treated; however, the urban literate are also known to often resort to this kind of treatment. The prestigious position of the healer, the similarity of cultural and social backgrounds, easy accessibility, and cultural beliefs play a great role in widespread acceptance of these native therapists. Different methods such as amulets, mantras, and even flogging are used by these healers, all of which work by suggestion. Improvement is generally short lasting (Sethi et al., 1977). Can these seemingly unconventional and often weird practices be labeled psychotherapy? They may not be congruent with the Western concept of psychotherapy, but definitely share certain characteristics, and more importantly, they heal (Varma, 1982b). A lot of attempts are thus being made to integrate these healers into the psychiatric services at the community level (NMHP—Progress Report, 1988).

There is not much difference from the West so far as biological treatments are concerned. The incidence of side effects with psychotropics seems to be more frequent, though certain adverse effects like tardive dyskinesia are reportedly less prevalent (Pandurangi, Ananth, and Channabasavanna, 1978). Electroconvulsive treatment (ECT) being a safe, cheap, and quick method of treatment is still widely used in about 15 percent of all functional psychotics, including schizophrenia.

The fact that schizophrenia has a better prognosis in developing countries is well known and this has been confirmed in various studies from India as well. A greater tolerance for chronic deficits of schizophrenia, a better system of social support, and a wider social network are cited as the various reasons. Affective disorders also seem to follow a more benign course with fewer episodes of shorter duration, and a larger proportion who recover completely after the first episode.

THE FUTURE

The practice of psychiatry in India is rapidly expanding despite numerous obstacles. Subspecialities like child psychiatry and community psychiatry have already carved a niche for themselves, others like forensic psychiatry have begun to grow. In this hectic pace of development it is important not to neglect the basic aspects of cross-cultural psychiatry. Even from this brief review it is clear that research needs to be conducted in many areas of this field. The immediate aim of this research would be to generate data which helps in constructing a dynamic model of transcultural psychiatry. The ultimate aim of any psychiatric practice in India, whatever form it takes, would be to ensure availability and accessibility of basic mental health care for all.

REFERENCES

Bhaskaran, K., & Saxena, B. N. (1970), Some aspects of schizophrenia in the two sexes. *Ind. J. Psychiat.*, 12:177–184.

Carstairs, G. M., & Kapur, R. L. (1976), *The Great Universe of Kota; Stress, Change and Mental Disorder in an Indian Village.* London: Hogarth Press.

Chakraborty, A., & Banerji, G. (1975), Ritual, a culture specific neurosis, and obsessional states in Bengali culture. *Ind. J. Psychiat.*, 17:211–216.

Dube, K. C. (1970), A study of prevalence and bio-social variables in mental illness in a rural and an urban community in Uttar Pradesh. *Acta Psychiat. Scand.*, 46:327–338.

————— Dube, S., & Kumar, A. (1982), Psychiatric syndromes in Ayurveda with description of epilepsy and alcoholism. In: *Readings in Transcultural Psychiatry,* ed. A. Kier & A. Venkoba Rao. Madras: Higginbothams Ltd.

Dutta, D., Phookan, H. R., & Das, P. D. (1982), The Koro epidemic in lower Assam. *Ind. J. Psychiat.*, 24:370–374.

Dutta Ray, S. (1962), Social stratification of mental patients. *Ind. J. Psychiat.*, 4:1–2.

Kala, A. K., & Wig, N. N. (1978), Content of delusions manifested by Indian paranoid psychotics. *Ind. J. Psychiat.*, 20:227–231.

Khanna, B. C., Wig, N. N., & Varma, V. K. (1974), General hospital psychiatric clinic—An epidemiological study. *Ind. J. Psychiat.*, 16:211–220.

Kulhara, P., & Varma, V. K. (1985), Phenomenology of schizophrenic and affective disorders in India—A review. *Ind. J. Soc. Psychiat.*, 1:148–167.

Mehta, P., Joseph, A., & Verghese, A. (1985), An epidemiological study of psychiatric disorders in a rural area in Tamil Nadu. *Ind. J. Psychiat.*, 27:153–158.

Nandi, D. N., Ajmany, S., Ganguli, H., Banerjee, G., Boral, G. C., Ghosh, A., & Sarkar, S. (1975), Psychiatric disorders in a rural community in West Bengal—An epidemiological study. *Ind. J. Psychiat.*, 17:87–99.

———— Das, N. N., Chaudhari, A., Banerjee, G., Datta, P., Ghosh, A., & Boral, G. C. (1980), Mental morbidity and urban life—An epidemiological study. *Ind. J. Psychiat.*, 22:324–330.

National Mental Health Programme for India (NMHP) (1988), *Progress Report 1982–1988*. Delhi: Ministry of Health.

Neki, J. S. (1973), Psychiatry in South-East Asia. *Brit. J. Psychiat.*, 123:257–269.

Pandurangi, A. K., Ananth, J., & Channabasavanna, S. M. (1978), Dyskinesia in an Indian mental hospital. *Ind. J. Psychiat.*, 20:339–342.

Sethi, B. B., Gupta, S. C., Mahendru, R. K., & Kumari, P. (1972), Migration and mental health. *Ind. J. Psychiat.*, 14:115–121.

———— Prakash, R., & Aurora, U. (1980), Guilt and hostility in depression. *Ind. J. Psychiat.*, 22:156–160.

————Sharma, M. (1982), Family factors in psychiatric illness. In: *Readings in Transcultural Psychiatry*, ed. A. Kiev and A. Venkoba Rao. Madras: Higginbothams, Ltd.

————Trivedi, J. K., & Sitholey, P. (1977), Traditional healing practices in psychiatry. *Ind. J. Psychiat.*, 19:9–13.

Singh, G. (1985), Dhat syndrome revisited. *Ind. J. Psychiat.*, 27:119–122.

Teja, J. S., Narang, R. L., & Aggarwal, A. K. (1971), Depression across cultures. *Brit. J. Psychiat.*, 119:253–260.

Thacore, V. R., Gupta, S. C., & Suraiya, M. (1971), Psychiatric clinic at the urban health centre, Alambagh, Lucknow. *Ind. J. Psychiat.*, 13:253–260.

Varma, V. K. (1982a), Linguistic competence and psychopathology—a cross-cultural model. *Ind. J. Psychiat.*, 24:107–114.

————(1982b), Present state of psychotherapy in India. *Ind. J. Psychiat.*, 24:209–226.

———— (1986), Cultural psychodynamics in health and illness. *Ind. J. Psychiat.*, 28:13–34.

———— (1988), Culture, personality and psychotherapy. *Internat. J. Soc. Psychiat.*, 34:142–149.

———— Bouri, M., & Wig, N. N. (1981), Multiple personality in India: Comparison with hysterical possession state. *Amer. J. Psychother.*, 35:113–120.

————Das, K., & Jiloha, R. C. (1985), Correlation of linguistic competence with psychopathology. *Ind. J. Psychiat.*, 27:193–200.

Venkoba Rao, A. (1973), Depressive illness and guilt in Indian culture. *Ind. J. Psychiat.*, 23:213–221.

———— (1984), Unipolar and bipolar depression: A review. *Ind. J. Psychiat.*, 26:99–105.

———— (1986), Indian and Western psychiatry: A comparison. In: *Transcultural Psychiatry*, ed. J. L. Cox. London: Croom Helm, pp. 291–305.

8.

Culture and Mental Illness among Jews in Israel

Yoram Bilu

A close look at Israel reveals an ethnically pluralistic society, marked by a strong historical consciousness and rich cultural differentiation. This ethnic diversity, tenuously contained within the modern framework of a Zionist state undergoing rapid social changes and continuous disruption by emergency conditions, appears as a fertile matrix for cultural influences on mental health.

In this review I will deal quite selectively with the relationships between mental illness in the Jewish sector and the three major cleavages in Israeli society, into which its wide ethnocultural variability is commonly reduced. These cleavages include the Jewish–Arab division and then, within the Jewish sector, the Ashkenazic (from Eastern Europe)–Sephardic (Asia and North Africa), and the secular–observant divisions. Arab and other non-Jewish groups are not included in the review. This does not reflect a political bias but rather the unfortunate fact (probably in itself politically related) that research on mental illness among these groups is almost nonexistent.

Given the limited scope, the review is far from exhaustive. Complementary material may be found in two earlier comprehensive essays which dealt with very similar subjects (Levav and Bilu, 1981; Sanua, 1989).

HISTORICAL AND CULTURAL BACKGROUND OF MENTAL ILLNESS IN ISRAEL

Jewish traditional views of mental disorders have been fashioned by references to this subject in the classical sources. The Bible, the Talmud, and other sacred texts, although lacking a systematically organized body of psychiatric knowledge, deal sporadically with mental disturbances, their diagnosis, classification, and treatment (Hes and Wollstein, 1964). Preoccupation with psychopathology is particularly noted in the Jewish mystical literature; for example, it is not by chance that cases of *dybbuk* possession, the most exotic variant of a Jewish culture-bound syndrome, started to appear in the sixteenth century in Kabbalistically oriented communities in the Mediterranean area and later spread to the mystically based Hasidic centers in Eastern Europe. The etiology and symptoms of *dybbuk* possession were clearly informed by mystical doctrines such as the transmigration of souls (Bilu, 1985a).

Military psychiatric facilities, developed during the War of Independence in 1948, were the nucleus for the public facilities which were organized by the Ministry of Health (Miller, 1981). The country was divided into three regions, the centers of which were the three main cities, Tel Aviv, Haifa, and Jerusalem. Each region was supposed to include three elements: mental health clinics, psychiatric hospitals, and rehabilitation centers ("work villages"). In 1972, a community model of mental health centers was introduced by the Ministry of Health but has not been fully implemented as yet.

EPIDEMIOLOGY OF MENTAL ILLNESS: GENERAL FINDINGS

Epidemiological data on mental illness in Israel have been obtained from two major sources: community studies and studies based on psychiatric case registry. Since these two types of study yield different rates of prevalence of psychopathology they will be discussed separately.

Community Studies

Aviram and Levav (1975) reviewed five community studies published in the 1960s and the 1970s. These studies were barely comparable in terms of their objectives, methods, and data sources, therefore the overall morbidity rates obtained in them were highly variable (between 5 and 50%). Nevertheless, the studies produced fairly consistent findings regarding major culture-linked variables such as sex, social class, and immigration.

In all of the studies, emotional disorders were higher amongst women than men. The gap was maintained for both the psychoses and the neuroses, but was reversed for personality disorders. Social class was also significantly associated with rates of psychopathology. In fact, an inverse relationship between socioeconomic variables and mental disorder was the most consistent finding in Israeli epidemiological studies. Higher prevalence rates of emotional disorders were also currently noted among immigrants when compared with native-born Israelis. These particular vulnerabilities of females, people of lower socioeconomic background, and immigrants were reestablished in more recent studies (e.g., Levav and Arnon, 1976; Levav and Abramson, 1984).

Against the central role that ethnic origin plays in Israeli society in shaping, demarcating, and preserving cultural differences, it should be noted that its association with mental disorder is not clear. Whether examined through generalized dichotomies (i.e., Ashkenazim vs. Sephardim), through specific categories referring to countries of origin (e.g., Iranians), or through middle-size aggregates (e.g., Eastern Europeans, North Africans), ethnicity appeared to be only tenuously related to psychopathology. It is true that in most studies Sephardim have usually appeared to be overrepresented on various measures of emotional distress (e.g., Maoz, Levy, Brand, and Halevi, 1966); but when social class was effectively controlled, this effect immediately subsided. Thus it appears that the higher morbidity rate of the Sephardim is more strongly associated with socioeconomic disadvantages, given their general underprivileged position in Israeli society, rather than with ethnicity per se (Levav and Abramson, 1984).

Studies Based on Case Registry

The existence in Israel of national register data encompassing all admissions to every inpatient psychiatric facility since the early 1950s has facilitated epidemiological research of treated cases. Following the computerization of these data, Rahav, Popper, and Nahon (1981) studied all the first admissions between 1950 and 1980. Interestingly, in this large-scale study (based on almost 70,000 cases) differential contributions of culture-linked variables were almost nonexistent. Despite the major political, economic, and social changes that the country had undergone in this 30-year period, the rate of admissions has remained quite stable, with only a small decrease in recent years, probably due to an increase in outpatient facilities. Moreover, in terms of countries of origin, there was little difference in regard to their contributions to the file; the most socially deprived settlements were *not* necessarily high on psychiatric morbidity, and sex distribution was about even.

These findings are clearly at odds with those derived from community studies. They portray mental illness in Israel as a relatively stable and persistent phenomenon, in which groups of different residential locations, immigration cohorts, cultural backgrounds, and ethnic origin are represented in roughly equal proportions. This picture of stability was augmented by another study which looked at morbidity rates of Israeli-born schizophrenic inpatients (Eaton and Levav, 1982). It was found that the rates were of the same order of magnitude as in the United States and in other Western countries.

In contrast, other epidemiological studies based on psychiatric admissions have reasserted the contribution of various culture-linked variables, such as immigration and social class, to differential morbidity rates of psychopathology (e.g., Halevi, 1963; Gershon and Liebowitz, 1975). In common with community studies, however, it has been found that the association between ethnicity and mental disorders is intricate and defies generalization. This intricacy calls for a closer look at the ethnic factor and its bearing on psychopathology in Israel.

EPIDEMIOLOGY OF MENTAL ILLNESS: EAST VS. WEST

As noted before, the recurrent finding of higher rates of psycho-pathology among Sephardim appears to be mediated by social class variables, that is, the existence in Israel of an asymmetrical status structure in which the Sephardim are socially disadvan-taged vis-à-vis the Ashkenazim (e.g., Samooha, 1978; Eaton, Lasry, and Segal, 1980). Seeking to explain the inverse relationship be-tween social class and rates of mental illness (particularly schizo-phrenia), this ethnically related social inequality was used in two studies conducted in Jerusalem (Rahav, Goodman, Popper, and Lin, 1986; Levav, Zilber, Danielovich, Eisenberg, and Turetsky, 1987), in which social class was controlled to test the rival hypoth-eses of social causation and social selection (Dohrenwend and Dohrenwend, 1969). Despite differences in the target populations and in methods, the data in both studies have favored the social selection hypothesis (even though social causation factors were also apparent). One major finding leading to this conclusion was the higher rates of morbidity among lower class Ashkenazim, the ethnically advantaged group, compared with lower class Seph-ardim.

In addition to socioeconomic variables, it appears that sex should also be taken into account in comparing rates of mental disorders between the two main ethnic sectors. Looking at first admissions, it was found that Ashkenazic women were clearly over-represented while Sephardic men were more vulnerable (Levav and Reitman, 1981). Various factors such as stress and depriva-tion, age structure and differential employment of psychiatric re-sources, appear to jointly contribute to this interaction between gender and ethnicity.

Is ethnic origin associated with differential prevalence rates of specific forms of psychopathology? Most studies reply in the affirmative. They present a recurrent pattern according to which Sephardim are overrepresented in schizophrenic disorders, while Ashkenazim have higher rates of affective disorders, particularly depression (e.g., Gershon and Leibowitz, 1975; Miller, 1979).

This common finding should be evaluated with caution, how-ever, since most of the studies that yielded it did not control social class variables (cf. Eaton and Levav, 1982). As mentioned before,

Levav et al. (1986) and Rahav et al. (1986), in well-controlled studies, have detected higher rates of schizophrenia among lower class Ashkenazim. It is interesting to note, however, that Rahav et al. have assumed that their most striking finding in this respect—a particularly high rate of schizophrenia among ultraorthodox Ashkenazic males—reflected in fact a preponderance of affective disorders in this group. This interpretation was based on the documented tendency of mental health practitioners to misdiagnose as schizophrenic strictly religious patients suffering from affective disorders. Historically, the association of depression with Ashkenazic Jews of East European extraction had been salient enough to give rise to the colloquial diagnostic label *melancholia agitata Hebraica* (Hollingshead and Redlich, 1958; Sanua, 1989).

Based on both community and case register studies, Sephardim appear to have higher prevalence rates of personality disorders, alcoholism, and drug addiction (Aviram and Levav, 1981; Snyder and Palgi, 1982). Since these disorders may be taken as indicators of "social pathology," it is reasonable to assume once again that socioeconomic factors play a more decisive role here than ethnicity per se. In accounting for the fact that Sephardim have higher rates of criminal behavior and prostitution, Eaton, Lasry, and Sigal (1980) emphasize that they constitute a socially disadvantaged group, exposed to more stressful events, and less equipped to cope with crisis situations in comparison with the Ashkenazim. The dire consequences of this underprivileged status are likely to be lower self-esteem and increased hostility against socially advantaged groups. In this vein, Landau (1975) has found that the homicide rate among Sephardim was twice as high as that among Ashkenazim (though significantly lower than that of non-Jews in Israel). By contrast, Ashkenazim showed higher levels of inward-oriented hostility (murder-suicide). Miller (1976) has demonstrated that suicide rates are higher among Ashkenazim, though Sephardim have higher rates of attempted suicide.

CULTURAL FORMS OF PSYCHOPATHOLOGY

In addition to differential rates of prevalence and incidence, ethnic group differences in psychopathology may manifest on the content level. A number of studies have undertaken to identify clinical pictures peculiar to or typical of Ashkenazim and Sephardim. Miller (1979), for example, compared Sephardim and Ashkenazim first admitted to inpatient facilities. He reported that the former were more emotional and dependent in their relationships, particularly with authority figures, tended to be more impulsive, and were more concerned with concrete experiences than with abstractions from reality. The fact that this study was based on clinical observations and interviews may cast doubt on the objectivity of these conclusions, particularly as they seem to echo pejorative stereotypical views of Sephardim prevalent in mainstream Israeli society. This predicament is common to other studies in which the ethnic origin of the subjects, quite visible during the psychiatric assessment, may influence its outcome.

Beyond symptomatology, noticeable differences between the two ethnic sectors were found in perceptions, images, and folk theories of mental illness. Rotenberg (1976), for example, who studied Ashkenazic and Sephardic inpatients with schizophrenic disorders, found that they maintained different belief systems concerning their problems. While Ashkenazic inpatients tended to perceive themselves as sick persons, suffering from an innate and incurable ailment (indicative self-labeling), their Sephardic counterparts tended to view themselves as basically healthy and attributed their predicament to external factors which could be eliminated (transmutive self-labeling). These ethnic differences were more noticeable early in the hospitalization. The longer the period of incarceration, the more dominant the indicative self-labeling became, irrespective of ethnic origin.

Rotenberg's hypotheses depict a dichotomous cultural demarcation in which the Ashkenazic perspective is identified with core-epistemological assumptions of the modern Western world whereas the Sephardic one is emblematic of the traditional. One might ask to what degree these two generalized categories cogently represent monolithic blocks of contrasting cultural worlds. This question, pertinent in fact to all the studies heretofore reviewed, is particularly bothering regarding the term *Sephardim*. Originally denoting Spanish Jews (who, following their expulsion from Spain in 1492, were dispersed throughout the Mediterranean countries and beyond), in Israel it has been expanded to include all the Jewish communities from Asia and North Africa. In view of the wide cultural differences between, say, Jews from Morocco, Yemen, Iran, and India, it appears that in lumping them together, researchers have created a rich ethnic amalgam, sometimes almost vacuous in terms of common cultural contents.

While in many epidemiological studies the broad ethnic categories of Sephardim (or "Orientals") versus Ashkenazim (or "Westerners") appear to prevail, other studies dealing with mental disorders have focused on specific, more culturally bounded groups. Since a detailed review of these studies appeared elsewhere (Levav and Bilu, 1980), the ensuing discussion is limited to more recent data which center selectively on three ethnic groups: Moroccans, Iranians, and Ethiopians.

Moroccan Jews—The Vicissitudes of Demonic Possession

The history of the Jews in Morocco and their arduous absorption in Israel after their massive immigration in the 1950s and 1960s is beyond the scope of this review. Suffice it is to say that as long-time residents of the Maghreb, they were heavily influenced culturally by the indigenous Arabs and Berbers, as clearly manifested in their distinctive ethnopsychiatry. This holds particularly true for the more traditional communities of southern Morocco. In terms of individual country of origin, Jews of Moroccan extraction constitute the largest ethnic group in Israel today.

Jewish Moroccan ethnopsychiatry, still in use in Israel, has been described in detail by Bilu (1977, 1979, 1980, 1985b). He has found that belief in traditional agents of disease, like demons (jnun) and sorcery (skhur) has not subsided entirely in the new country. Rather it has undergone a very selective attenuation differentially affecting the diverse cultural modes of psychopathology which the newcomers brought with them from Morocco.

Demonic illnesses are a case in point. The classificatory system of these ailments is dichotomous, in accord with the two modalities of demonic attack—external blow and internal penetration. The former group of disorders, generically designated *tsira,* includes symptoms of anxiety of a conversive and somato-form nature, while the latter, *aslai,* is characterized by dissociation which may take the classical form of possession. While possession illnesses are rapidly vanishing from the Israeli scene, it seems that the external blow disorders are alive and well in Israel despite the changing cultural circumstances. This relative resilience of *tsira* as against the fragility of *aslai* has to do with the fact that in the former the demon is assigned a participational mode while in the latter its status is merely explicative (cf. Crapanzano, 1973). In other words, possession illnesses, in which the symptoms are meticulously molded by the culture, cannot be "enacted" without a deep involvement in the traditional core beliefs and the exis-tence of models close by. These prerequisites are hardly attainable under the corrosive influence of the modern mainstream culture.

Demonic illnesses without possession, by contrast, are cul-ture-bound only insofar as their alleged etiology is concerned. They survive, and even thrive, in the modern setting because the demon-cum-explanatory agent might be often resorted to in times of plight, after modern means had been employed and found ineffective. Ironically, it is the very existence of an hegemonic medical system that contributes to and sharply demarcates the realm of traditional illnesses ("that which physicians can't cope with") and thus sustain them as autonomous diagnostic catego-ries. These "benefits of attenuation" (Bilu, 1985b) are reflected in many other aspects of Jewish Moroccan ethnopsychiatry.

Beyond the partial (but tenacious) persistence of culturally informed disorders among Moroccan Jews, with their correspond-ing theories of causation and healing roles (Bilu and Hasan-Ro-kem, 1989), there is some evidence that psychiatric patients of this ethnic background have a distinctive pattern of coping with their problems, whether or not with culturally based manifesta-tions. Thus Minuchin-Itzigsohn, Ben-Shaul, Weingrod, and Krasi-lowski (1984) have characterized Moroccan patients who seek help in mental health clinics as tending to view socioeconomic problems as the source of their ailments. Accordingly, they expect the clinic to give them instrumental help and are likely to reject psychodynamically oriented treatment. The fact that they view their suffering as caused by objective life circumstances reduces the stigma they might otherwise feel.

Iranian Jews—"The Persian Syndrome"

In Israeli psychiatry, Iranian Jews, whether those who came before the establishment of the State of Israel in 1948 or newcomers who fled the Khumeini Revolution, have been notorious for high morbidity rates (Maoz, Levy, Brand, and Halevi, 1966) and peculiar symptomatology, barely responsive to treatment (Basker, Beran, and Kleinhauz, 1982). Typically, patients from this ethnic group were sent to a psychiatric clinic after the health system failed to find any organic basis for their somatic complaints (Minuchin-Itzigsohn et al., 1984). The transactions in the clinic with Israeli mental health practitioners, replete with cultural misunderstandings and miscommunications resulting from incongruent explanatory models, are often sealed with the informal label *Parsitis*, a pejorative and highly stereotypical term indicating an ostensibly untreatable, peculiarly Iranian culture-bound syndrome.

In what appears to be the only full-length book on culture and mental health in Israel, Pliskin (1987) has sought to decipher the "silent boundaries" (i.e., the cultural constraints on diagnosis), which leave Israeli practitioners frustratingly incapable of dealing with the strange-looking symptoms of their Iranian patients. She shows how Iranian ways of communicating are related to both the hierarchical social organization of Iranian society and the ethnopsychological concept of the individual as internally sensitive and externally clever. Under stressful conditions, which the immigration to Israel has no doubt exacerbated, Iranian Jews often succumb to *narahati*, a culturally patterned emotion of being ill-at-ease, which they fight to keep private and well-concealed. The symptoms that often ensue are framed in culturally distinctive ways, grounded in traditional conceptions of the body and sickness. To the biomedically trained Israeli practitioners these symptoms, which usually take odd somatic forms, make no sense. In labeling them *Parsitis*, they account for their failure to effectively deal with the problems at hand by vaguely ascribing them to an obscure and persistent ethnic mentality. Parsitis, thus, is an ethnic stereotype posing as a diagnosis.

Ethiopian Jews—Eating Arrest Disorder

Approximately 20,000 Jewish immigrants from Ethiopia arrived in Israel between 1979 and 1991. For many of them, the crisis of acculturation was aggravated by the terrible ordeals they had to undergo on their way to Israel. A particular group at risk includes children and adolescents who were separated from their families (still stranded in Ethiopia). Many of these youngsters have developed clinical pictures akin to posttraumatic stress disorder (PTSD) (Arieli, 1987; see also Ratzoni, Apter, Blumensohn, and Tyano, 1988). One particular set of eating problems which recurs among Ethiopian youth deserves special attention, given its resemblance to anorexia nervosa. In view of the notion that the latter is the Western culture-bound syndrome par excellence, it is intriguing to note that it is also manifested in a group which is culturally the least Westernized in present-day Israel.

Ben-Ezer (1990), in a culturally sensitive analysis, unravels the psychocultural bases of the disorder of eating arrest among the Ethiopians. As in Pliskin's (1987) work on the Iranians, the symptomatology is placed in its proper semantic field by highlighting the cultural perception of the abdomen as the container of all emotions. Given this perception, an acute sensation of being filled with agony and pain which cannot be contained any longer might be translated into an eating arrest disorder. These uncontainable troubles are related to earlier persecutory experiences and their derivatives (e.g., survivor's guilt) as well as to present acculturation problems aggravated by differences in appearance and culture. Ben-Ezer convincingly shows that despite the similarity to anorexia, none of the criteria of the DSM-III-R (APA, 1987) for the latter are met by the Ethiopian disorder (e.g., no weight phobia or disturbance in body image are noticed).

This selective presentation does injustice to a number of valuable works in which mental disorders in other ethnic groups were discussed. One excellent example is Palgi's thorough analysis of Jewish Yemenite ethnopsychiatry (Palgi, 1981).

RELIGION AND MENTAL ILLNESS

The secular–religious dichotomy, often presented as one of the main cleavages in Israeli society, is more accurately portrayed as a wide spectrum of varying degrees of religious commitment. In looking for noticeable effects of religiosity on psychopathology, the natural target for investigation should be the small minority (5 to 10% of the Jewish population) of the strictly observant or ultraorthodox community. This group constitutes a distinct subculture, quite estranged from mainstream Israeli society, in which Jewish Law is the sole guideline for behavior in every aspect of daily life. Most of the data on the subject at hand have been collected in the densely populated ultraorthodox communities of northern Jerusalem.

As noted before (Rahav et al., 1986), there is some indication that this group is overrepresented in the distribution of treated mental illness, particularly affective disorders. One plausible explanation is genetic transmission among the reclusive and highly inbred members of the community. Fairly scant evidence suggests that this higher morbidity rate recurs in other ailments such as Down's syndrome (Sharav, 1985).

Some of the risk factors peculiar to growing up in an ultraorthodox community are specified by Goshen-Gottstein (1987). She maintains that boys are more vulnerable at a younger age, due to high expectations for emotional and cognitive maturity, and excellence in the realm of study, while girls have higher rates of mental illness from the onset of puberty, when their ritual impurity becomes apparent and their sexuality is harshly supressed.

Religion may affect the content of mental disorders. A series of studies examined the manifestations of obsessive compulsive disturbances among the ultraorthodox (Greenberg and Chir, 1984; Greenberg, Witztum and Pisante, 1987; Greenberg, 1987; Greenberg and Witztum, 1991). While the compulsive rituals of the patients are replete with religious contents, centering around topics such as dietary laws and prayers, clear-cut criteria exist which differentiate them from normative religious rituals (e.g., the compulsive patient is racked with distressing doubts, forbidden by the Law). It is clear that in these cases the religious commitment was incorporated into a preexisting problem rather than being a causal factor.

The incorporation of religious content into psychotic disorders has been analyzed by other researchers. Weil (1990) has shown how orthodox patients use various religious symbols and figures to articulate personal conflicts. Perez (1977) described the messianic delusions of psychotic inpatients, Jews as well as non-Jews. Witztum, Buchbinder, and Van der Hart (1990) and Bilu, Witztum, and Van der Hart (1990) examined cases in which persecutions by demons and angels—core beliefs in Jewish mysticism—have fashioned depressive syndromes.

Religious penitents ("born-again Jews") appear as a group at risk among the ultraorthodox, given the high prevalence rates of schizophrenic and affective disorders among them (Witztum, Greenberg, and Buchbinder, 1990; Witztum, Greenberg, and Dasberg, 1990). In two-thirds of the treated patients, however, psychiatric difficulties had preceded the religious transformation. In spite of these problems most of the patients were married and sought professional help only five years on average after the religious change. Religious change appears therefore as having a stabilizing effect on potentially disturbed converts, though this effect is not permanent.

The accumulated experience of the above mentioned researchers has led to the formulation of guidelines for culture-sensitive therapy, in which religious idioms and rituals and the assistance of esteemed religious figures (e.g., the patient's rabbi) are employed in concert with conventional modes of treatment (see Bilu et al., 1990; Witztum, Greenberg, and Buchbinder, 1990).

While cultural and religious contents are strongly present in various mental disorders of particular ethnic or observant groups, the term *culture-bound syndromes* should be applied with caution in present-day Israel. Most of the disturbances discussed above can be placed within the standard psychiatric classification. It is interesting to note that the classical forms of spirit possession, like the *dybbuk* (see Bilu, 1985a) or "evil spirit disease" (Bilu, 1980), perhaps the genuine culture-bound syndromes in Judaism, have disappeared from both Ashkenazic and Sephardic communities in modern Israel. No less interesting is the fact that clinical cases bearing similarity to non-Jewish culture-specific syndromes (e.g., Koro) have been documented in Israel, but the numbers are too small to allow sound conclusions (Modai, Munitz, and Eizenberg, 1986; Kumar, 1987).

STRESS, TRAUMA, AND MENTAL ILLNESS

The traumatic history of the Jewish people in this century and the wearisome cycle of bloodshed and hostilities in which the State of Israel has been engulfed since it was established in 1948, have left their mark on various facets of the Israeli collective experience. As stress-enhancing factors, these historical and political circumstances have direct bearings on mental health.

The Holocaust

More than forty-five years after the massive destruction of the Jewish people by the Nazis, the effects of the trauma are still felt as an increased risk to health among various groups in Israel. Dasberg (1987), in a comprehensive review, summarizes these effects. As might be expected, the survivors (called "the first generation") pay the highest psychological toll in terms of emotional distress (e.g., depression, anxiety, interpersonal difficulties, PTSD). With advancing age, late effects increase rather than abate. The erstwhile child survivors, now approaching midlife, are the most vulnerable subgroup among the first generation. Although socially successful, they run the risk for later decompensation of precariously balanced, life-long personality disturbances.

The offspring of the survivors, the second generation, constitute another vulnerable group. Studies indicate that they are detrimentally affected by the traumatic family milieu created by their mourning and demanding parents or by parents who deny the past and become cognitively constricted. Recent studies have shown that even the third generation is not spared these adverse effects. The potential vulnerability of the survivors' offspring becomes especially apparent when they are exposed to additional stress. Unfortunately, the political turmoil in the Middle East constitutes a fertile matrix for multiple stress.

War-Related Stress

The dire consequences of the Israeli–Arab conflict—recurrent wars, border conflicts, terrorist attacks on civilians, and the Palestinian uprising—create conditions of tension with potentially adverse effects on emotional well-being. Although these risk factors appear ubiquitous, certain groups in Israeli society are more exposed to them. A recent spate of studies has documented these effects in both military and civilian populations. The awareness of combat stress reactions and PTSD among soldiers has been growing since the traumatic 1973 War and was translated into ramified scientific investigation after the 1982 Lebanon War. These studies have examined vulnerability-enhancing variables (personal and situational), stress inoculating factors, and effective treatment methods (Milgram, 1986; Solomon, Noi, and Bar-On, 1986; Solomon, Oppenheimer, Elizur, and Waysman, 1990).

Another line of investigation has examined the long-term adjustment of various vulnerable groups in the civilian sector, such as survivors of terrorist attacks (Milgram, 1986; Dreman, 1989). Of these groups bereaved parents appear to be particularly at risk in terms of rates of mortality and psychopathology (Auslander, 1987).

In addition to ethnic and religious variables, stress-related variables emanating from particular historical and political conditions should also be viewed as part of the intricate web of sociocultural factors affecting mental health in present-day Israel.

REFERENCES

American Psychiatric Association (1987), *Diagnostic and Statistical Manual of Mental Disorders*, 3rd ed. rev. (DSM-III-R). Washington, DC: American Psychiatric Press.

Arieli, A. (1987), Crisis intervention in an absorption center for young Ethiopians (Hebrew). *Harefua*, 112:109–112.

Auslander, G. K. (1987), Bereavement research in Israel: A critical review of the literature. *Israel J. Psychiat.*, 24:33–51.

Aviram, U., & Levav, I. (1975), Psychiatric community in Israel: An analysis of community studies. *Acta Psychiat. Scand.*, 52:295–311.

———— ———— eds. (1981), *Community Mental Health in Israel* (Hebrew). Tel-Aviv: Gomeh, Cherikover.

Basker, E., Beran, B., & Kleinhauz, M. (1982), A social science perspective on the negotiation of a psychiatric diagnosis. *Soc. Psychiat.*, 17:53–58.

Ben-Ezer, G. (1990), Anorexia nervosa or an Ethiopian coping style? *Mind & Human Interaction*, 2:36–39.

Bilu, Y. (1977), General characteristics of referrals to traditional healers in Israel. *Israel J. Psychiat.*, 15:245–252.

———— (1979), Demonic explanations of disease among Moroccan Jews in Israel. *Cult., Med. & Psychiat.*, 3:363–380.

———— (1980), The Moroccan demon in Israel. *Ethos*, 8:24–39.

———— (1985a), The taming of the deviants and beyond: Dybbuk possession and exorcism in Judaism. *The Psychoanalytic Study of Society*, 11:11–32.

———— (1985b), The benefits of attenuation: Continuity and change in Jewish Moroccan ethnopsychiatry in Israel. In: *Studies in Israel Ethnicity: After the Ingathering*, ed. A. Weingrod. New York: Gordon & Breach.

———— Hasan-Rokem, G. (1989), Cinderella and the saint: The life story of a Jewish Moroccan female healer in Israel. *The Psychoanalytic Study of Society*, 14:227–266.

———— Witztum, E., & Van der Hart, O. (1990), Paradise regained: Miraculous healing in an Israeli psychiatric clinic. *Cult., Med. & Psychiat.*, 14:105–127.

Crapanzano, V. (1973), *The Hamadsha: A Study in Moroccan Ethnopsychiatry*. Berkeley: University of California Press.

Dasberg, H. (1987), Psychological distress of Holocaust survivors and their offspring in Israel, 40 years later: A review. *Israel J. Psychiat.*, 24:243–256.

Dohrenwend, B. P., & Dohrenwend, B. S. (1969), *Social Status and Psychological Disorder: A Causal Inquiry*. New York: Wiley.

Dreman, S. (1989), Children of victims of terrorism in Israel: Coping and adjustment in the face of trauma. *Israel J. Psychiat.*, 26:212–220.

Eaton, W. W., & Levav, I. (1982), Schizophrenia, social class, and ethnic disadvantage: A study of first hospitalization among Israeli-born Jews. *Israel J. Psychiat.*, 19:289–302.

———— Lasry, J. C., & Sigal, J. (1980), Ethnic relations and community mental health among Israeli Jews. *Israel Ann. Psychiat.*, 17:165–174.

Gershon, E. S., & Liebowitz, J. H. (1975), Sociocultural and demographic correlates of affective disorders in Jerusalem. *J. Psychiat. Res.*, 13:37–50.

Goshen-Gottstein, E. (1987), Mental health implications of living in an ultra-orthodox community. *Israel J. Psychiat.*, 24:145–166.

Greenberg, D. (1987), The behavioral treatment of religious compulsions. *J. Psychol. & Judaism*, 11:41–47.

———— Chir, B. (1984), Are religious compulsions religious or compulsive: A phenomenological study. *Amer. J. Psychother.*, 38:524–531.

———— Witztum, E. (1991), The treatment of obsessive-compulsive disorder in strictly religious patients. In: *Obsessive-Compulsive Disorders*, ed. M. T. Pato & G. Zohar. Washington, DC: American Psychiatric Press, pp. 157–172.

—— —— Pisante, J. (1987), Scrupulosity: Religious attitudes and clinical presentations. *Brit. J. Med. Psychol.*, 60:29–37.

Halevi, H. S. (1963), Frequency of mental illness among Jews in Israel. *Internat. J. Soc. Psychiat.*, 9:268–282.

Hes, J. P., & Wollstein, S. (1964), The attitudes of the ancient Jewish sources to mental patients. *Israel Ann. Psychiat.*, 2:103–116.

Hollingshead, A. B., & Redlich, F. K. (1958), *Social Class and Mental Illness*. New York: Wiley.

Kumar, H. V. (1987), Koro in an Israeli man. *Brit. J. Psychiat.*, 150:133.

Landau, S. (1975), Pathologies among homicide offenders: Some cultural profiles. *Brit. J. Criminol.*, 15:157–166.

Levav, I., & Abramson, J. H. (1984), A community study of emotional distress in Jerusalem. *Israel J. Psychiat.*, 21:19–35.

—— Arnon, A. (1976), Emotional disorders in six Israeli villages. *Acta Psychiat. Scand.*, 53:387–400.

—— Bilu, Y. (1980), A transcultural view of Israeli psychiatry. *Transcult. Psychiat. Res. Rev.*, 17:7–56.

—— Reitman, E. (1981), Application of epidemiological data in selecting target group in community psychiatry. In: *Community Mental Health in Israel* (Hebrew), ed. U. Aviram & I. Levav. Tel-Aviv: Gomeh, Cherikover.

—— Zilber, N., Danielovich, E., Eisenberg, E., & Turetsky, N. (1987), The etiology of schizophrenia: A replication test of the social selection vs. the social causation hypothesis. *Acta Psychiat. Scand.*, 75:183–189.

Maoz, B., Levy, S., Brand, N., & Halevi, H. S. (1966), An epidemiological survey of mental disorders in a community of newcomers in Israel. *J. College Gen. Practitioners*, 11:267–284.

Milgram, N., ed. (1986), *Stress and Coping in Time of War*. New York: Brunner/Mazel.

Miller, L. (1976), Some data on suicide and attempted suicide of the Jewish population in Israel. *Ment. Health & Soc.*, 3:178–181.

—— (1979), Culture and psychopathology of Jews in Israel. *Psychiatric J. U. Ottawa*, 4:302–306.

—— (1981), Community intervention and the historical background of community mental health in Israel. In: *Community Mental Health in Israel*, ed. U. Aviram & I. Levav. Tel-Aviv: Gomeh, Cherikover.

Minuchin-Itzigsohn, S. D., Ben-Shaul, R., Weingrod, A., & Krasilowski, D. (1984), The effects of cultural conceptions on therapy: A comparative study of patients in Israeli psychiatric clinics. *Cult., Med. & Psychiat.*, 8:229–254.

Modai, I., Munitz, H., & Eizenberg, D. (1986), Koro in an Israeli male. *Brit. J. Psychiat.*, 149:503–506.

Palgi, P. (1981), Traditional coping devices with mental problems among Yemenites in Israel. In: *Community Mental Health in Israel*, ed. U. Aviram & I. Levav. Tel-Aviv: Gomeh, Cherikover.

Perez, L. (1977), The messianic psychotic patient. *Israel Ann. Psychiat.*, 15:364–374.

Pliskin, K. L. (1987), *Silent Boundaries: Cultural Constraints on Sickness and Diagnosis of Iranians in Israel.* New Haven, CT: Yale University Press.

Rahav, M., Goodman, A. B., Popper, M., & Lin, S. P. (1986), Distribution of treated mental illness in the neighborhoods of Jerusalem. *Amer. J. Psychiat.*, 143:1249–1254.

——— Popper, M., & Nahon, D. (1981), The psychiatric case register in Israel: Initial results. *Israel J. Psychiat.*, 18:251–267.

Ratzoni, G., Apter, A., Blumensohn, R., & Tyano, S. (1988), Psychopathology and management of hospitalized Ethiopian immigrant adolescents in Israel. *J. Adol.*, 11:231–236.

Rotenberg, M. (1976), Self-labeling theory: Preliminary findings among mental inpatients (Hebrew). *Megamot*, 22:449–466.

Samooha, S. (1978), *Israel: Pluralism and Conflict.* Berkeley: University of California Press.

Sanua, V. D. (1989), Studies in mental illness and other psychiatric deviances among contemporary Jewry: A review. *Israel J. Psychiat.*, 26:187–211.

Sharav, T. (1985), High-risk population for Down syndrome: Orthodox Jews in Jerusalem. *Amer. J. Ment. Deficiency*, 89:559–561.

Snyder, C. R., & Palgi, P. (1982), Alcoholism among the Jews in Israel. *J. Studies on Alcohol*, 4:623–654.

Solomon, Z., Noi, S., & Bar-On, R. (1986), Risk factors in combat stress reactions: A study of Israeli soldiers in the 1982 Lebanon War. *Israel J. Psychiat.*, 23:3–8.

——— Oppenheimer, B., Elizur, Y., & Waysman, M. (1990), Trauma deepens trauma: The consequences of recurrent combat stress reaction. *Israel J. Psychiat.*, 27:233–241.

Weil, L. (1990), *Phenomenology of Mental Disorders in Ultra-Orthodox Population.* Unpublished Ph.D. dissertation. Hebrew University, Jerusalem.

Witztum, E., Buchbinder, J. T., & Van der Hart, O. (1990), Summoning a punishing angel: Treament of a depressed patient with dissociative features. *Bull. Menninger Clinic*, 54:524–537.

——— Greenberg, D., & Buchbinder, J. T. (1990), "A Very Narrow Bridge": Diagnosis and management of mental illness among Bratslav Hasidim. *Psychotherapy*, 27:124–131.

——— ——— Dasberg, H. (1990), Mental illness and religious change. *Brit. J. Med. Psychol.*, 63:33–41.

9.

Culture and Mental Illness in South Korea

Kwang-iel Kim

CULTURAL AND HISTORICAL BACKGROUND

The Koreans are an ancient and homogenous ethnic group with a unique alphabet and language, distinct from both Chinese and Japanese. Korea is traditionally an agrarian society with a 5000-year history. South Korea is a materialistic and open society, whereas the North is socialistic and closed. Thus the focus of this chapter will be only on South Korea, which is drastically changing from a traditional society to an industrial one, resulting in serious acculturational problems.

Korea is a multireligious society. Historically, the indigenous religion involved the worship of nature, and it was followed by shamanism. Buddhism and Confucianism were introduced to Korea in the fourth century B.C., and Christianity in 1794, and these have become the three major religions. There are currently 250 new religious cults in Korea, but even today when modernization is in vigorous progress, religious attitude is mostly influenced by shamanism. The psychopathology of the patients differs little according to religious affiliation. Ancestor worship, filial piety, family ties, *jeung* (an emotive term referring to a special interpersonal bond), and individual and family prestige are the main keys to understanding the Korean mind.

Indigenous concepts of mental illness are derived from shamanism and traditional medicine. Like all illness, mental illness was believed to result from an improper relationship with the spirits which brought spirit intrusion, soul-loss, and violation of taboos. Mental illness was treated with magicoreligious rituals in the shamanistic society (Kim, 1973). In traditional medicine, emotional problems and mental illness are attributed to the disharmony of internal organs according to theories of Yin-Yang and the five elements. Each organ is believed to have its specific symbolic emotional or mental function: the heart is the site of pleasure, ideation, and spirit; the liver is the site of anger, courage, and soul; the lungs, of worry, sorrow, and an inferior spirit; the gall bladder, of decision making and power; the spleen, of idea and will; and the kidneys, of fear and energy. In this context, all mental problems are interpreted as having originated from the dysfunction of a particular organ or organs. For example, depression is ascribed to a dysfunction of the liver and the kidneys; anxiety, to a dysfunction of the heart; and mental confusion, to the heart and spleen (Kim, 1973). Eventually, mental illness was treated by treating the corresponding organs.

In shamanism all emotional ailments are ascribed to the intervention of supernatural beings, whereas in traditional medicine, the body is regarded as the source of the problem (Kim, 1973).

Although Kraepelin-oriented psychiatry was introduced to Korea in 1910, psychiatrists were rare and remained largely alien to the majority of Koreans. After liberation from the Japanese occupation in 1945, dynamic psychiatry was introduced by a significant number of American-trained Korean psychiatrists, followed by biological psychiatry, which is now an integral part of psychiatric practice in South Korea. Today there are 1,400 practicing psychiatrists and psychiatric residents, comprising one psychiatrist to every 32,143 people, and 16,160 psychiatric beds, or one bed to every 2,815 people.

PUBLIC KNOWLEDGE AND ATTITUDE TOWARD MENTAL ILLNESS

Mental illness in Korea is perceived as deviant and harmful behavior. A survey reported that a dangerous paranoid schizophrenic was recognized as mentally ill by 83 percent of the public, whereas a withdrawn simple schizophrenic was recognized by 50 percent, and alcoholism by 34 percent (Kim, Seo, Park, Lee, and Kim, 1989). According to another survey, alcoholic behavior, neurotic and psychosomatic symptoms, suicidal behavior, calm and withdrawn way of life such as depression and simple schizophrenia, are seldom regarded as psychiatric problems. Rather, they are considered normal or as somatic illnesses (Kim, Won, Zin, Kim, Chang, Lee, Hong, and Ohm, 1973).

Twenty-six percent of the public are afraid of mental patients and 49 percent are ashamed of family members who are mentally ill. Forty percent agree that family care is more effective in the treatment of mental illness than hospitalization (Kim, Seo, Park et al., 1989).

Cultural barriers filter out only the unmanageable patients with detrimental, excited behavior while allowing alcoholics and calm, withdrawn patients to remain in society.

ILLNESS BEHAVIOR

Projection of inner psychic problem onto the soma, and onto supernatural beings and other people seem to be the principal psychopathological traits of Korean patients.

A strong somatizing tendency is evident, resulting from disease concepts of traditional medicine, traditional suppression of verbal and nonverbal expressions of hostility in the large family, and in conventional social life (Kim, 1973). Actually, about two-thirds of psychiatric patients initially complain of emotional ailments in the form of somatic dysfunction. Depression is frequent but usually masked by somatic symptoms. Somatization disorder and classical conversion disorder are common among female psychiatric patients.

Traditional and elderly persons still project their emotional problems onto the supernatural so that they frequently visit a fortuneteller or a shaman. In more modern social circles, this projecting tendency has shifted from supernatural beings to other people or to social or political regimes, manifesting paranoid symptoms with social and political themes. Consequently, many psychiatric patients visit internists, neurosurgeons, traditional physicians, shamans, and faith healers, while some other psychotic young people may simply develop antigovernment delusions.

Nowadays, illness in Korean patients and their families is characterized by syncretism; among psychiatric outpatients, those who have been previously treated by shamanistic devices were 17 to 23 percent, by faith healing 11 to 15 percent, and by traditional medicine 60 to 65 percent. Sixty-six percent of them have been treated by multiple methods such as shamanistic rites, faith healing, over-the-counter medication, traditional medicine, and modern medicine (Lee, Hwang, and Yiu, 1973; Rhi, 1973). Regarding illness behavior, five cohorts were identified: *the folk-oriented people, the syncretic people, the religious people, those who were negative toward modern medicine,* and *those who believed in modern medicine.* All cohorts except *the latter* prefer to follow various therapeutic regimens simultaneously (Hwang, Kim, and Song, 1988).

Above all, Korea has a multiple health care system: modern medicine, traditional medicine, and other quasi-medical systems such as chiropractice, acupuncture, psychological therapy institutes, stuttering correction institute. These are government-authorized. Thus, patients and their families are usually puzzled and confused by the multitude of choices when seeking help.

EPIDEMIOLOGY

A nationwide epidemiological survey was carried out in 1986, using the Diagnostic Interview Schedule (DIS) (Lee, Kwak, Rhee, Kim, Han, Choi, and Lee, 1986). The lifetime prevalences are summarized in Table 9.1.

Compared with the findings of New Haven and St. Louis (Myers, Weissman, Tischler, Holzer, Leaf, Orvaschel, Anthony, Boyd, Burke, Kramer, and Stoltzman, 1984), rates of alcohol abuse and dependence are drastically higher in Korea, and drug abuse and dependence is apparently lower, while DIS disorder rates as a whole, except substance use disorders, are lower. Schizophrenia, affective disorders, and phobia rates are lower and cognitive disorder rates are higher.

TABLE 9.1
Lifetime Prevalence Rate of DIS/DSM-III Disorders in Korea*

DIS disorders	Seoul (%)	Rural (%)
Any DIS Disorder Covered	39.81	41.05
Any DIS Disorder Except Tobacco Dependence	31.80	22.02
Any DIS Disorder Except Substance Use		
Disorders	13.36	13.46
Substance Use Disorders	31.75	31.98
Alcohol Abuse	12.95	10.65
Alcohol Dependence	8.76	11.74
Tobacco Dependence	19.92	20.96
Drug Abuse/Dependence	0.88	0.49
Schizophrenic/Schizophreniform Disorders	0.34	0.65
Schizophrenia	0.31	0.54
Schzophreniform Disorder	0.03	0.11
Affective Disorders	5.52	5.11
Manic Episode	0.40	0.44
Major Depression	3.31	3.47
Dysthymia	2.42	1.89
Anxiety/Somatoform Disorders	8.17	8.51
Phobia(sum)	5.89	5.97
Agoraphobia	2.08	3.62
Social Phobia	0.53	0.65
Simple Phobia	5.37	4.67
Panic Disorder	1.11	2.60
Agoraphobia with Panic Attack	0.65	1.27
Obsessive Compulsive Disorder	2.29	1.90
Somatization Disorder	0.03	0.18
Anorexia	0.03	0.00
Antisocial Personality Disorder	2.08	0.91
Gambling	1.02	0.98
Cognitive Impairment Mild	4.60	8.77
Cognitive Impairment Severe	0.16	1.85

Source: Lee, Kwak et al. (1986)

Alcohol abuse and antisocial personality disorder occur at higher rates in Seoul than rural areas. On the other hand, rates of alcohol dependence, agoraphobia, panic disorder, and cognitive impairment are higher in the rural areas. The male population manifests higher prevalence of alcoholic disorders, antisocial personality disorder, and gambling, while the female population manifests higher prevalence in affective disorders, phobia, panic disorder, and cognitive impairment.

ACCULTURATIONAL PROBLEMS

Alcohol consumption has rapidly increased during the past two decades in proportion to the economic improvement: annual consumption per capita for those aged 15 and over was 9.05 liters of absolute alcohol, and that of male adults was 18.4 liters in 1988. The public neglects drinking as a social and medical problem (Kim, 1990). Drug abuse by youngsters, with a close relationship to delinquent behavior, has recently become a serious social issue, even if its prevalence is still lower than that of Western society. Amphetamines, cocaine, marijuana, antianxiety drugs, and other analgesics are the main drugs of abuse. Inhalation of butane gas and toluene-based glue is a serious social and psychiatric problem amongst adolescents.

Quite recently, youngsters' delinquent behavior such as violence, rape, kidnapping, vandalism, running away from home, robbery, and murder have drastically increased and are more brutal and carried out by groups. The collapse of traditional values and social tolerance of violence are attributed to this increase in delinquent behavior.

The doors to high schools and colleges are so narrow that students are pressed to study hard. Ninety-five percent of high school graduates and 98 percent of junior high school graduates want to get a higher education. In 1991, 1 million students applied to colleges, but the nationwide capacity for college freshmen is only 270,500. Each year, there are 1 million young people who cannot enter colleges and high schools and who are unemployed. Educational fever occasionally results in friction between students and their parents. Some vulnerable students try to escape the situation by committing suicide, passive aggressive sabotage of their studies, depression, and acting out. Other vulnerable students suffer from "the senior syndrome" in which various transient neurotic and psychosomatic symptoms or psychotic episodes are manifest.

In the summer of 1979, an epidemic mass hysteria broke out among junior school students in five rural communities. This outbreak was attributed to the collapse of traditional family support to children and adolescents due to rapid acculturation of the rural community: All adults, both men and women, spend less time at home in order to improve their economic condition (Kim, Kim, and Kim, 1984).

Daughter-in-law/mother-in-law conflict has become more overt due to different values; younger women do not want to live with elderly parents who follow the traditional ways of living. The main conflictual area of one-third of women admitted to psychiatric facilities was reported to be related to this issue (Kim and Nam, 1978).

The elderly person is easily frustrated by loneliness, role deprivation, along with collapse of traditional regard for the elderly and the protective environment once provided by the family. Previously, senile psychosis was regarded as a natural phenomenon of the aged and was accepted. Now, family members are unwilling to care for them, and they are often sent to hospitals or nursing homes.

SOME CLINICAL FEATURES

Even though admission rates for alcoholism and senile psychosis are still low (5–10%, 2–3% respectively), admission rates have increased during the past two decades, probably due to increased public knowledge and the collapse of the traditionally supportive milieu (Kim, 1990).

Admission rates for hysteria are high and symptoms are classic. This high rate has been attributed to the low level of medical knowledge, traditional repression of sexuality, the disease concept of traditional medicine that facilitates projection toward the soma as the source of psychic conflict, and the traditional inhibition of verbalization and expression of emotion (Hahn, 1964). But during the past two decades, hysteria rates have decreased and the symptoms have become less dramatic. This is possibly due to improvements in medical knowledge, sexual liberation, and changes in the familial and social role of women.

Depression is common and has recently increased in the clinical setting: 10 to 30 percent of outpatients, 10 to 13 percent of inpatients. The increase is partly due to the increase of reactive depression and partly due to changes in help-seeking behavior from intrafamilial resolution to the professional route. Somatic symptoms are initial and superficial complaints, but guilt feelings and suicidal ideation are also apparent. One transcultural survey reported that guilt feelings and suicidal ideation were more prevalent than in the United States, Britain, and India (Kim, 1977). The guilt feelings are toward the family and community rather than toward God (Kim and Nam, 1984). There are no geographic and religious differences in the manifestations.

Regarding schizophrenia, the common symptom has much changed during the past fifty years; during the Japanese occupation prior to 1945, the most common symptom was excitement and a delusion of poverty; during the five years after liberation from the Japanese occupation, grandiose delusions with a political theme dominated; after the Korean War (1950–1953) political themes such as "communist" and "spy" were common; during the two decades after the military coup (1961), "secret agent" and "high official" were common themes; while "reunification" and persecution by various social and political regimes have recently been the main themes of delusion. These reflect sociopolitical changes and turmoil in Korea over the past fifty years. A thinly disguised sexual theme is prevalent, reflecting conflict between the rigid traditional sexual morality and the recent sexual liberalism (Chang and Kim, 1973). On the other hand, delusions about family and neighbors are constant, reflecting the family and community-oriented traditional culture.

Sex perversions including homosexuals are hardly seen in clinics. It is unclear whether they themselves are rare; however, many professionals attribute the low incidence to the assignment of distinctly different roles to men and women from childhood and strict social sanctions against perversions (Hahn, 1970).

Taijinkyofu (interpersonal fear), a possible culture-bound syndrome, is prevalent in Korea and in Japan (Lee, 1988) and is rare in China and the Philippines, according to a transcultural survey (Kitanishi, Kim, and Liu, 1991). This is attributed to the traditional overconcern about the opinions of others.

Hwa-byung (a fire or anger syndrome) is a mixture of various neurotic and psychosomatic symptoms of traditional people reacting to a stress-ridden situation mostly in an interpersonal context. The course is relatively short and quickly disappears soon after resolution of the stress (Lee, 1977). Actually, neurotic patients in rural areas manifest various mixtures of neurotic and psychosomatic symptoms (Lee and Kim, 1975). This can be regarded as a local name for a mixed form of neurotic condition rather than as a culture-bound syndrome.

Shin-byung (a divine illness), a possssion syndrome, often occurs in the course of a prolonged psychosomatic illness, neurosis, or psychosis. The possessed person has a "revelation" through a dream, a hallucination, or a feeling in which one is persuaded to become a shaman. The possessor is usually a dead ancestor (animal possession is extremely rare). With the person's conversion into a shaman, the patient then becomes "cured" of the ailment. The occurrence of *shin-byung* is decreasing (Kim, 1972).

The Western classification system can hardly be applied to the above three syndromes.

CULTURE-RELEVANT APPROACHES

There is no difference between Korean and Western countries in dosage and side effects of psychoactive drugs.

Psychotherapy, individual or familial, analytic or supportive, is effective. Research and therapeutic application of *Tao*, an important cultural inheritance, have been active and seem to be a promising area for developing a culture-relevant model of psychotherapy. *Tao* aims at developing a self that perceives the inner and outer world realistically and tries to liberate itself from all forms of emotional bondage, pathological or existential. *Tao* itself is not a psychotherapeutic system but a philosophical teaching. But, there are strong psychotherapeutic elements in *Tao* such as the attitude, process, and methods of developing insight into one's mind. In applying the principles of *Tao* to psychotherapy, practitioners understand and treat not merely the pathological condition, but also help patients to discover and cultivate their health potential (Rhee, 1968).

FUTURE PERSPECTIVES

A serious problem for psychiatry involves the poor care delivery system and the nonmedical institute for mental patients. About

60 percent of psychotic patients are still confined in the institutes without psychiatric care. The mental health act has not yet been enacted in Korea. Another problem, as well as in other branches of medicine in Korea, is the multiple and disorganized care system, even though the national medical insurance system, covering the whole population, was established in 1987 (Kim, 1989).

A study of cultural psychiatry in Korea can be interesting and productive, since it is a country where the forces of tradition and rapid modernization are likely to be sensitively reflected. Despite the rich rewards of cultural psychiatric study in this country, little has been done in transcultural research or the developmental approach. Cooperative studies on an international level are on the way. Active research in these areas will be a task for the future.

REFERENCES

Chang, S. C., & Kim, K. I. (1973), Psychiatry in South Korea. *Amer. J. Psychiat.*, 130:667–669.

Hahn, D. S. (1964), A clinical and anthropological study of hysteria in Korea. *Neuropsychiatry* (Seoul), 3:9–21.

——— (1970), Sexual deviation in Korea. *Neuropsychiatry* (Seoul), 9:25–34.

Hwang, K. H., Kim, K. I., & Song, S. S. (1988), Lay people's attitude toward illness behavior. *Neuropsychiatry* (Seoul), 27:80–95.

Kim, E. Y., Kim, M. J., & Kim, K. I. (1984), Mass hysteria among middle schools in the Korean rural communities 1976. *Mental Health Res.* (Seoul), 2:159–172.

Kim, K. I. (1972), "Shin-byung": A culture-bound depersonalization syndrome. *Neuropsychiatry* (Seoul), 9:47–56.

——— (1973), Traditional concepts of disease in Korea. *Korea J.* (Seoul), 13:12–18.

——— (1977), Clinical study of primary depressive symptom, part III: A crosscultural comparison. *Neuropsychiatry* (Seoul), 16:53–60.

——— (1989), Mental health law in Korea. *Ment. Health Res.* (Seoul), 8:212–214.

——— (1990), Alcoholic disorders in Korea. *Ment. Health Res.* (Seoul), 9:131–147.

——— Nam, J. H. (1978), Mother-in-law/daughter-in-law conflict among psychiatric inpatients. *Neuropsychiatry* (Seoul), 17:27–32.

——— ——— (1984), Clinical study of primary depressive symptom, part VI: Pattern of guilt. *Ment. Health Res.* (Seoul), 2:186–197.

——— Seo, H. H., Park, Y. C., Lee, S. T., & Kim, G. Y. (1989), Public knowledge and attitude toward mental illness. *Ment. Health Res.* (Seoul), 8:118–132.

——— Won, H. T., Zin, S. T., Kim, M. J., Chang, H. I., Lee, K. N., Hong, W. S., & Ohm, Y. S. (1973), Korean attitude toward abnormal behaviors. *Neuropsychiatry* (Seoul), 12:41–52.

Kitanishi, K., Kim, K. I., & Liu, X. (1991), A transcultural study of interpersonal fear. Typescript.

Lee, C. K., Kwak, Y. S., Rhee, H., Kim, Y. S., Han, J. H., Choi, J. O., & Lee, Y. H. (1986), The epidemiological study of mental disorders in Korea–By DIS-III Korean version. *Seoul J. Psychiat.*, (Seoul), 11(suppl.):121–141.

Lee, H. Y., Hwang, I. K., & Yiu, J. M. (1973), Treatment methods before psychiatric admission. *Neuropsychiatry* (Seoul), 12:59–69.

Lee, J. H., & Kim, K. I. (1975), Preliminary survey on the neurotic cases in a Korean rural community. *Neuropsychiatry* (Seoul), 14:15–24.

Lee, S. H. (1977), A study of the "Hwa-byung" (Anger syndrome). *J. Korea Gen. Hosp.*, 1:63–69.

——— (1988), Social phobia in Korea. *Seoul J. Psychiat.* (Seoul), 13:125–153.

Myers, J. K., Weissman, M. M., Tischler, G. L., Holzer III, C. Z., Leaf, P. J., Orvaschel, H., Anthony, J. C., Boyd, J. M., Burke, Jr., J. D., Kramer, M. K., & Stoltzman, R. (1984), Six month prevalence of psychiatric disorders in three communities. *Arch. Gen. Psychiat.*, 41:959–967.

Rhee, D. S. (1968), Philosophical backgrounds for psychotherapy and counseling in Korea. In: *A Collection of Psychological Papers in Commemoration of the 60th Birthday of Prof. Tae Rim Yun.* Seoul: Sookmyung University Press.

Rhi, B. Y. (1973), A preliminary study of medical acculturation problems in Korea. *Neuropsychiatry* (Seoul), 12:97–109.

10.

Culture and Mental Illness in Singapore: A Sociocultural Perspective

Kok Lee-Peng and Tsoi Wing-Foo

Singapore is an island city of 626 square kilometers, situated in South East Asia. Modern Singapore was founded in 1819 by Sir Stamford Raffles as a colony of Britain, and it became an independent country in 1965. During the next twenty-five years it developed rapidly into an industrialized republic and is at present a commercial, communication, and financial center in this region with a per capita income of about US $10,000 in 1990. Singapore's population is made up of three main ethnic groups which has been maintained at a fairly constant level: Chinese 77 percent, Malays 15 percent, Indians 6 percent, and others (mainly Caucasians, Eurasians, and Arabs) 2 percent.

PSYCHIATRIC SERVICES

The psychiatric services of Singapore are provided mainly by Woodbridge Hospital (the only mental hospital, with 2500 beds) whose staff also run most of the outpatient and rehabilitation services in the country. Other important psychiatric facilities include (1) the University Department of Psychiatry which has a twenty-eight-bed psychiatric ward in a general hospital; (2) a twenty-four-bed private psychiatric ward, and a forty-five-bed private psychiatric hospital; and (3) voluntary organizations which cater to the mentally disordered, mentally retarded, and substance abusers. Traditional healers are also consulted by psychiatric patients.

EPIDEMIOLOGICAL SURVEY

Three epidemiological surveys of mental disorders in the general population have been carried out in Singapore. (1) A General Health Survey, 1978; (2) a Mental Health Survey in a suburb of Singapore, 1981; (3) a General Population Survey by the Singapore Association of Mental Health, 1989. The latest survey of 1153 respondents (about half male and half female) using a modified General Health Questionnaire with twenty-eight items and a two-thirds cutoff point, showed a prevalence rate of 18 percent for minor psychiatric morbidity. All three surveys showed that the Indians consistently had the highest prevalence of psychiatric morbidity (a mean of 23%), followed by the Chinese (15%), and the Malays (14%).

SCHIZOPHRENIA

Schizophrenia constitutes about 60 percent of all new admissions and about 70 percent of all the inpatients at Woodbridge Hospital (Tsoi and Chen, 1979).

A study of 423 unselected first admission schizophrenic patients in 1975 revealed the following. There were: 248 (59%) males (mean age 26 years) and 175 (41%) females (mean age 29 years); 80 percent were Chinese, 9 percent Malays, and 10 percent other races, showing that the Malays were underrepresented as the racial breakdown for Singapore in 1975 was Chinese 76 percent, Malays 15 percent, other races 9 percent. The Malays who were natives of the country generally had better social support than the other two groups and were more likely to seek traditional treatment rather than admission to a hospital. The mean duration of illness before admission was 17.8 months. There were no differences in the clinical presentation between the four racial groups. Their most frequent symptoms were sleep disturbance (55%), talking to oneself (43%), laughing to oneself (40%), aggressive or assaultive behavior (32%), abnormal or unconventional behavior (30%), social withdrawal (24%), "talking nonsense" (21%), crying to oneself (21%), and restlessness or hyperactivity (21%).

The subjects were divided into four groups: (1) paranoid schizophrenia; (2) typical schizophrenia; (3) atypical/undifferentiated schizophrenia; (4) simple schizophrenia.

The cohort was followed up, and at the end of fifteen years in 1990, seventy-two (17.1%) had died—40 (9.5%) from suicide and 32 (7.6%) from natural causes. The paranoid group had the lowest, and the simple type, the highest suicide rate. The surviving patients were followed up in 1980 and 1990 and at the end of the fifth and fifteenth year, about 30 percent had recovered fully, 30 percent recovered partially, and 40 percent had not recovered. Their outcome showed that schizophrenia stabilized after the fifth year. Simple schizophrenia and a long duration of illness predicted a poorer outcome, whereas paranoid schizophrenia and the Malay race were associated with a better outcome.

SUICIDE

Suicide data in Singapore from 1894 to 1989 showed that the suicide rate was low (4 to 8 per 100,000 per year) before 1905. After that the five yearly rates fluctuated around 10 per 100,000 except for the period just before (1936–1940) and during World War II (1941–1945) when it was 15.5 and 13.1 per 100,000 respectively.

The first comprehensive study of suicide in Singapore by Murphy (1954), showed a steady increase in the suicide rates since 1948. The rates were lowest among Malays and highest in Indians.

Later studies by Hassan and Tan (1970) and Chia and Tsoi (1972) showed that the rate of those who committed suicide by jumping increased steadily, and was highest in the old city center area.

Chia (1978) confirmed most of the findings of earlier studies.

Mental illness (29%), physical illness (26%), and interpersonal problems (23%) were found to be the main causative factors. Physical illness was the most frequent cause for suicide among aged males and mental illness the most frequent cause for suicide in young adults. In addition, for males aged 25 to 44 and females aged 16 to 24 job problems and interpersonal problems respectively were important causes.

The latest study by the authors covering a period of ten years from January 1, 1980 to December 31, 1989, showed that there were 2889 suicides (1690 males and 1199 females). The suicide rates rose with age from 3.3 per 100,000 for the age group 10 to 19 years to 72 per 100,000 for ages 60 years and above. The suicide rate for the Chinese (12.7 per 100,000) was similar to that for the Indians (13.2 per 100,000) but much higher than that for the Malays (2.8 per 100,000). The Chinese were older (mean age 47.4 years) than the rest of the other races (mean age 38.1 years). The methods and causes were similar to previous studies. Jumping was associated with a younger age, being of the Malay or Chinese race, and hanging with an older age, being of the Indian or other races. The Indians had higher rates for self-immolation and throwing themselves under trains. Mental illness and interpersonal problems were more prevalent among the younger subjects (age 49 and below) and Chinese, while physical illness was more common among the older subjects (age 50 and above) and Malays. Of the individual causative factors, the commonest were schizophrenia 25 percent, depression 15 percent, debts, alcohol, pain, and respiratory diseases (3–4% each).

ATTEMPTED SUICIDE

Attempted suicide has also been studied by examining the records of all such admissions into all government general hospitals in Singapore for the years 1971, 1980, and 1986 (Chia and Tsoi, 1974; Tsoi and Kok, 1982; Kok, 1988). The rates rose progressively from 55 to 70 to 92 per 100,000 during these periods. For 1986, there were 2376 cases (886 males and 1498 females), with a rate of 104 per 100,000 (male 75, and female 134 per 100,000). The rate was highest in the age group 20 to 29 years (157 per 100,000), followed by the group 30 to 39 years (129/100,000), and 40 to 49 years (92 per 100,000). As in suicide, Malays had the lowest rate, followed by Chinese (107), Indians (223), and others (238).

Kok (1988), in a study of 364 cases of attempted suicide admitted to a general hospital in one year, found that the commonest method of attempted suicide by far was by drug and substance ingestion (95%), followed by jumping and hanging (4%), and the rest (1%) resorted to a variety of methods including stabbing, cutting, jumping, hanging, drowning, self-immolation, and gasing. The reasons given for suicidal attempts were relationship problems (50%), illness (28%), insomnia (10%), work problems (10%), and financial problems (3%). The majority were single, less than 10 percent were married. Suicide attempters were found to be significantly more neurotic, rigid, and less extroverted than controls.

SUBSTANCE ABUSE DISORDER

The common drugs of abuse in Singapore are heroin, opium, cannabis, tranquilizers, and volatile substances. Heroin is the most serious drug of abuse, but the number of abusers has declined from 13,000 in 1977 to 9,000 in 1988. Of those arrested in 1988, 91 percent abused heroin, 11 percent tranquilizers, 5 percent cannabis, and 3 percent opium. The number of new addicts decreased from 860 per month in 1977 to 454 per month in 1988. The proportion of those addicted in the age group who were under 20 years was 31 percent in 1977 compared to 10 percent in 1988. The majority came from the lower socioeconomic group and 95 percent were school dropouts. Most were unemployed or had casual jobs (Poh, 1989). The racial breakdown showed that Malays were overrepresented and their rates had increased from 2.28 per 100,000 in 1983 to 6.94 per 100,000 in 1988. The corresponding rates for other races were 1.19 and 1.97 per 100,000.

Inhalation of volatile substances has become increasingly popular among adolescents because of the easy availability and relatively low prices of such substances as paint thinner, glue, petroleum products, spray paints, nail polish remover. In 1980 only twenty-four subjects were found to be abusing inhalants, but this number increased about thirtyfold to 763 in 1984. The racial breakdown for inhalant abuse was Chinese 67 percent, Malays 23 percent, Indian 9 percent, and others 0.2 percent, showing again that the Malays were overrepresented (Lim, 1985), as Singapore Malays aged 19 made up only 14.8 percent of the population.

Alcoholism is an uncommon condition in Singapore although the consumption of alcohol has been rising over the past few years. The rate of alcohol abuse in the population is not known, but in a study by Kua (1986) Indians were overrepresented among patients hospitalized for alcoholism (39%) compared with Chinese (61%), and Malays (0%), as the racial breakdown for Singapore was Indian (6%), Chinese (77%), Malay (15%). The ratio of males to females was 7 to 1. Women were younger than men, were less heavy drinkers, had fewer physical problems, and resorted to drinking because of relationship problems with their husbands or boyfriends.

EPIDEMIC KORO

Gwee and Lee (1969) described a Koro epidemic in Singapore in which a total of 454 males and 15 females were affected. It was a predominantly male Chinese phenomenon as there were only four Malay men (0.9%) and six Indian men (1.3%) among the subjects. The epidemic was triggered off by a newspaper report that some people, as a result of eating the flesh of pigs innoculated with antiswine fever vaccine, had developed Koro. Further newspaper reports on the subject increased the spate of rumors and Koro cases started to be seen at the hospitals. The majority of the subjects were educated and it was postulated that Koro, being an entity closely linked to cultural beliefs, was transmitted via the printed word at the onset and would affect those with some education.

EPIDEMIC HYSTERIA

Unlike Koro, epidemic hysteria is a female phenomenon. Kok (1975) described an outbreak of epidemic hysteria in a large television assembly factory and two other factories. The outbreak started at 7:00 P.M. when a female worker suddenly started screaming and fainted. This triggered off a spate of trance and seizure cases over the next few days. A total of eighty-four persons were involved. All but one were females, and all but one were Malays.

Another study of epidemic hysteria in two Singapore factories in 1981 showed a similar pattern except that there were more Indians and a few Chinese. Those who were affected had significantly higher levels of anxiety, hypochondriasis, and phobia than the controls. One of the precipitating factors was unhappiness among the workers at not being given time off on the eve of a public holiday (Chan, 1979; Kok, Tsoi, Chan, and Phoon, 1981).

Many of the subjects believed that the attacks were caused by supernatural agents (*jinns* or *hantus*). A common belief among the Malays is that when a person's spirit or *semangat* is weak or lowered, she becomes affected by devils (*hantus*). This lowering of the spirit may be caused by physical illness, a shock, emotional problems, the sight of blood, or menstruation.

TRANSSEXUALISM

Ratnam and Sundarason (1973) performed the first male to female sex reassignment surgery in Singapore on February 15, 1972. Since then there has been a steady stream of people applying for sex reassignment surgery.

Psychiatric investigation by Tsoi, Kok, and Long (1977) showed that, compared with the controls, the subjects had a less happy life during childhood and school. Their occupations and activities were those of the opposite sex. The onset of their sexual inversion started around the age of 8 to 10 years; they became friends with their first homosexual partner at age 16 to 17 years, and were first intimate at age 19 to 20 years. They became fully developed transsexuals (cross-dressing and living the life of an opposite sex member) at age 21 for males and age 16 for females. The Singapore transsexuals were similar to those reported elsewhere, but they had less psychiatric illness, less electroencephalographic abnormalities and no heterosexual tendencies. Sex reassignment surgery was carried out on forty-three males, of whom twenty-five were followed up and all had good adjustments.

For the females the figures were thirty-eight operated on, twenty-two followed up, and twenty-one (95%) with good adjustments.

REFERENCES

Chan, O. Y. (1979), Epidemic hysteria—high risk factors in Singapore factory workers. *Occupational Health & Safety*, 48:58–60.

Chia, B. H. (1978), *Suicide in Singapore*. Unpublished doctoral dissertation. National University of Singapore.

———— Tsoi, W. F. (1972), Suicide in Singapore. *Singapore Med. J.*, 13:91–97.

———— ———— (1974), A statistical study of attempted suicides in Singapore. *Singapore Med. J.*, 15:253–256.

General Population Survey. Singapore Association of Mental Health (1989), Typescript.

Gwee, A. L., & Lee, Y. K. (1969), The Koro epidemic in Singapore. *Singapore Med. J.*, 10:234–242.

Hassan, R., & Tan, K. L. (1970), Suicide in Singapore: A sociological analysis. *Southeast Asian J. Sociol.*, 3:13–26.

Kok, L. P. (1975), Epidemic hysteria (a psychiatric investigation). *Singapore Med. J.*, 16:35–38.

———— (1988), *Attempted Suicide by Drug Overdose*. Unpublished doctoral dissertation. National University of Singapore.

———— Tsoi, W. F., Chan, M., & Phoon, W. (1981), Mass hysteria in 2 Singapore factories. (Psychological aspects.) Typescript.

Kua, E. H. (1986), Alcohol related hospitalization in Singapore. *Singapore Med. J.*, 25:392–395.

Leong, A. P. K., Chua, E. C., Loy, T. J., & Foo, E. C. B. (1983), A preliminary survey of mental health in a new town in Singapore. *Singapore Med. J.*, 24:90–94.

Lim, Y. C. (1985), Inhalant abuse in Singapore. Paper presented at a Symposium on Inhalant Abuse.

Ministry of Health (1978), General Health Survey. Typescript.

Murphy, H. B. M. (1954), Mental health in Singapore—Suicide. *Med. J. Malaya*, 9:1–45.

Poh, G. E. (1989), Current drug scene. In: *Selected Readings on Drug Abuse*. Singapore: Singapore Antinarcotic Association.

Ratnam, S. S., & Sundarason, R. (1973), Treatment of the male transsexual. Paper presented at 46th General Scientific Meeting, Singapore, Royal Australasian College of Surgeons.

Tsoi, W. F. (1988), *A Psychiatric Investigation of Transsexualism in Singapore.* Unpublished doctoral dissertation. National University of Singapore.

―――― Chen, A. J. (1979), New admissions to Woodbridge Hospital 1975 with special reference to schizophrenia. *Ann. Acad. Med., Singapore,* 8:275–290.

―――― Kok, L. P. (1982), Suicidal behaviour in Singapore for the year 1980. *Singapore Med. J.,* 23:299–305.

―――― ―――― Long, F. Y. (1977), Male transsexualism in Singapore: A description of 56 cases. *Brit. J. Psychiat.,* 131:405–409.

11.

Mental Illness in an Islamic-Mediterranean Culture: Turkey

Can Tuncer

Turkey, which straddles two continents and has a population of more than 50 million, is indeed a bridge between Asia and Europe. Anatolia, its ancient name, means "orient," to the east of Europe, and constitutes the mainland part of Turkey. Anatolia has been the cradle of a variety of civilizations, with prehistoric archaeological findings as old as 6000 B.C. Amongst the civilizations of Anatolia, the Hittites were influential between 1400 and 1200 B.C. They were followed by the Phrygians, the Ionians, the Romans, and the Byzantine Empire, which adopted Christianity and prevailed in Anatolia from the fourth century A.D. until the arrival of the Turks in the tenth and eleventh centuries (Ozturk and Volkan, 1971). During the ninth and tenth centuries, the Turks adopted Islam. They initially occupied Central Asia, and then, during the eleventh and twelfth centuries, Seljuk Turks settled in Anatolia and founded the Seljuk Empire. In 1299, the Ottoman Empire was established and lasted until 1923, when the Turkish Republic was founded.

Acknowledgments: I wish to thank Associate Professor Harry Minas, Director, Victorian Transcultural Psychiatry Unit, for reviewing the manuscript and his comments.

I am grateful to Clare Lonergan for her secretarial assistance.

169

HISTORY OF PSYCHIATRY IN TURKEY

Aesculapian temples, functioning as healing centers during the sixth century B.C., were widespread in Greece, Western Anatolia, and the Aegian Islands. Aesculapian temples in Anatolia, especially in Pergamon and Ephesus, were amongst the most famous healing centers of the time. Such temples were situated away from population centers, usually near rivers or mineral springs. Suppliants would be purified by bathing in the sea, river, or spring; they would fast or undertake other dietary regimens. During sleep in the temple indications of cure would be divinely sent, and afterwards dreams would be interpreted (Koptagel-Ilal and Kazancigil, 1981). These practices would be accompanied by prayer and sacrifice, music and exercise (Osler, 1921). Reminders of these Aesculapian methods may be found in some traditional practices to be found in contemporary Turkey. Echos of animist beliefs (the worshipping of earth, sky, and water [Volkan, 1975]) of the Turks of Central Asia may also be found.

Yusuf Has Hacip's book *Kutadgu-Bilig*, published in 1069, describes the *efsuncus* (Unver, 1943). Their status was said to be below that of the *otaci* (physician), who cured disorders and pain with medicine while *efsuncus* treated maladies which were caused by *jinns* (Ozturk, 1964; Volkan, 1975; Sari, 1981). Avicenna, also known as Ibni Sina, was, according to Turkish textbooks on psychiatry (Adasal, 1969; Songar, 1980), a Turk who was born in Bokhara and later settled in Ispahen (980–1073). His famous *Canon* consisted of twelve volumes, in which he discussed some psychiatric disorders and in fact described mania and depression as illness. One of the important contributions of Avicenna was his connection of mind and body, an example of which was one of his case studies describing the effects of love on the pulse (Gruner, 1930).

Turkish culture, coming from Central Asia, Arabian civilizations, and Islamic medicine, influenced the attitude of Seljuks toward mentally ill people. Aesculapian methods of dealing with the mentally ill persisted in Anatolia during the Seljuk and Ottoman eras (Koptagel, 1971). During the Seljuk period several hospitals were built, such as those in Kayseri (1205), Sivas (1217),

Kastamonu (1275), and in Amasya (1308), which accepted responsibility for the care of the mentally ill (Volkan, 1975). In addition, *tekkes* (houses of sufic belief) were established all over the country and were also useful for the care and treatment of the mentally ill. Those *tekkes* have roots which may be traced to the Aesculapian temples of Anatolia (Koptagel, 1971; Volkan, 1975). It was said that the *tekke* was established as a refuge from the corruption of society (Y. N. Ozturk, 1988). In these houses (*tekkes*) beliefs and practices were generally based on religious sufic philosophy. They provided mentally ill people with aid and support based on the basic principle of sufism—the concept of love and unity with the eternal love object (Koptagel-Ilal and Kazancigil, 1981).

During the Ottoman era, in 1470, Ottomans established a hospital for mentally ill patients in Istanbul. During the reign of Emperor Sultan Bayezid II (1481–1512), a second mental hospital in Edirne was established in 1484. In these hospitals the highly developed care for the mentally ill included singers and musicians (Volkan, 1975; Guvenc, 1986). Another mental hospital was built in 1539 in Manisa. The first neuropsychiatric clinic in Turkey was opened in 1898 in Istanbul by Rasit Tahsin, who had been a student of Kraepelin. The Turkish Neuropsychiatric Society was founded in 1914. After the establishment of the Republic of Turkey in 1923, with the creation of new university medical schools and the development of departments of psychiatry, psychiatric activities were gradually separated from neurology. Professor Uzman, regarded as the founder of modern Turkish psychiatry and also influenced by Kraepelin, was the first chairman of the psychiatric department at Istanbul University. Until 1973, medical doctors qualified as "specialists in neurology and psychiatry." Since 1973, psychiatry and neurology have been formally recognized as separate specialties. They have separate training programs, with a four-year postgraduate training program in psychiatry. In 1987 there were approximately 320 specialist psychiatrists and 372 neurologists (Coskun, 1987). There are now five regional mental hospitals, with a total of 6139 psychiatric beds for all Turkey (Coskun, 1987).

BELIEFS AND ATTITUDES TOWARD MENTAL ILLNESS

Beliefs concerning the causes and care of mental illness range from the very traditional and supernatural to naturalistic conceptions influenced by scientific medicine. Before Islam, Turks living in north and central Asia regarded mental illness as being caused by spirits. Such spirits have a variety of names in different Turkish communities. For example, the spirit named *kut*, when it leaves the body, and the bad spirit called *black kormos*, when it occupies the brain, could each cause mental illness. A variety of practices for dealing with such spirit-caused mental illness also existed. In order to replace the escaping spirit there was a ritual of "lead pouring." In order to expel a bad spirit from the body a bird was flown near the patient so that the spirit might occupy the bird and free the person who had been inhabited by the spirit. Amulets with special properties were also used against mental disorders amongst the pre-Islamic Turks (Bayat, 1989).

The Muslim religion accepts spiritual beings such as *jinns* (equal to demons), angels, and fairies. The *jinns* are able to take on different forms in different places such as in forests, rocks, caves, and chimneys. The *jinns* may be overactive, mobile, aggressive, and punitive. Children sometimes are raised on tales of the frightening aspects of *jinns*. Villagers often believe that mental illness is a result of being possessed or mixed up by *jinns*. The *jinns* may be seen accidentally or appear after violation of certain taboos, such as failure to take a ritual cleansing bath after sexual activity, or improper behavior toward parents or to God. The result may be a "strike" by the *jinns* or "possession" by the *jinns* leading to aphonia or schizophrenic reaction, mania, and other illnesses (Ozturk, 1964).

The evil eye is a belief that Turks share with Greeks and other people of the Mediterranean, the Balkans, and the Middle East (Volkan, 1975; Dionisopoulis-Mass, 1976; Spooner, 1976). Many illnesses, both mental and physical, as well as failures in life, may be attributed to the evil eye. Certain people (generally those with blue or green eyes) are believed to have the potential of evil eyes. Villagers frequently hide their babies from the eyes of others in order to prevent such evil influences (Ozturk, 1964). Terms frequently used for the evil eye are *to eye* or to *eye strike, the bad eye,* and *the look* (Spooner, 1976). If one wishes to prevent one's eyes from unintentionally having an evil influence one must say *masallah* (God protection), which counteracts the evil eye (Ozturk, 1964).

Mental illness may also occur as a result of sorcery which, unlike the evil eye which is generally involuntary, is intentionally malevolent magic. It may cause the inability to concentrate, physical weakness, sexual impotence, loss of love, hallucinations, and confusional states. The sorcery may be carried out by a sorcerer with special knowledge (which may involve tying of knots, hiding amulets near the intended victim) hired by enemies such as a rival, a spouse, or an unknown person (Ozturk, 1964).

The traditional person's beliefs concerning illness may reflect religious attitudes, such as all goodness and all suffering comes from God (Volkan, 1975). "God gave an illness" is a common expression. Praying may serve as both a preventive and therapeutic measure against mental illness. Of course if praying is done by men of religion, such as *hodjas* (the priests of Muslim religion who, in the past, were both priest and teacher), it is believed to be more effective (Ozturk, 1964). Praying may be accompanied by sacrifices, visiting holy places such as the tombs of saints or *hodjas,* and springs, fountains, and caves which may be the sites of ancient churches or temples, and which are believed to have special healing powers. Such practices are contemporary remnants of ancient Anatolian culture.

Special words or prayers or *surahs* from the Koran are also widely used to ward off *jinns.* Amulets (*muskas*), the history of which goes back to ancient times, are an expression of a widespread belief in the power of written material, particularly when this is from the Koran. A *muska* is an amulet inscribed by the *hodja* for the treatment or prevention of mental disorder or other illness, evil, and sorcery. They may also be used for the purpose of sorcery. The *muska* consists of a small scroll upon which various *surahs* from the Koran are inscribed, as well as ritualistic signs and numerical configurations. The scroll is folded into a cloth of various colors or leather, and is worn like a necklace or sometimes fastened with a safety pin under the arms or over the chest. It is possible to see three or more amulets worn by the same patient.

There are some common folk treatments such as prayer,

breathing, animal sacrifice, fumigation, reading special phrases from the Koran, tying pieces of cloth on sacred places such as the *odjak* (hearth), *yatir,* and tombs of *hodjas* and saints. Melting lead and pouring it into a cup which is held over the person's head is an example of a method of exorcism of the *jinns,* of sorcery, or the evil eye (Ozturk, 1964). This procedure is sometimes applied by older members of the family such as grandparents. (The majority of the *hodjas* applying such "treatments" have no religious training or function, and these kinds of "treatment procedures" by *hodjas* are regarded as illegal.) The *odjak* (hearth) may be a living specialist *hodja*'s place, or a tomb or another place which has the influence to ward off evil and illness. Particular *odjaks* are believed to have particular effectiveness for specific disorders, such as malaria *odjak,* rabies *odjak,* jaundice *odjak,* and mental illness *odjak* (Ozturk, 1964; Sari, 1981).

The *yatir* (laying one) is like an *odjak* place except it is the tomb of a spiritually gifted *hodja.* Many villages have their own *yatirs.* The villagers have the belief that the buried *hodja* has the power to cure illness. When the *yatir* is visited there may be prayer and animal sacrifice. Rituals similar to those which may be performed at an *odjak* may also be performed at the *yatir.*

Karaca Ahmet Tekke, a famous spiritual leader who lived in the fourteenth century, had a special importance in the literature of the folk treatment of mental illness in Turkey. There are various holy places in Turkey bearing his name. In these holy places healing procedures are similar to those in the Aesculapian temples in ancient Anatolia, including careful selection of the patients, bathing in holy water, sleeping in a holy place, staying at that place for a period of time, and special dietary regimens (Sari, 1981; Bayat, 1989).

In Turkey there is a long history of humane treatment of the mentally ill, unlike the treatment to which such people were subjected in medieval Europe. Community attitudes toward the mentally ill have always been supportive.

PREVALENCE OF MENTAL ILLNESS

In Turkey, the university and state hospitals use ICD-9 (WHO, 1978) or DSM-III-R (APA, 1987) as the major diagnostic systems.

For hospital patient statistics, ICD-9 is widely used. Between 1980 and 1986 2 percent of all hospital beds were occupied by psychiatric inpatients. Between 1959 and 1962, 1586 inpatients of a medical school psychiatric clinic in Ankara were investigated. Approximately two-thirds of the patients had psychotic disorders and one-third had neurotic disorders. Amongst the psychotic and neurotic groups schizophrenia and anxiety were the leading diagnoses respectively. Thirty-one percent of patients were female and 57 percent were between the ages of 20 to 39 years (A. K. Ozbek, 1962). Between 1961 and 1974, schizophrenia accounted for between 20 and 60 percent of all inpatients in various psychiatric hospitals in Turkey (Kuey, Ustun, and Gulec, 1987).

SCHIZOPHRENIA

Schizophrenia is the most common diagnosis amongst inpatients of the Istanbul Bakirkoy Mental Hospital, the most common subtype being paranoid schizophrenia. Delusional content covers the full spectrum from religious to bizarre delusions. In a study of Turkish-born people living in foreign countries and diagnosed as suffering from schizophrenia, the most common delusions were delusions of persecution, reference, jealousy, grandeur, and religious delusions (Tuncer, Sener, Oral, and Karamustafalioglu, 1987). Differences have been identified in the symptom patterns exhibited by urban and rural patients with schizophrenia. Urban patients were more frequently anxious, tense, rigid, perseverating, and depersonalized than rural patients. Rural patients manifested more frequent behavioral outbursts, pressured thought, depressed mood, and somatic concerns than urban ones. Rural patients were often withdrawn, disoriented, confused, or delirious and more frequently exhibited deficiency in communication than urban patients. Concerning the rural schizophrenics, flight of ideas and lapses of consciousness were more frequent than amongst city dwellers (Chu, Lee, Sallach, Cetingok, and Klein, 1986). Klein, Person, Cetingok, and Itil (1978) compared the attitudes of families of Turkish schizophrenics with those of American schizophrenics in Missouri. It was reported that in Missouri, patients' families were less willing to take patients home from the hospital and more ready to initiate readmission, whereas in Turkey, families were very keen to have patients discharged from hospital, leading to difficulties keeping patients in inpatient treatment for a sufficient period. Family and patients pressed for discharge as soon as even a slight improvement was achieved.

Reviewing the past thirty years, many studies showed that therapeutic dose ranges of various psychotropic drugs vary among different groups, with European patients generally receiving lower dosages of neuroleptics than comparable American patients (Keh-Ming, Poland, and Lesser, 1986). Patients from non-Western countries, including Turkey, were clinically improved at a much lower dosage level of neuroleptics as compared to Americans and Europeans (Itil, 1975).

DEPRESSION

The prevalence rate of depressive symptoms is 20 percent and of clinical depression 10 percent. The risk factors associated with depression are being over 40 years of age, female, widowed, nuclear family, and low socioeconomic status (Kuey and Gulec, 1989). A comparative study in Istanbul revealed that elderly people living in nursing homes manifested depressive symptoms more frequently than the elderly who lived with their families (Eker, 1982).

In Turkish patients, depression is more likely than in Western patients to present with somatic symptoms (Basoglu, 1984). Depression and simple forms of schizophrenia are less likely to be regarded as illness, and more likely to be dealt with by traditional nonmedical means of support such as advice from religious people and from family members. In urban areas the medical approach is more widely accepted than in rural areas (Savasir, 1969). In those who are depressed, suicidal thoughts are common (40%) (Gogus, 1984). Turkey has a low suicide rate (2–2.5 per 100,000) (Fidaner and Fidaner, 1988) as compared with Hungary (45/100,000), Denmark (32/100,000), Greece (3/100,000), and Britain and Holland (10/100,000) (WHO, 1982). Suicide is more common in those who are over 35 years old, males (particularly those who are divorced or widowed), and more common in un-married, divorced, or widowed women than in married women.

The low suicide rate may be related to the fact that Turkey is a Muslim country. Islamic teachings regard suicide as sinful. In 1986 the prescription of benzodiazipines and also some other anxiolytic drugs was restricted and only available by special prescription. This regulation is thought to have reduced the male suicidal rate (Fidaner and Fidaner, 1988).

ALCOHOL AND DRUG ADDICTION

The traditional alcoholic beverage in Turkey is the spirit *raki* (*aslan sütü*: lion's milk); however, the consumption of beer is increasing. Amongst 3236 alcoholic patients studied at the Istanbul Bakirkoy Mental Hospital, Alcohol and Substance Treatment and Research Centre during 1985 and 1987, the initial drink was *raki* in 39.3 percent, beer in 36.3 percent, and wine in 10.8 percent. Age at which drinking commenced was 54.3 percent between 15 and 20 years; 57.9 percent commenced drinking at home and in the context of family functions, such as home, picnics and weddings; 54.5 percent ceased drinking during Ramadan and other religious days (Tuncer and Karamustafalioglu, 1989). In Western societies men have a three to four times greater rate of alcoholism than women (Donovan, 1986). In the Turkish sample alcoholism is almost thirty times as common in males as in females, with 96.7 percent of alcoholics being male (Tuncer et al., 1989).

Cannabis is by far the most widely abused substance (40.2%), amongst the drug addicts (Karamustafalioglu, Tuncer, and Beyazyurek, 1989; Tuncer, Ersul, Beyazyurek, and Karamustafalioglu, 1987).

SOMATIZATION

Kuey, Ustun, and Gulec (1987) reported that somatoform disorders and neurosis were more frequently diagnosed in females and psychosis, alcoholism and drug addiction, and personality disorders were commonly diagnosed in male patients. Somatization and conversion disorders are relatively frequent in the female population (Koptagel-Ilal, Tuncer, and Ozer, 1981; Ozturk, 1987), as in some other Mediterranean countries (Van Moffaert and Vereecken, 1989). In Van Moffaert and Vereecken's overview (1989), it was reported that amongst female Mediterranean patients feelings of anxiety are generally expressed as somatic symptoms, commonly heart palpitations. In an Istanbul study of social factors in somatic symptomatology, it was found that palpitations and headache were more prominent in female than in male patients (12.7% and 9.3% respectively) (Koptagel-Ilal, Tuncer, and Ozer, 1981). The overt, exaggerated clinical findings may falsely cause the diagnosis of histrionic disorder (Van Moffaert and Vereecken, 1989). It is also known that these types of exaggerated responses may be seen in Arabic cultures (El-Islam, 1982).

ORGANIZATION OF MENTAL HEALTH SERVICES IN TURKEY

The university hospitals, mental hospitals, and general state hospitals are the main facilities provided and funded by the state for psychiatry service. Only some of these twenty-two university hospitals have outpatient psychiatric units, and this is also true for some state general hospitals (Coskun, 1987). There are three private psychiatric hospitals in Istanbul which generally provide psychogeriatric units as well. Mental hospitals, such as Bakirkoy Mental Hospital in Istanbul, have local community mental health units (Ruh Sagligi Dispanserleri), staffed by psychiatrists, psychologists, psychiatric nurses, social workers, and sometimes occupational therapists. They may also provide family visits. Also as part of a mental hospital activity "day hospital" (caring for the outpatients especially for rehabilitation during the day), occupational therapy facilities are available.

Alcoholics and drug addicts are generally treated at the divisions of psychiatric clinics. The Alcohol, Drug Addiction Research and Treatment Centre was established in 1983 as a separate unit at the Istanbul Bakirkoy Mental Hospital campus.

The full range of somatic and psychotherapeutic treatment

modalities is widely available in Turkey. Patients from rural areas frequently regard injections as having greater therapeutic efficacy than tablets. Psychotherapy is not readily accepted by the more traditional, and is sometimes regarded as "just talking." These features are similar to those seen in Arabic culture (El-Islam, 1982). Amongst the psychotherapeutic approaches, behavior therapy, group therapy, and psychodrama are especially becoming popular amongst the new generation of psychiatrists. Even though patients from time to time seek treatment from *hodjas*, these kinds of treatments are regarded as illegal. Concerning the alcoholic population, there are also Alcoholics Anonymous groups available.

REFERENCES

Adasal, R. (1969), Klinik Psikiyatri (Clinic Psychiatry). Ruh Hastaliklari, Ankara Universitesi Yayinlarindan, Ankara.

American Psychiatric Association (1987), *Diagnostic and Statistical Manual of Mental Disorders*, 3rd ed. rev. (DSM-III-R). Washington, DC: American Psychiatric Press.

Basoglu, M. (1984), Symptomatology of depressive disorder in Turkey. A factor-analytic study of 100 depressed patients. *J. Affect. Disord.*, 6:317–330.

Bayat, A. H. (1989), Turk dunyasinda ozellikle Anadolu tibbi Folklorunda akil hastaliklarinin tedavi yollari ve kaynaklari (Forms of treatment in mental illness and their origins in Turkish world especially in Anatolian medical folklore). In: *Turk Halk Hekimligi Sempozyumu Bildirileri*, Ankara Universitesi Basimevi, Ankara.

Chu, C. C., Lee, A. Y., Sallach, H. S., Cetingok, M., & Klein, H. E. (1986), Symptom differences between urban and rural schizophrenics in Turkey. *Internat. J. Soc. Psychiat.*, 32:65–71.

Coskun, B. (1987), Turkiyede ruh sagligi hizmetleriyle ilgili varolan kaynaklar, bu konudaki guclukler-ve cozum yollari (Current sources associated with mental health services in Turkey and their difficulties, ways of solutions). *Toplum ve Hekim*, 4:11–15.

Dionisopoulos-Mass, R. (1976), Greece. The evil eye and bewitchment in a peasant village. In: *The Evil Eye*, ed. C. Maloney. New York: Columbia University Press.

Donovan, J. M. (1986), An etiologic model of alcoholism. *Amer. J. Psychiat.*, 143:1–11.

Eker, E. (1982), Senil demans hastalarinda depresif semptomlarin objektif ve subjektif olculmesi ve kurumlarda yasayan yaslilarin temel duzey depresyon durumlari ile karsilastirilmasi (Measurement of depressive symptoms objectively and subjectively, their comparison with the basic-level depression status in the elderly living in nursing homes). Dissertation for associate professorship, Istanbul Universitesi Cerrahpasa Tip Fakultesi, Istanbul.

El-Islam, M. F. (1982), Arabic cultural psychiatry. *Transcult. Psychiat. Res. Rev.*, 19:5–24.

Fidaner, H., & Fidaner, C. (1988), *Intihar Yazilari* (Papers on Suicide). Ankara.

Gogus, A. K. (1984), *The Prevalence of Suicidal Thoughts and Behaviour in a Population of Psychiatric Outpatients.* Unpublished doctoral dissertation. Ankara University, Ankara, Turkey.

Gruner, O. C. (1930), *A Treatise on the Canon of Medicine of Avicenna,* spec. ed. Birmingham, AL: The Classics of Medicine Library, 1984.

Guvenc, O. (1986), Turklerde ve dunyada Muzikle ruhi tedavinin tarihcesi ve gunumuzdeki durumu (History of music therapy in Turkey and the world, its current status). *Symposium* No. 2–3.

Itil, T. M. (1975), Transcultural psychopharmacology from the EEG point of view. In: *Transcultural Neuropsychopharmacology,* ed. T. M. Itil. Istanbul: Bozak.

Karamustafalioglu, O., Tuncer, C., & Beyazyurek, M. (1989), Psychosocial factors influencing drug addiction. Paper presented at Symposium on Psychiatry Today: Accomplishments and Promises. *VII World Congress of Psychiatry Abstracts,* ed. C. N. Stefanis, C. R. Soldatos, & A. D. Rabavilas. Excerpta Medica International Congress Series. Amsterdam: Elsevier Science Publishers.

Keh-ming, L., Poland, R. E., & Lesser, I. M. (1986), Ethnicity and pharmacology. *Cult., Med., & Psychiat.,* 10:151–165.

Klein, H. E., Person, T. M., Cetingok, M., & Itil, T. M. (1978), Family and community variables in adjustment of Turkish and Missouri schizophrenics. *Comprehen. Psychiat.,* 19:233–240.

Koptagel, G. (1971), Rehabilitation of the mentally handicapped in Turkey. Past and present. *Soc. Sci. & Med.,* 5:603–606.

Koptagel-Ilal, G., & Kazancigil, A. (1981), Historical background of scientific thinking and the concept of psychosomatic medicine in the Middle East. In: *Proceedings of the 13th Conference on Psychosomatic Research,* ed. G. Koptagel-Ilal & O. Tuncer. Istanbul: Bozak basimevi.

———— Tuncer, C., & Ozer, C. (1981), Effects of social environment on psychosomatic symptomatology in a transitional society. In: *Proceedings of the 13th Conference on Psychosomatic Research*, ed. G. Koptagel-Ilal & O. Tuncer. Istanbul: Bozak basimevi.

Kuey, L., & Gulec, C. (1989), Depression in Turkey in the 1980's: Epidemiological and clinical approaches. *Clin. Neuropharmacol.*, 2 Supp. SI–SII.

———— Ustun, T. B., & Gulec, C. (1987), Turkiyede ruhsal bozukluklar epidemiyolojisi arastirmalari uzerine bir gozden gecirme calismasi (Overview on epidemiological studies of mental disorders in Turkey). *Toplum ve Hekim*, 44:16–30.

Osler, W. (1921), *The Evolution of Modern Medicine*. New Haven, CT: Yale University Press.

Ozbek, A. K. (1962), Uc sene icinde klinigimize yatan psikoz-ve psikonevroz vakalarinda cinsiyet hastalik taksimi bolgelere gore-dagilis meslek ve yas fakforlerinin rolu. Ihtisas tezi (Distribution of sex, disorder, regions and effects of profession and age over the inpatients of psychoses and neuroses of our clinic). Ankara Universitesi Psikiatri Klinigi Ankara.

Ozturk, O. M. (1964), Folk treatment of mental illness in Turkey. In: *Magic, Faith and Healing*, ed. A. Kiev. New York: Free Press of Glencoe.

———— (1987), Turkiyede Ruh Sagligi Sorunlarina genel bir bakis (A general overview of mental health problems in Turkey). *Toplum Hekim*, 44:5–10.

———— & Volkan, V. D. (1971), The theory and practice of psychiatry in Turkey. *Amer. J. Psychother.*, 25:240–271.

Ozturk, Y. N. (1988), *The Eye of the Heart*. Istanbul: Redhouse Press.

Sari, N. (1981), Halk hekimliginde ve Osmanli-Tip Yazmalarinda akil ve sinir hastaliklarinin tedavisi (Treatment of mental and neurological disorders in folk medicine and Ottoman medical literature). *Symposium*, 3:72–84.

Savasir, Y. (1969), *Research on the Attitudes and Beliefs Towards Mental Disorders and Patients*. Dissertation for associate professorship in psychiatry. Hacettepe University, Ankara.

Songar, A. (1980), *Psikiyatri-Psikobijoloji ve Ruh hastaliklari* (Psychiatry, Psychobiology and Mental Disorders). Istanbul: Serhat Yayinevi.

Spooner, B. (1976), Arabs and Iran. The evil eye in the Middle East. In: *The Evil Eye*, ed. C. Maloney. New York: Columbia University Press.

Tuncer, C., Sener, A. I., Oral, T., & Karamustafalioglu, O. (1987), Yurtdisinda Psikiyatrik bozukluk gosteren vakalarin incelenmesi (Investigation of cases manifesting psychiatric disturbances in foreign countries). In: *Proceedings of XXIII. National Psychiatry and Neurological Sciences Congress, Bakirkoy Mental and Neurological Diseases Hospital,* Istanbul, September 14–18.

———— Ersul, C., Beyazyurek, M., & Karamustafalioglu, O. (1987), Madde bagimlisi hastalarda bir demografik calisma (Demographic study of drug addicts). In: *Proceedings of XXIII. National Psychiatry and Neurological Sciences Congress, Bakirkoy Mental and Neurological Diseases Hospital,* Istanbul, September 14–18.

———— Karamustafalioglu, O. (1989), Cultural study of drinking patterns in alcoholics. In: *Psychiatry Today: Accomplishments and Promises. VII World Congress of Psychiatry.* Abstracts, ed. C. N. Stefanis, C. R. Soldatos, & A. D. Rabavilas. Excerpta Medica International Congress Series. Amsterdam: Elsevier Science Publishers.

Unver, A. S. (1943), *Tip tarihi* (History of Medicine). Istanbul Universitesi, Yayinlari, Istanbul.

Van Moffaert, M., & Vereecken, A. (1989), Somatization of psychiatric illness in Mediterranean migrants in Belgium. *Cult., Med. & Psychiatry,* 13:297–313.

Volkan, V. D. (1975), Turkey. In: *World History of Psychiatry,* ed. J. G. Howells. New York: Brunner-Mazel.

World Health Organization (1978), *Mental Disorders: Glossary and Guide to Their Classification in Accordance with the Ninth Revision of the International Classification of Diseases* (ICD-9). Geneva: World Health Organization.

———— Working Group (1982), *Changing Pattern in Suicide Behaviour. Euro Reports and Studies No. 74.* Copenhagen.

PART IV

Australia, Latin America, and South Pacific

12.

Psychiatry in Multicultural Australia

Iraklis Harry Minas

Australia is the largest island continent and also the most sparsely populated, with a population density of 2.1 persons per square kilometer. It is a highly urbanized society, with 85 percent of the population living in urban centers, most people being concentrated in the major cities of the eastern seaboard—Melbourne, Sydney, and Brisbane (Tan and Lipton, 1988). Australia is a federation with three tiers of government, federal, state, and local. Public responsibility for health care is divided between the Commonwealth and state governments, which have varying responsibilities for the funding and provision of services (Davis and George, 1988).

Australian dominant culture is firmly rooted in British traditions and institutions, with American influence being of increasing importance in the post-World War II period. Several core cultural values, shared with other "Anglo" societies, are worthy of mention since they are not core values of an increasing proportion of the population and are relevant to any consideration of health, illness, and health service planning and delivery. These include an emphasis on individualism, a time orientation which focuses on the future, a profound conviction that, given sufficient knowledge and enterprise, nature can be both understood and subjected to man's will, an emphasis on activity in the face of difficulties, and a positivist orientation to the nature and sources of knowledge. Such values are often so deeply imbedded in the frame of reference of health service planners and clinicians that they are taken for granted and their relevance to a particular patient or to Aboriginal or immigrant communities is not questioned. That such values are cultural products, and that they are not values necessarily shared by all, still comes as something of a surprise to many involved in the planning and delivery of health services.

Another central Australian cultural value is what is locally referred to as "a fair go," the widely expressed belief that fairness is an essential characteristic in human interaction. This value is reflected in Australia's democratic traditions, in its relative lack of rigid class distinctions which allows considerable social mobility, and in its capacity to accommodate people from virtually every corner of the globe in great numbers and over a relatively short period of time, with very little social disruption. Although the children of immigrants have fared well in the Australian education system and labor market, unfamiliarity with Australian processes and practices, lack of English language proficiency, cultural difference, and prejudice continue to be associated with social disadvantage (Office of Multicultural Affairs, 1989). In relation to minority communities, especially the Aboriginal communities, the belief that everybody is entitled to a fair go is, unfortunately, more honored in the breach than in the observance. The national policy of multiculturalism seeks to provide a framework whereby maintenance of cultural traditions, beliefs, and practices by minority communities does not preclude equal treatment in education, work, and human services such as health services.

In relation to other areas of health, mental health has low priority, both in terms of funding of services and in funding of research. Beginning not long after the establishment of the first lunatic asylum in the early 1800s, there has been a cycle of public scandals arising out of the neglect of the mentally ill, followed by judicial and other inquiries, brief flurries of interest and reform, followed again by longer periods of neglect. The last several years have seen psychiatric scandals in almost every state, with inquiries in the three most populous states in the last few years. The most important of these is the inquiry currently being conducted by the Human Rights and Equal Opportunity Commission into the human rights of people with mental illness. We are currently in the midst of a period of enthusiasm for reform, a situation which provides important opportunities for improving mental health services. One important change which is undoubtedly occurring is a shift away from a monocultural health system to one which is beginning to recognize the cultural and linguistic diversity of the population and to acknowledge that it is the responsibility of the health system to attend appropriately to the diverse mental health needs of such a population. This is in the context of a significant change in Australian culture from a society which generally regarded cultural, linguistic, and racial diversity as a threat to Australian values and institutions to one where such pluralism is beginning to be seen as both desirable and as a national asset. This cultural shift, most clearly articulated in Australia's national policy of multiculturalism, is beginning to find its way into more specific areas, such as state and national mental health policies and educational programs.

PREVALENCE OF PSYCHIATRIC DISORDERS AND AN OVERVIEW OF PSYCHIATRIC SERVICES

The prevalence of the common psychiatric disorders in the general Australian community is within the ranges reported from different sites of the United States Epidemiologic Catchment Area Studies (Andrews, 1991). The most commonly used classification system in clinical practice is DSM-III-R (APA, 1987), although all official statistics are collected using ICD-9 (APA, 1987). There are seventy-four psychiatric beds and ten psychiatrists per 100,000 population (Andrews, 1991), with the numbers of beds varying considerably across states and across urban and rural centers. Patients of state services are characterized by socioeconomic disadvantage, with more than half on pensions, unemployment, or other social security benefits. Although most admissions are to state inpatient units, 77 percent of psychiatric consultations occur in a private setting, with 23 percent occurring in public hospitals or clinics (Andrews and Hadzi-Pavlovic, 1988). Two-thirds of psychiatrists are in predominantly private practice and one-third in predominantly public practice, while many work in both public and private settings. Private psychiatric practice is largely publicly funded through the Medicare system, which is a universal health insurance program, funded by a levy on taxable income. In any one year, approximately 1 percent of the population consults a private psychiatrist, and approximately 14 percent of general practitioner consultations are attributable to mental illness (Jorm and Henderson, 1989).

CULTURAL AND LINGUISTIC MINORITIES

Australian Immigration

Aboriginal communities have occupied the Australian continent for tens of thousands of years and now constitute 1 percent of the population. Apart from the original inhabitants, Australia is a nation of immigrants and the descendants of immigrants. Although its institutions are of British origin, and most of the population is of British descent, its people have come from over 100 different countries, speaking nearly as many languages. Since the 1940s the population has doubled, from 7.6 million in 1947 to 17 million in 1991, with over 40 percent of this increase directly due to immigration (Castles, 1989). The proportion of the population born in non-English speaking countries has increased considerably during this period. In 1947 90.2 percent of the population was Australian-born, with 7.9 percent having migrated from English-speaking countries and 1.9 percent from non-English speaking countries. In 1986 the corresponding figures were 79.2, 9.2, and 11.6 percent. The countries from which immigrants have come have changed further over the past couple of decades, with an increasing proportion coming from non-English speaking countries, particularly from Asia (Betts, 1988).

Mental Health of Aboriginal Communities

In considering the mental health status and mental health service needs of Aboriginal communities it is essential to have some understanding of the history of 200 years of contact between Aboriginals and Europeans which "was catastrophic for the Aborigines.

They were dispossessed of their land by disease and by violence, the authority of their elders collapsed, together with the cultural practices that had sustained them for at least 30,000 years" (Kamien, 1978, p. 44, cited in Reser, 1991). It is also necessary to be aware of the serious social and economic disadvantages which currently apply to these communities. The average life expectancy for Aboriginal people is approximately twenty years less than that of other Australians; infant mortality is three times the Australian average; unemployment rates are approximately six times the national average; and average income approximately half that of other Australians. A large proportion of Aboriginal families live in substandard accommodation and imprisonment rates are approximately twenty times those of other Australians. Aboriginal people suffer substantially higher rates of "life-style" (e.g., diabetes) and communicable diseases (Humes, 1991).

Recent studies of psychiatric morbidity amongst adults attending Aboriginal primary care health services in Melbourne and Sydney (McKendrick, 1987, 1988; Aboriginal Medical Service Co-operative, 1991), demonstrated substantially higher prevalence of psychiatric disorder and psychological morbidity than in the general Australian population. A number of socioeconomic variables were associated with increased risk of morbidity, including low socioeconomic status, a high degree of geographic mobility, lack of social supports, unemployment, and adverse childhood experiences. The particular features of childhood history that were most important were a history of separation from biological parents, neglect, and institutionalization. It should be noted that it was still common practice until the 1960s to remove Aboriginal children from their families and place them with white foster families or in institutions. In an analysis of inpatient and outpatient referrals seen by the Victorian Aboriginal Mental Health Network (see below) 44 percent of outpatients and 56 percent of inpatients had been brought up in institutions or in non-Aboriginal foster homes (McKendrick, Thorpe, Cutter, Austin, Roberts, Duke, and Chiu, 1990). The authors of the report of the Sydney study concluded that "mental health problems are a common problem among urban Aboriginal patients attending primary health care practitioners and a large number of these problems are associated with reality factors—with inescapably difficult life situations" (Aboriginal Medical Service Co-operative, 1991, p. 29).

With some notable exceptions, the quality of the epidemiological data concerning Aboriginal mental health is generally poor.

> Twenty-five years of ethnopsychiatric research has not resulted in an accurate or valid picture of the nature or incidence of Aboriginal mental health problems, or a genuine understanding of the constituent features of positive mental health. . . . [However] the situation at the beginning of the 1990s is very different: there exists a more helpful and available cross-cultural mental health literature; there are many social scientists as well as medical professionals working in the general area of indigenous mental health; and Aboriginal communities are both increasingly concerned about mental health issues and committed to finding solutions to community-defined health problems. This augurs well for what will hopefully be a spectrum of community-based mental health initiatives in many Aboriginal communities. . . . The contemporary picture is emphatically not one, however, of a destroyed Aboriginal culture, of a "sick" society which somehow cannot take "advantage" of acculturation and "development" opportunities. Aboriginal culture is alive, dynamic, and pervasive throughout remote and urban Australia. . . . Aboriginal culture is the change agent operating in Aboriginal communities, it informs and makes sense out of the present, it provides continuity to the past, it bonds people and communities, and, as a frame of reference and provider of identity, it is a powerful adaptive and therapeutic force [Reser, 1991, pp. 277–279].

Mental Health of Immigrant Communities

Data from the Australian Health Survey (Australian Bureau of Statistics, 1986) suggest that the point prevalence of mental disorders is substantially higher in many (although not all) non-English speaking background (NESB) immigrant communities than in the Australian-born and than in English speaking background

(ESB) immigrants. The point prevalence of mental disorders per 10,000 population amongst the largest country-of-birth groups was as follows: Australia 35.7; United Kingdom and Ireland 32.3; Italy 67.8; Greece 57.3; Yugoslavia 65.9; other European 55.6; Asia 28.0. Earlier work by Krupinski and his colleagues (Jayasuriya, Sang, and Fielding, 1992) demonstrates that overall prevalence is very variable across country-of-birth groups and also that the diagnostic distribution of disorders varies widely across immigrant communities.

Burvill, McCall, Stenhouse, and Reid (1973) reported that, overall, immigrants had slightly higher mean standardized suicide rates than the Australian-born. In a more recent study of suicide in New South Wales (NSW Bureau of Crime Statistics and Research, 1990) the rates of suicide per 10,000 population for some of the largest country-of-birth groups were as follows: Australia 1.14; England 1.04; Italy 1.50; Yugoslavia 4.41; Vietnam 2.06. The countries of birth of immigrant groups with high suicide rates were the same as those countries where the native populations also have high rates, and immigrant groups with rates lower than the Australian-born came from countries with low suicide rates, suggesting that enduring cultural patterns may play a greater role in determining suicide rates than the stresses associated with immigrant status.

Extensive work done at the Victorian Mental Health Research Institute by Krupinski and colleagues in the 1960s and 1970s demonstrated increased prevalence of major mental disorders amongst the post-war Eastern European refugees (then referred to as Displaced Persons) who settled in Australia (Jayasuriya et al., 1992). From a large prospective follow-up study of young Indochinese refugees carried out in Melbourne (Krupinski and Burrows, 1986) it was reported that the prevalence of psychiatric disorder at initial assessment was approximately twice that of a comparable (age and sex) Australian group. At two-year follow-up, the prevalence had declined to approximately half that of the Australian-born population. This finding needs to be seen in the context of a study of consecutive referrals of Vietnamese patients to a bilingual outpatient service (Klimidis, Lien, and Minas, 1991) which reported that the mean duration of residence in Australia prior to onset of psychiatric disorder was approximately four years. This is in accord with the earlier work referred to with Eastern European refugees which showed that the peak incidence of mental disorder was a number of years after arrival (Jayasuriya et al., 1992).

Work focusing on patterns of service use of state psychiatric services in Victoria shows that, in general, immigrant communities substantially underutilize mental health services, despite the probably greater prevalence of disorders in those communities (Minas, 1991a). Similar findings have been reported from New South Wales (McDonald, 1991). The rate of underutilization of community mental health services is even greater than that for inpatient hospital services (Minas, 1991a). It is necessary to add the caveat that the patterns of utilization are quite complex, and that general statements about immigrants, rather than about specific subgroups, may be quite misleading. For example, underutilization is generally most marked in the smaller, more recently arrived, and more culturally distinct communities, whereas a number of communities, such as the Yugoslav, German, and Polish, utilize inpatient and community services at rates greater than that of the Australian-born.

NESB immigrants are significantly more likely to be admitted as involuntary patients than are the Australian-born or patients from English speaking countries, there is more likely to be police involvement in the admission of NESB patients than in the Australian-born or in the ESB communities, and there is a lower rate of self-referral in the NESB group (Minas, 1991a). There are significant differences in the diagnostic distributions of Australian-born, ESB, and NESB inpatients, with a higher rate of psychosis diagnosed in the NESB group as compared with the ESB and Australian-born groups. This does not mean, of course, that the prevalence of psychosis is necessarily higher in NESB people in general. It may merely indicate that NESB patients with nonpsychotic disorders are, for a number of reasons, less likely to be admitted to a psychiatric hospital than are such Australian-born and ESB patients.

Australia is experiencing a rapid increase in both the absolute numbers of elderly people and in the proportion of the population which the elderly constitute. Although the total Australian population is expected to grow by 24 percent between the years 1986 and 2006, the population aged 65 and over is expected to increase by 44 percent, with the numbers of those over 75 years increasing at an even more rapid rate (Ames, 1991). The increase in the proportion of elderly people in ethnic communities is occurring at three times the rate of that in the Australian-born. In some communities, such as the Greek, Italian, Hungarian, and those from the Baltic states, over 30 percent of the people will be over age 65 by the year 2000. This situation will present particular challenges for mental health services. There are very few studies of the prevalence of mental disorders in elderly immigrants. In one such study of elderly Italian immigrants (Chiu, Berah, and McKenzie, 1989) 35 percent of the sample had case levels of psychiatric disorder, a level higher than that for the Australian community. This is consistent with evidence that social factors, such as generally smaller social networks and lower incomes, result in increased vulnerability to the development of psychiatric disorders amongst the ethnic aged (McCallum and Shadbolt, 1989).

There have been very few studies of treatment approaches, and outcomes of psychiatric treatment, in immigrants. In a study of rates of electroconvulsive treatment (ECT) of 474 consecutively admitted general hospital psychiatric inpatients (Minas, 1983) it was found that NESB immigrants were treated with ECT at substantially higher rates than either the Australian-born or ESB immigrants. Amongst the possible explanations for these findings are the following: (1) NESB immigrants may be admitted to hospital later in the illness episode and with more severe illness; (2) it may be only those with the most severe illness who accept psychiatric hospitalization; (3) language and cultural differences, and differences in illness expression, may lead to misinterpretation of the nature and the severity of illness; (4) the lack of a common language between patient and clinician generally precludes the effective use of psychological therapies and promotes a reliance on drugs and other physical treatments, such as ECT. In a study of the drug treatment of Turkish patients prior to their referral to a Turkish-speaking psychiatrist (Minas, Szmukler, Demirsar, and Eisenbruch, 1988) it was found that drug treatment was common, regardless of diagnosis, and that there was a poor match between diagnostic category and the classes of drugs which patients were receiving, suggesting that treatment with inappropriate classes of drugs was not uncommon.

Next to nothing is known about the quality of treatment outcomes for those members of NESB communities who come into contact with mental health services. One might expect, however, that outcomes for non-English speaking patients would be worse than for others, since the range of treatment modalities which are essentially language-based (such as the psychotherapies, family therapy, rehabilitation programs, and so on) are not generally available to this group of patients. A further issue of relevance here is the nature of the cross-cultural clinical process itself. Even when the patient and clinician speak the same language and are from the same cultural background, inadequate clinical communication may occur, leading to problems in the diagnostic and treatment process. This is much more likely to occur when patient and doctor do not speak the same language, come from different cultural backgrounds, and bring to the clinical encounter radically different conceptions concerning the nature of health and illness and what constitutes an appropriate response in the presence of illness. Such discrepancies may lead to inaccurate diagnosis, inappropriate and even harmful or dangerous treatment.

There is, particularly in the large cities where most immigrants settle, a profusion of practitioners of traditional healing arts from virtually all the great religions and many of the world's cultures. Immigrants who seek the assistance of traditional practitioners in dealing with illness most often also attend orthodox Western practitioners at the same time. Beyond this anecdotally based information there is very little known about the types of traditional healers, their practices, the frequency with which immigrants seek their services, and so on. Such practitioners and their practices in Australia have not been systematically studied. There have been no attempts, as have occurred in other places around the world, to establish a dialogue between orthodox and traditional practitioners. The one exception is the interest by anthropologists and psychiatrists in Aboriginal traditional healers who have, from time to time, been invited to assist in the treatment of Aboriginal patients. This has been more likely to occur in remote rather than in urban areas.

RESPONSES TO DIVERSITY

Education of Health Professionals

Although there has been some improvement in recent years in the education of health professionals in the cultural aspects of psychiatric assessment and treatment, mental health professionals are generally ill-prepared by their training for working sensitively and effectively with people who speak little English and who come from a culture which has values and beliefs different to those of the host culture (Tham, Klimidis, and Minas, 1991). This is amongst the most important areas for change if inequalities in standards of mental health care are to be reduced. The number of NESB students in health-related university courses has increased gradually over the past couple of decades. Approximately 60 percent of currently enrolled first-year medical students in Australian universities have at least one parent born in a non-English speaking country. This change will have a long-term effect on the profile of the health professions in Australia, more accurately reflecting the cultural diversity of the Australian population. Approaches are required which will capitalize on the linguistic and cultural knowledge of these students, and which will more adequately prepare them for work in a diverse society.

Psychiatric Services Policies

In recent years, there has been increasing recognition by governments that non-English speaking communities have specific health needs, and that these needs have largely been ignored in the past. This recognition is increasingly finding its way into federal and state mental health policy statements (e.g., Office of Psychiatric Services, 1992), which charge mental health agencies with the responsibility of recognizing and appropriately responding to the specific mental health needs of cultural and linguistic minorities, and outline strategies whereby this may be achieved. Such policy developments represent the beginnings of major change in the culture of the mental health service system, and have occurred in the context of the federal policy of multiculturalism. The challenge now is to transform such statements of intent into programs which will deliver mental health services of a comparably high quality to all citizens, regardless of racial or ethnic background, proficiency in English, or cultural affiliation. One of the major impediments to the achievement of such goals is the grossly inadequate level of research in the area of defining the mental health service needs of Aboriginal and NESB communities, in the investigation of the appropriateness and effectiveness of educational and service systems, and in the development of service models and treatment approaches which are responsive to identified mental health care needs (Minas, 1991c). Even the most cursory review of research studies carried out in Australia shows that the most common exclusion criterion for sample selection is "subjects with an inadequate knowledge of English." This is understandable given the complexities and increased research costs involved in attempting to secure a sample which is truly representative of the Australian community. However, this one research issue has the effect of perpetuating inequalities. Research results are not representative of the whole Australian community and cannot be generalized to NESB communities. What is known concerning the mental health needs and treatment responses of the majority community is almost invariably not known about NESB communities. This is particularly important in epidemiological studies, in studies of the efficacy of new treatment strategies, and in studies producing data relevant to the planning and evaluation of new service approaches. The lack of reliable and comprehensive data concerning NESB communities continues to perpetuate the situation where services informed by research findings may be appropriate to the majority community but may be entirely inappropriate to NESB communities. It also has the effect that any deficiencies in services in relation to minority communities cannot be demonstrated because, when the effectiveness of the services is evaluated, then NESB service users who do not speak adequate English are again likely to be excluded from study.

Examples of Specialist Services

A number of specialist services have been established in recent years. The Multicultural Psychiatry Centre in Perth, Western Australia, has been providing psychiatric services in a multitude of languages and conducting educational programs for almost a decade. The Victorian Transcultural Psychiatry Unit was established in 1988 by the Victorian Health Department with responsibility for contributing to the development of appropriate policies and programs for improving the quality of psychiatric services available to NESB communities (Minas, 1989). As well as carrying out direct clinical work, the Unit has developed research and teaching programs in the area of transcultural psychiatry. In its research work the Unit is combining epidemiological methods with anthropologically informed approaches to the investigation of needs and the development of programs (Minas, 1991b, 1991c). In the area of Aboriginal mental health, a number of innovative, community-based and community-controlled mental health services for Aboriginal communities have been developed in recent years. One such service is the Victorian Aboriginal Mental Health Network (McKendrick et al., 1990). Evaluation of this service has demonstrated the major positive changes which occur in patterns of service utilization when the community is integrally involved in the design, implementation, and control of a service which is appropriate to the needs of that community. In 1988 the Service for the Treatment and Rehabilitation of Trauma and Torture Survivors was established in Sydney (Reid, Silove, and Tarn, 1990). This followed the publication of a report which investigated the prevalence of past experience of torture and trauma among recently arrived refugees (Reid and Strong, 1987). It was conservatively estimated that 10 percent of refugees from countries in which torture is known to occur, and who were admitted to Australia under the Special Humanitarian program, were likely to have been subjected to torture. Subsequent experience during the development of the service suggests that the figure may be substantially higher, particularly amongst people from some countries, such as Cambodia. A service with broadly similar aims, the Victorian Foundation for Survivors of Torture, has been established in Melbourne (McGorry, 1988) and others have been established in Adelaide, Brisbane, Perth, and Hobart.

CONCLUSION

Australian mental health services are currently undergoing a period of substantial change in a number of areas. The most significant change in relation to Australia's minorities is that the culture of the mental health system (in which I include government health departments, tertiary institutions which educate mental health practitioners, research funding bodies, mental health service agencies, clinicians, and the patients and families using mental health services) has begun to change in important ways. The most fundamental of these changes are:

1. A recognition of the diversity of needs of a diverse population;
2. An acknowledgment that it is the responsibility of the system to respond appropriately and flexibly to identified needs;
3. The increasing involvement of the communities for which the services exist in the shaping of service structures and priorities; and
4. The increasing attention being paid to health promotion and illness prevention in mental health research, education, and practice.

There is reason to be hopeful that these beginnings will be built upon so that race, cultural affiliation, and lack of English proficiency cease to serve as markers for disadvantage in the area of mental health.

REFERENCES

Aboriginal Medical Service Co-operative (1991), *N.S.W. Aboriginal Mental Health Report*. Sydney, Australia: Aboriginal Medical Service Co-operative.

American Psychiatric Association (1987), *Diagnostic and Statistical Manual of Mental Disorders*, 3rd ed. rev. (DSM-III-R). Washington, DC: American Psychiatric Press.

Ames, D. (1991), Geriatric psychiatry in a culturally diverse society. In: *Cultural Diversity and Mental Health*, ed. I. H. Minas. Melbourne, Australia: RANZCP-VTPU.

Andrews, G. (1991), The Tolkien report: A description of a model mental health service. Typescript.

——— Hadzi-Pavlovic, D. (1988), The work of Australian psychiatrists, circa 1986. *Austral. & NZ J. Psychiatry*, 22:153–165.

Australian Bureau of Statistics (1986), *Australian Health Survey 1983: Illness Conditions Experienced*. Canberra: Australian Government Publishing Service.

Betts, K. (1988), *Ideology and Immigration: Australia 1976 to 1987*. Melbourne: Melbourne University Press.

Burvill, P., McCall, M. G., Stenhouse, N. S., & Reid, T. A. (1973), Deaths from suicide, motor vehicle accidents and all forms of violent deaths among migrants in Australia, 1962–66. *Acta Psychiatrica Scand.*, 49:28–50.

Castles, I. (1989), *Overseas Born Australians 1989: A Statistical Profile*. Canberra: Australian Bureau of Statistics.

Chiu, E., Berah, M., & McKenzie, A. (1989), Psychiatric morbidity in elderly Italian migrants residing in Australia. In: *Program and Abstracts of the Fourth Congress of the International Psychogeriatric Association*. Tokyo: IPGA.

Davis, A., & George, J. (1988), *States of Health: Health and Illness in Australia*. Sydney: Harper & Row.

Humes, G. (1991), Aboriginal mental health: Past neglect and present needs. In: *Cultural Diversity and Mental Health*, ed. I. H. Minas. Melbourne: RANZCP-VTPU.

Jayasuriya, L., Sang, D., & Fielding, A. (1992), *Ethnicity, Migration and Mental Illness: A Critical Overview of Australian Research*. Canberra: Australian Government Publishing Service.

Jorm, A. F., & Henderson, A. S. (1989), The use of private psychiatric services in Australia: An analysis of Medicare data. *Austral. & NZ J. Psychiatry*, 23:461–468.

Kamien, M. (1978), *The Dark People of Bourke: A Study of Planned Social Change*. Canberra: AIAS.

Klimidis, S., Lien, O., & Minas, I. H. (1991), Vietnamese presenting to a bilingual psychiatric service: Demographic and diagnostic characteristics. In: *Cultural Diversity and Mental Health*, ed. I. H. Minas. Melbourne: RANZCP-VTPU.

Krupinski, J., & Burrows, G. (1986), *The Price of Freedom: Young Indochinese Refugees in Australia.* Sydney: Pergamon Press.

McCallum, J., & Shadbolt, B. (1989), Ethnicity and stress among older Australians. *J. Gerontol. Soc. Sci.,* 44:S89–96.

McDonald, R. (1991), *New South Wales Hospitalization of NESB Migrants with Mental Disorders: A Preliminary Report.* Typescript.

McGorry, P. D. (1988), The sequelae of torture and implications for health services in Australia. In: *Mental Health of Ethnic Communities,* ed. E. Chiu & I. H. Minas. Melbourne: St. Vincent's Hospital.

McKendrick, J. (1987), *A Psychosocial Survey of an Urban Aboriginal General Practice Population.* Diploma in Psychological Medicine Thesis. University of Melbourne.

——— (1988), Psychiatric morbidity in urban aboriginal adults: A cause for concern. In: *Mental Health of Ethnic Communities,* ed. E. Chiu & I. H. Minas. Melbourne: St. Vincent's Hospital.

McKendrick, J. H., Thorpe, M., Cutter, T. N., Austin, G., Roberts, W., Duke, M., & Chiu, E. (1990), A unique mental health network for Victorian Aboriginal people. *Med. J. Australia,* 153:349–351.

Minas, I. H. (1983), The treatment of Australian-born and immigrant psychiatric disorders. *Med. J. Australia,* 1:152.

——— (1989), Facing a culturally diverse community: The Victorian Transcultural Psychiatry Unit. *RANZCP News & Notes,* 18:14–15.

——— (1990), Culture and mental health. In: *The Health of Immigrant Australia: A Social Perspective,* ed. J. Reid & P. Trompf. Sydney: Harcourt Brace Jovanovich.

——— (1991a), Mental health services for immigrant communities. Paper presented at the annual meeting of The Federation of Ethnic Community Councils of Australia, Sydney.

——— (1991b), Epidemiology and mental health services research in a multicultural society. Paper presented at the conference I Servizi di salute mentale in una societa multiculturale, Milan, Italy.

——— (1991c), Psychiatric services research in a culturally diverse society. In: *Cultural Diversity and Mental Health,* ed. I. H. Minas. Melbourne: RANZCP & VTPU.

——— Szmukler, G., Demirsar, A., & Eisenbruch, M. (1988), Turkish patients presenting to the Royal Park Ethnic Psychiatry Service, 1985–86. In: *Mental Health of Ethnic Communities,* ed. E. Chiu & I. H. Minas. Melbourne: St. Vincent's Hospital.

NSW Bureau of Crime Statistics and Research (1990), Crime and Justice Bulletin. Contemporary Issues in Crime and Justice, No. 8.

Office of Multicultural Affairs (1989), *National Agenda for a Multicultural Australia: Sharing Our Future.* Canberra: Australian Government Publishing Service.

Office of Psychiatric Services (1992), *Policy and Strategic Directions for Public Psychiatric Services in Victoria*. Melbourne: Office of Psychiatric Services, Health Department, Victoria.

Reid, J., Silove, D., & Tarn, R. (1990), The development of the New South Wales Service for the Treatment and Rehabilitation of Torture and Trauma Survivors (STARTTS): The first year. *Austral. & NZ J. Psychiatry*, 24:486–495.

———— Strong, T. (1987), *Torture and Trauma: The Health Care Needs of Refugee Victims in New South Wales*. Sydney: NSW Department of Health and Cumberland College of Health Sciences.

Reser, J. P. (1991), Aboriginal mental health: Conflicting cultural perspectives. In: *The Health of Aboriginal Australia*, ed. J. Reid & P. Trompf. Sydney: Harcourt Brace Jovanovich.

Tan, E-S., & Lipton, G. (1988), *Mental Health Services in the Western Pacific Region*. Melbourne: St. Vincent's Hospital.

Tham, G., Klimidis, S., & Minas, I. H. (1991), Psychiatric nurses: Their awareness of cultural factors in patient management. In: *Cultural Diversity and Mental Health*, ed. I. H. Minas Melbourne: RANZCP & VTPU.

13.

Cultural Factors, Religious Beliefs, and Mental Illness in Bali: Indonesia

Luh Ketut Suryani

CULTURAL BACKGROUND

Bali is a province in the Republic of Indonesia. It is a relatively small island, 5808.8 square kilometers in size. The population in 1990 was 2,777,356, which is only 1.5 percent of the total population of Indonesia, the fifth largest country in the world. Males and females are about equally represented. The chief occupation is farming.

The major religion is Hinduism which encompasses 93 percent of the population. In 1988 Suryani studied the effects of sociocultural influences from outside of Bali on Balinese culture and found that although the Balinese are exposed to many outside cultural influences, no major changes have occurred in predominant Balinese sociocultural patterns and customs. There have been some changes in social systems, such as in marriage and child rearing, but there have been few changes in socialization practices. Suryani (1988) found no changes in Balinese religious philosophy, religious rituals, in the status of male siblings within the family, or in the system of inheritance. These examples indicate that values, cultural beliefs, and practices probably have changed little. Outside sociocultural factors appear to have had little influence on Balinese traditions, or they have been adapted to them.

The Hindu religion practiced by the Balinese is unique. It originated in Java and was strongly influenced by local Balinese customs and Buddhism. Balinese Hindus believe in five principles (*panca srada*): (1) a supreme god (*Sang Hyang Widi Wasa*); (2) existence of an eternal soul (*atman*). Mental activity, including thinking, emotions, behavior, and personality are determined by the soul. All human mental and physical activities, including mental illness are functions of the soul; (3) every deed has rewards or consequences (*karma pala*), of which illness may be one; (4) reincarnation (*punarbawa*) or rebirth into the world. This is repeated until one attains the perfect life, at which point it ends because one is unified with God; and (5) eventual unity (*moksa*) with God. These principles are practiced in daily life and influence and guide constructs and practices of traditional healers.

The belief in reincarnation guides the daily life of the Balinese. The events of a person's current life are considered to be related to their previous life. The Balinese believe that what happens in the present is caused, in part and often, by deeds of one's past life. One's current life is oriented to expiate past undesirable deeds, and work toward a better future life.

It is common practice for families to take a newborn infant to a spiritual medium healer (*balian metuun*) to find out which ancestor's soul possesses the child and to discover thereby the nature of the child's personality. During this visit, the spiritual medium healer (*balian*) becomes possessed by the soul of the ancestor and tells the family what the soul needs in order to carry out its new life successfully. This might be a puppet performance or making an offering of a roasted pig to expiate a sin, or to protect against greed or a bad personality. The chief purpose of this visit is to strengthen the family's hope that the life of the infant will be a success.

BALINESE HINDU CONCEPTS OF ILLNESS

Balinese believe that three factors are highly important for well-being, happiness, and health: (1) the microcosmos (*buana alit*) which is the individual or the soul and is a manifestation of God; (2) the macrocosmos (*buana agung*) which is the universe; and (3) God (*Sang Hyang Widi Wasa*). They strive to keep these three factors in equilibrium, a concept called *tri hita karana*. This is practiced in daily living whether at home, at the market, or at the office, all of which have small temples.

Balinese Hindus believe that they will become vulnerable to illness if these three factors are not in equilibrium. Mental disorders can be caused by both natural factors (e.g., bone fracture and infection) including genetics and changes in bodily physical balance (i.e., becoming hot or cold); and by supernatural factors, for example, being under a spell. Examples of the latter include *bebai* in which an evil spirit is made by a sorcerer which receives power from God and inflicts it on someone, and witchcraft (*guna-guna*); being under the curse of ancestors; activity of the gods; having an unfavorable birth date; being assigned an unfavorable or unsuitable name; being poisoned (*cetik*) by someone; or suffering from black magic (*leak*).

Disorders classified as being caused by the supernatural are known by the general title of "Bali Illness." The Balinese continue to believe that most mental disorders are caused by spirit possession or by a curse of an ancestor or the gods. Furthermore, they consider that such disorders are curable and that patients will function normally when they recover. With this orientation, recovered patients can resume family functions similar to those that existed before they became ill. The family feels no disgrace over illnesses due to these causes. In contrast, families feel disgraced when members have the mental disorder regarded as insanity (*buduh*) because of their belief that this kind of sickness is genetic and incurable.

The concepts of diagnosis of mental illness held by families and patients change over time. Table 13.1 shows concepts of mental illness diagnosis held by 113 acutely psychotic patients and their families at first examination by psychiatrists and then one year later. Initially 12 percent believed the patient had *buduh* but after one year none believed they had *buduh*, and the number who believed they had "Bali Illness" increased considerably from 6 to 33 percent (Suryani, 1988).

TABLE 13.1

Concepts of Mental Illness Diagnosis Held by 113 Acutely Psychotic Patients and Families at First Examination by a Psychiatrist and One Year Later

Diagnosis	First Exam.		Exam. 1 year later	
	N	%	N	%
"Nervous illness"	72	64	37	33
Buduh	14	12	0	0
Mental illness	20	18	31	27
"Bali illness"	7	6	37	33
Don't know	0	0	8	7
Total	113	100	113	100

SERVICES FOR MENTAL DISORDERS

People with mental disorders in Bali are cared for by medical physicians, by traditional healers (*balian*), priests (*pemangku*), and trained high priests (*pedanda*).

There are two psychiatric hospital service centers which deal with mental disorders. The Bangli Mental Hospital has a 225-bed capacity which primarily treats chronic patients. It integrates its services with ten different medical health centers and six general hospitals throughout Bali. It employs two psychiatrists, three general medical physicians, and ninety paramedical personnel. In 1990, the Bangli Mental Hospital cared for 859 inpatients and served 3512 outpatients. The Department of Psychiatry at Wangaya General Hospital in Denpasar has a 20-bed capacity and generally treats acute patients. In 1990, the Department of Psychiatry at Wangaya Hospital cared for 421 inpatients and served 3227 outpatients (766 new patient visits and 2461 old patient visits). The unit employs five staff psychiatrists, five psychiatry residents, and one staff psychologist.

The number of *balians* in Bali is estimated at 2500, 73 percent of whom work mainly as farmers and 27 percent of whom are wholly limited to *balian* practice (Leimena and Thong, 1983). There are several types of *balians* who deal with mental disorders: (1) 45 percent are *Balian Usada*, *balians* who have learned to treat from the *lontar* (traditional Balinese teachings); (2) 10 percent are *Balian Ketakson, balians* who treat with trance; (3) 19 percent are *Balian Matuun, balians* who function as trance mediums possessed by God spirits; and (4) 25 percent are self-taught spiritualists (*kebatinan*). All *balians* tend to specialize in mental problems. Most *balians* consider their work as a type of social service rather than as a trade or commercial occupation. They generally become *balians* because of feelings of responsibility or because family members were traditionally *balians*. Balinese regard the traditional *balian* healer as able to understand and treat problems arising from supernatural causes and able to restore equilibrium of the three factors. They believe doctors are able to treat only diseases caused by natural factors. For example, if a family member has a mental disorder manifested primarily by behavioral and emotional symptoms, they usually go first to the *balian* for treatment.

A variety of complaints ranging from physical to psychological symptoms are brought to *balians* who use a variety of techniques to diagnose and treat, including the healer and/or client going into trance, white magic to counteract black magic, smoke treatment (*madusdus*), holy water, medicinal concoctions, and massage. The *balian* prays for the power to heal. Then he or she chants, blesses the offering brought by the client, and may examine and treat the patient by touch in a variety of ways. Generally the client's family members are in attendance. The *balian* may inform the client and family of the nature of the problem arising from natural or supernatural causes and may give a diagnosis such as "*Bali illness*," a disorder caused by the supernatural. The priests and high priests heal through special ceremonies such as purification (*melukat*) as well as techniques used by *balians*.

Most patients with physical and behavioral symptoms seek treatment by and are treated only by traditional healers. Most patients who manifest more severe mental illnesses, such as psychoses, however, who are not cured by traditional healers, eventually come to psychiatrists for treatment. They are either brought by their family directly or are referred by traditional healers.

Suryani (1988) found that most patients (76%) who come under the care of psychiatrists in the two public psychiatric hospitals in Bali had been seen by traditional healers before referral to psychiatrists. Eighty percent of patients and families continued to follow traditional healing rituals during psychiatric hospitalization, and contacted the healers again following discharge. Patients and families with cultural concepts of mental disorders (e.g., supernatural causes such as black magic) complied with Western psychiatric treatment, including neuroleptic medication, but after recovery maintained their cultural beliefs of illness and traditional healing practices (i.e., healing ceremonies).

In Bali, the integrated practice of psychiatry and traditional healing takes several forms: (1) The traditional healer comes into the hospital to treat the patient along with the treatment received by the psychiatrist. This has been the practice of only one psychiatrist in Bali. (2) The traditional healer refers the patient to a psychiatrist while maintaining continuity of therapy. (3) Patients in the psychiatric hospital leave the hospital temporarily to attend purification ceremonies by a traditional healer. This practice is followed at the two existing public mental hospitals in Bali. (4) The psychiatrist discusses the meaning of traditional healers' work with the patient and refers the patient to traditional healers or allows the patient to see healers while maintaining continuity of psychiatric treatment.

MENTAL DISORDERS IN BALI

The Balinese manifest a wide range of mental disorders classified in DSM-III-R (APA, 1987) and ICD-9 (WHO, 1977) with several exceptions, and there are differences in prevalence from Western data. The childhood disorders of attention deficit disorder and conduct disorders are relatively infrequent. Juvenile delinquency rates are strikingly low. So far, no cases of multiple personality disorder (MPD) have been seen in Bali. Possibly this is due to the fact that child abuse, which tends to be associated with MPD, is virtually unknown in Bali. Other disorders that have not yet been seen in Bali are bulimia, anorexia nervosa, and alcoholic psychosis. Drug abuse is rare. Major depression, phobias, obsessive compulsive disorder, and borderline personality disorder are relatively uncommon. The incidence of schizophrenia is also relatively low (Jensen and Suryani, 1992). Suicide attempts in Bali differ from Western cases in that most occur in a trance state (Suryani, 1991).

More common disorders are somatization disorder, panic disorder, generalized anxiety disorder, acute psychosis, and bipolar disorder, manic. Many of these differences in prevalence are a reflection of culture. Several culture related disorders in Bali include *amok, latah,* and the trance disorder, *bebainan.*

BEBAINAN

Bebainan is a culture-related illness which Balinese believe to be caused by the ill individual's soul being possessed by a malignant spirit called *bebai* (Suryani, 1984). The term *bebai,* which in old Balinese means evil spirit, refers to both the malignant spirit and its material representation. Most first attacks occur between the ages of 16 and 30.

Bebainan is not clearly associated with the physical state of the sufferer: most attacks had not been preceded by abnormal temperature, illness, or a severe accident causing physical discomfort. Witnesses as well as the victims generally insist that the episodes of *bebainan* almost invariably were sudden, albeit not always completely unexpected.

Several triggering conditions or events were found (Suryani, 1984): (1) *kajeng kliwon* (74%) a day which comes every fifteen days by the Balinese calendar. It is a potentially fearful time because on this day the evil spirits abound and persons with bad intentions may easily be possessed and disturb others. Persons with mental illness generally date the onset of their symptoms to that day; (2) emotional stress (70%); (3) physical exhaustion (41%); the morning after a sleepless night (33%); (4) other Balinese holidays (30%); and (5) menstruation (11%). No reason was indicated in 15 percent of the cases.

The prodromal symptoms of *bebainan* include: (1) feelings of confusion (76%); (2) a cold feeling beginning in the legs and spreading to the rest of the body (63%); (3) feeling empty, with a loss of desire or will (59%); (4) ringing in the ears (57%); (5) a feeling that the surrounding environment has gone dark (44%); (6) stomachache (37%); (7) feeling of fear upon seeing certain things (7%); (8) a feeling of stiffness in the body (4%). After experiencing these symptoms, the victims reported suddenly losing control of themselves. Some cried out, cried ceaselessly for no reason (82%); some spoke giving voice to the *bebai* that they felt possessed them (44%), while others were silent (11%) or ran *amok* (11%). Only 7 percent of the respondents were aware of the events that occurred during an attack, while the others (93%) felt themselves to be totally out of control.

In the majority of cases, *bebainan* attacks last only fifteen minutes to one hour, while some of the attacks last longer than one hour. Suryani (1984) found that after an attack, 63 percent of victims reported sleeping soundly, while the remainder reported restlessness and difficulty in sleeping. Feelings of calm after an attack were reported by 59 percent, while the remainder reported feeling anxious, a feeling of seeming to be in the clouds and emptiness, and not knowing what to do next. Only after one or two days did individuals report returning to normal functioning.

From a psychiatric standpoint, then, the most compelling characteristics of *bebainan* are its sudden onset and the temporary character of its impact. During an attack, the victim suffers a severe impairment of consciousness and sense of identity and a loss of control over motor functions. These symptoms disappear completely at the cessation of the attack. Consequently, the illness can best be considered a type of dissociative disorder. More specifically it is a manifestation of trance with possession.

ACUTE PSYCHOSIS

About 60 percent of psychiatric patients admitted to Wangaya Hospital suffer from acute psychosis. The acute psychosis disorders are important to classification because they are the predominant form of severe psychiatric disorder in developing countries. They currently fall into a confusing variety of diagnostic categories. Acute psychoses were never specifically defined or clearly conceptualized in DSM-III-R (APA, 1987) or ICD-9 (WHO, 1977).

The criteria developed for diagnosis of acute psychosis (Suryani, 1988) are: (1) acute onset (abrupt onset of psychotic symptoms with less than one week of prodromal symptoms); (2)

absence of personality disorder; (3) marked symptoms of delayed sleep and confusion or disorientation, each with at least one of the following: hallucinations (visual and auditory), delusions (persecution, control, or religious), severe psychomotor excitement (overagitation or overactivity), and lability of mood; (4) good and rapid response to neuroleptics (generally in less than one week); and (5) complete functional recovery within three months (return to normal social and occupational functioning and use of spare time). Presence of an identifiable stressor is usual but not essential, and recurrence of acute psychosis does not preclude the diagnosis.

The amount of exposure to sociocultural influences from outside Bali was correlated with symptoms. Patients who had more experience with outside influences showed greater agitation and overactivity. Patients who had less influence showed more negative symptoms such as lack of initiative, blunted affect, apathy, and weak emotional rapport.

All acute psychoses are treated immediately on admission to the hospital, beginning with low doses of neuroleptics which are increased daily if symptoms continue: haloperidol 1.5 mg up to a maximum of 10 mg/day; trifluperazine 2.5 to 15 mg per day; or chlorpromazine 100 to 900 mg per day.

Classification of the acute psychiatric disorders constitutes a problem. In ICD-9 they are included under acute schizophrenic episode, schizoaffective type, other schizophrenia, unspecified schizophrenic, schizophreniform psychosis, paranoid state unspecified, and other nonorganic psychoses (depressive type, excitative type, reactive confusion, acute paranoid reaction, psychogenic paranoid psychosis, other and unspecified reactive psychosis, and unspecified psychosis).

Suryani (1988) identified three arguments for conceptual separation of the acute from the more chronic psychoses: (1) The management of the patient is different. Most acutely psychotic patients need neuroleptics for only a short time and need supportive psychotherapy directed toward the goal of restoring adaptive abilities and capacity. Family therapy is important to help them understand the patient's problem and to deal with recurrence. Patients with longer lasting psychosis (i.e., more than three months) need longer neuroleptic treatment and also rehabilitation and education to facilitate resumption of occupational and social functioning. (2) The economics are different. Acute psychotic patients may be admitted to the hospital for only a few days and then receive medication and psychotherapy as outpatients. More chronic patients stay longer in the hospital and require more services. (3) The attitudes associated with labels make a difference. The doctor, patient, family, and employer will generally give more attention to the acute psychotic patient and will seek others to help cure the patient. Further, the family is more accepting of the patient because they think he or she will be cured. The physician will try another course of neuroleptic treatment if the patient does not respond. In Bali, patients considered to have had acute psychosis will not lose their job because they are not stigmatized. On the other hand, the Balinese believe that disorders classified in the West as schizophrenia cannot be cured and will be progressive.

PSYCHIATRIST, TRADITIONAL HEALER, AND CULTURE INTEGRATED IN CLINICAL PRACTICE IN BALI

Psychiatrists and traditional healers have vastly different premises, theories, methods, techniques, and modalities of treatment which are aimed at some of the same symptoms and problems, but also at some different ones. Integrated care by a psychiatrist and a traditional healer means that they work with the same patient in an informal agreement, each providing treatment compatible with their particular abilities, knowledge, and theory. What would appear as two modalities or treatment processes in conflict is averted by genuine belief in the validity and value of each. From the point of view of psychiatrists, this might be termed clinical acculturation in practice. To accomplish this, the psychiatrist and the traditional healer need not be in direct contact nor is it necessary for them to communicate with each other regarding their treatments (Suryani and Jensen, 1991). Each should not attempt to influence or change the other's methods and treatments. This situation is not only an ideal but has been attained in reality in the case of an epidemic of mass hysteria in schoolchildren in Bali (Jensen and Suryani, 1992).

REFERENCES

American Psychiatric Association (1987), *Diagnostic and Statistical Manual of Mental Disorders*, 3rd ed. rev. (DSM-III-R). Washington, DC: American Psychiatric Press.

Jensen, G. D., & Suryani, L. K. (1992), *The Balinese People: A Reinvestigation of Character*. Singapore: Oxford University Press.

Leimena, S. L., & Thong, D. (1983), Pengobatan Traditional di Bali. In: *Traditional Healing Practices*, ed. K. Setyonegoro & W. M. Roan. Jakarta: Directorat of Mental Health.

Suryani, L. K. (1984), Culture and mental disorder: The case of *Bebainan* in Bali. *Cult., Med. & Psychiat.*, 8:95–113.

———— (1988), *Psikosis Akut pada Orang Bali yang Beragama Hindu di Bali*. Unpublished doctoral dissertation. Suatu Studi Pendekatan Kliniko-Sosiobudaya.

———— (1991), Percobaan Bunuh Diri: Tinjauan Psikiatri. Typescript.

———— Jensen, G. D. (1991), Psychiatrist, traditional healer and culture integrated in clinical practice in Bali. *Med. Anthropol.*, 13:301–314.

World Health Organization (1977), *Manual of the International Statistical Classification of Diseases, Injuries, and Causes of Death (ICD-9)*. Geneva: WHO.

14.

Social and Cultural Psychiatry of Jamaicans, at Home and Abroad

William Wedenoja

Jamaica is a verdant and mountainous island in the Caribbean with 2.5 million people. It gained its independence from Britain in 1962. The island was inhabited by perhaps 60,000 Indians when Columbus landed in 1494. By 1655, when the British took it from Spain, there were few if any of the original inhabitants left. The production of sugar cane on plantations dominated the economy until the twentieth century. About 750,000 slaves were brought in from Africa, and their descendants make up about 96 percent of the population today. The remainder are of British, East Indian, Chinese, and Lebanese ancestry.

Jamaica is blessed with a lovely climate, great beauty, and substantial reserves of bauxite. The life expectancy (71 years) and the literacy rate (73%) arc high. But it has many of the typical problems of the Third World, including extreme inequality, high unemployment and underemployment, a per capita GNP of only $960 (U.S.) per annum, and rapid urbanization. Crime is a serious problem in the major city, Kingston, and the homicide rate has risen dramatically since the 1960s.

The social structure has been characterized as a color–class pyramid, with the small number of white citizens being predominantly upper class, a somewhat larger mulatto or "brown" middle class, and a predominantly black lower class (Henriques, 1968).

The middle- and upper-class family is generally nuclear and patriarchal. Common law unions, illegitimacy, and matrifocal (mother-headed) households are common in the lower class, where legal marriage is idealized and comes relatively late in life. Men and women often pursue relatively separate lives, even in marriage. Conjugal relations tend to be fragile, but close ties are maintained with one's kindred (close relatives).

THE CULTURE

Jamaica was a British colony for over 300 years, during which time it absorbed many English customs, values, and traditions, but its African heritage is still evident. The middle and upper classes identify with modern Western culture, whereas the lower class, particularly in rural areas, has a Creole (indigenous, syncretic, Afro-European) culture. For example, the elite speak a Jamaican variant of British English whereas the black majority speak an indigenous language known as Jamaican Creole.

Jamaicans are extremely religious and largely Christian fundamentalists. The elite belong to the Anglican, Methodist, Presbyterian, and Catholic churches. Many if not most of the poor and an increasing number of middle-class Jamaicans go to Pentecostal churches, which have experienced phenomenal growth since the Second World War. Indigenous cults with a strong African influence such as Kumina, Pukkumina, and Zion Revival are waning.

Religious worship is often highly emotional. Pentecostal sects and indigenous cults encourage dramatic convulsive performances, which are interpreted as divine possession, and they practice spiritual healing, attributing illness and misfortune to demonic interference.

Jamaicans believe in a wide range of signs, taboos, spells, and charms. Dreams are important portents of the future. There is a strong belief in "duppies" (ghosts), which can trouble the living, and the ability of "obeahmen" (sorcerers) to control ghosts and "set hand" on the living. Misfortune and illness are often blamed on Obeah. People worry about "grudgeful" or "bad minded" people working Obeah on them. One source of protection is the "scientist" or "professor" who practices a form of magic called "DeLaurence."

The famous Rastafarian movement came to prominence in the 1960s (Owens [1976] is an excellent account). "Rastas" believe that Haile Selassie, the former emperor of Ethiopia, whom they call "Jah" (God), is the messiah of black people. Marijuana is smoked frequently as a sacrament. The ideology of the Rastafarians is profound, but it probably sounds bizarre—if not delusional—to the uninitiated.

SOCIALIZATION AND PERSONALITY

Communal involvement, social interaction, spontaneity, and innovativeness are important values for Jamaicans (Alleyne, 1984), who have "a highly interpersonal view of the world, one in which the social nexus is a primary determinant of an individual's perspective on life" (Jones and Zoppel, 1979, p. 451). There is, however, a lot of tension and conflict in this social nexus. Suspicion, mistrust, envy, and malicious gossip are endemic, at least in small communities (Cohen, 1955). And many women regard men as unreliable, untrustworthy, and sexually obsessed (Brody, 1974).

The most extensive and incisive study of Jamaican personality is *Personality and Conflict in Jamaica*, which identified an "extrapunitive" attitude: "The individual himself never offends, it is always someone else who does something to him or 'puts something on him' " (Kerr, 1963, p. 167).

The main thesis of the book is that the "white bias" of the culture leaves very deep scars (a negative identity), which can cripple an individual with strong feelings of inferiority, insecurity, and powerlessness. There is evidence, for example, that black Jamaicans evaluate the body according to Caucasian norms and are dissatisfied with some of their physical features (Phillips, 1973). In addition, Jamaicans experience a "paradox of normalcy" in that the family structure of many if not most does not conform to the patriarchal, Eurocentric ideals of the culture and is, by implication, "abnormal" (de Chesney, 1986).

The nucleus of a lower-class family is usually a mother, her children (who often have different fathers), and the maternal grandmother. Fathers are often secondary if not peripheral, partly because separations are frequent but also because child-rearing is not a role expectation of men. The mother-child bond is strong, particularly with sons, who are expected to help their mother throughout life. There is a lack of independence training, and dependency is encouraged.

Children are desired. They are a measure of a man's virility. Having a baby transforms a girl into a woman, and the status of motherhood is held in high regard. Women often think that having a baby for a man will tie him to her. But the Jamaican family is not child-centered. For example, children are rarely given toys or taken on outings.

Child-shifting is common because many mothers work or migrate. The mother's mother often takes on full responsibility for child-rearing. Children are sometimes shifted to the mother's sister too, and occasionally even to friends or neighbors. This instability is to some extent counteracted by strong ties to, and the support and affection of, many members of the child's kindred.

Parents tend to be domineering, authoritarian, and strict disciplinarians. They stress obedience, submission, and respect for elders and are particularly concerned about "rudeness" and cleanliness. Punishment takes the form of nagging, threats, criticism, and "floggings." Parents are much more restrictive, even overprotective, with girls than with boys.

PSYCHIATRIC SERVICES

A lunatic asylum was established in Kingston in 1838 and replaced by a new facility, Bellevue Hospital, in 1863. Virtually all psychiatric care was provided by Bellevue until 1948, when an outpatient clinic was established at Kingston Public Hospital. The patient population reached a peak of 3123 in 1959.

In 1958 a consultant recommended decentralization of psychiatric services and the development of inpatient and outpatient services at rural hospitals. Implementation of this plan began in 1964 with the creation of a Department of Psychiatry at the University of the West Indies, which began to provide inpatient and outpatient services in 1965. Five psychiatric nurses were trained and placed in rural parishes as mental health officers in 1969.

The country was divided into three psychiatric service regions outside of the Kingston area in 1973. Outpatient clinics were established at seventeen hospitals across the island, with inpatient services at several regional hospitals. The immediate result was a dramatic reduction in the number of patients at Bellevue, financial savings, and a "marked improvement in the quality of care for the acutely mentally ill patient" (Hickling, 1976).

Another innovative program of the time was a very popular radio call-in psychiatry program that began in 1975 and did much to inform the public about the nature of mental illness and about the availability of psychiatric services (Hickling, 1992).

The election of a democratic socialist government in 1972, and the development of worker participation programs, inspired major changes at Bellevue. The goal was to change the hospital from "an authoritarian custodial system" to a "therapeutic community." Management of the institution was democratized and work therapy and large group psychotherapy were emphasized. A carpentry and repair workshop, vocational arts and crafts workshops, and a horticultural center were established. Patients cleaned and repaired old buildings, painted walls, landscaped the grounds, reared chickens, and grew crops. Staff and patients met regularly in "ethnohistorical" sessions to explore and analyze the history of the institution. They produced "sociodrama" pageants, rooted in the culture and employing poetry, dance, and music, as a form of rehabilitation. Public performances were staged in a new hospital theater and around the country in an effort to remove the stigma of mental illness (Hickling, 1988, 1989).

Many of the innovative programs at Bellevue were discontinued by a new and conservative government in 1982. The seventeen psychiatric clinics are, however, still functioning and they served 2093 new patients and 5607 old patients in 1988. The Community Psychiatric Service provides largely medical rather than psychological treatment, and it focuses on psychosis. Bellevue Hospital, which is situated on 120 acres near downtown Kingston, has about 1400 beds today. Additional psychiatric care is provided by private practitioners and private hospitals.

ETHNOPSYCHIATRY

In Jamaican culture, the term *madness* refers to unusual and unintelligible behavior such as "talking foolishness," giving away money to strangers, and setting fire to a house (typically one's parents' home). A "madman" is always a deviant, but not necessarily psychotic. Generally, treatment is not sought unless a madman becomes troublesome, destructive, or violent.

Misfortune and afflictions, including mental disorders, are often blamed on duppies and Obeah. "Madness" is also attributed to "nerves" (which are said to be "broken down" by excessive work, study, worrying, brooding, and thinking), as well as to bad living (immorality can "sick" the body), upbringing, economic conditions, and "ganja" (marijuana) smoking.

The mentally ill are highly visible. Indigent patients, most of whom have absconded from Bellevue, are common on the streets of Kingston. They are often theatrical and acquire colorful names such as "Walkabout," "Good News," and "Bag an' Pan." Children sometimes tease and ridicule "madmen." In rural areas, adults generally treat them with kindness and sympathy or at least tolerate and look after them. In urban areas, on the other hand, the public (particularly the middle class) is constantly pressing for their removal. The police have authority to detain the mentally ill, who may be sent to Bellevue on order of a judge after medical certification, but removal is primarily the responsibility of mental health officers.

The main resort of the lower-class majority for counseling, catharsis, and emotional support is charismatic churches and traditional healers. Hundreds of people practice a form of healing called Balm (described by Barrett [1976]). Perhaps a majority of healers are women, and most are associated with an Afro-Christian religion called Zion Revival.

The ability to heal with Balm is regarded as a "spiritual gift," and diagnosis is based on a spiritual "reading" of the patient. "Temporal" (natural) illnesses are treated with "bush" (herbs) and common drugs, but most illnesses are believed to be at least partly spiritual. The Balm healer specializes in spiritual afflictions, and she is the main resort for protection from duppies and

Obeah. Spiritual treatment includes a bath, prayers, candles, protective amulets ("guards"), and a "shouting" ritual to remove "destruction" (sin or the influence of duppies and demons).

Most of the cases seen by healers seem to involve somatized anxiety and depression caused by problems in living. A few Balm healers specialize in the treatment of "madness," but most now see few cases of psychosis, perhaps because it is increasingly being perceived as a medical problem by the populace.

Healers are often effective counselors. They are particularly important in reducing anxiety over bewitchment. One advantage they have over the psychiatrist is, of course, a shared world view with the patient about the nature and causes of illness. Another is the confidence that Jamaicans have in traditional healers and "bush" treatment. In addition, I have argued that Balm healing is a ritualized extension of mothering which involves maternal transference and meets an emotional need for attachment under stress (Wedenoja, 1989). The Jamaican elite and health professionals generally look down on Balm as ignorant superstition, and it operates on the fringes of the law.

EPIDEMIOLOGY

Royes (1962) reported a first admission rate of 450 per 100,000 for a twelve-year period (1949–1969)—an average of 37.5 per annum. He also conducted a community survey, which indicated a prevalence of 492 cases per 100,000 in 1960.

A recent comparison of psychiatric admissions in 1971 and 1988 shows a 49 percent decrease from 136 per 100,000 to 69 per 100,000 (Hickling, 1991a). The rate for males was 82 and that for females 55 in 1988. This is far lower than the rates of 320 for males and 485 for females reported for native English in the United Kingdom in 1981 (Cochrane and Bal, 1989).

There are, of course, many problems with cross-national comparisons. Although the data above suggest that the overall rate of mental disorders in Jamaica is low, much if not most of the difference might be accounted for by the greater availability of treatment in England. A comparison of rates of schizophrenia would be more legitimate.

The rate of (all) admissions for schizophrenia in Jamaica declined from 60 per 100,000 in 1971 to 35 in 1988. The rates of 86 for males and 52 for females in 1971 are comparable to those of 68 for males and 72 for females for England in the same year, although the sex ratio is different, and the Jamaican rates of 43 for males and 26 for females in 1988 are much lower than the rates of 63 for males and 60 for females in England in 1981 (Hickling, 1991a).

The diagnostic profile for psychiatric admissions to Jamaican hospitals in 1988 was schizophrenia and paranoid psychoses 50 percent, affective disorders 18 percent, other psychoses 17 percent, neuroses and personality disorders 5 percent, and alcoholism and other substance abuse 5 percent (Hickling, 1991a). Passive dependence is the most common personality disorder (Allen, 1985).

More males than females are admitted to psychiatric wards. But a majority of psychiatric patients (about 55%) are female. This is because schizophrenia, alcoholism, organic disorders, and personality disorders are more common in males, and depression and anxiety in females (Marriott, 1973; Hickling, 1975).

About three-fourths of all patients are 40 years of age or less, with about two-thirds under age 35. The age at onset is generally younger in males than in females. Burke (1974) calculated the age at onset for schizophrenia as twenty-six for males and twenty-nine for females, and for affective disorders as thirty-five for males and forty-five for females. The rate of disorder for males peaks in the 25 to 30 age group, and declines precipitously after age 40, whereas the female rate peaks in the 30 to 35 age group, remains constant from 35 to 50, then declines gradually (Wedenoja, 1981).

The prevalence of syphilis in the population is about 20 percent. Burke (1972a,b) found that 43 percent of admissions to Bellevue had significant physical pathology. In particular, 17 percent had latent syphilis and 8.5 percent neurosyphilis, with a high incidence of dementia as the main feature.

"Rum shops" are plentiful and drinking is a major form of recreation for men, but alcohol (which is usually consumed in company) is only a minor problem for psychiatry. A community survey in Kingston found that heavy drinking was associated with higher social class, and estimated the prevalence of alcoholism at 5 percent (Beaubrun, 1966). The number of patients treated for alcohol-related disorders is small. The great majority are male and upper class, and whites are overrepresented.

Marijuana is used extensively, for smoking and as a tea, by about two-thirds of the population. The elite believe it causes antisocial and violent behavior. Many Jamaicans, including physicians, also believe it leads to mental disorders, and the diagnosis "ganja psychosis" is often used. Some Jamaican psychiatrists believe that marijuana can "trigger" manic or hypomanic disorders, depression, and schizophrenia in susceptible individuals, but others think it may play a protective role.

The suicide rate, which Burke (1985) calculated as 1.4 per 100,000 per annum in 1975 and 1976, is extremely low by global and even by Caribbean standards (the U.S. rate was 12.2 in 1982). It has declined significantly in recent years, with only twelve cases in 1988 (.51 per 100,000). Burke found a sex ratio of four males to one female in 1975 to 1976, in contrast to a ratio of 12:1 in 1969 to 1970. The rate increases with age for both sexes, and is highest in the 65+ age group. The main methods are hanging for men and poisoning and drowning for women. About one-quarter of all cases had a history of mental illness.

Approximately 70 percent of all children are born to fatherless families, 63 percent are fostered out, and 37 percent experience a mother–child separation of over six months. Migration is the main factor in separation, which is associated with emotional and conduct disorders (Wray and McLaren, 1976). Antisocial behavior is almost invariably associated with numerous separations from a parent, especially when separation occurs in the first five years of life (Feldman and Marriott, 1970), whereas psychoneurosis (mainly feelings of guilt and depression) is associated with late separation (Burke, 1980).

Fifty-two percent of schoolchildren in a sample were behaviorally disturbed, as measured by the Rutter Scale, with roughly half showing neuroticism and half conduct disorders. There was a higher rate of disturbance in boys than girls, in urban than rural areas, and in poor and working-class rather than well-off families. The rate of hyperactivity—24 percent—was high, with boys outnumbering girls 2:1 (Wray, Barnaby, and McLaren, 1980).

EMIGRATION

Emigration has been an increasingly significant facet of Jamaican life since 1881, when thousands began to go to Panama to build the canal. There was a massive exodus to Britain from 1948 to 1968. Emigration to the United States increased dramatically in 1967, and many also emigrated to Canada in the 1970s. Today, there are roughly 500,000 Jamaicans in the United States, 300,000 in Britain, and 100,000 in Canada.

Little research has been done on Jamaicans and other British West Indians in Canada or the United States. I have been able to locate only five brief articles on mental health, four of which deal with counseling or psychotherapy. On the other hand, there are over 100 articles on mental disorders among British West Indians (the majority of whom are Jamaicans) in England.

The main focus of the psychiatric research on West Indians (or Afro-Caribbeans) in Britain is epidemiology. The rate of admission for all psychiatric disorders for first generation migrants from the British West Indies is only slightly higher than that for native British. Migrants have low rates of depression, neuroses, personality disorders, and alcohol and drug abuse but a dramatically higher rate of schizophrenia. Admission of West Indian males for schizophrenia is extremely high in the 16 to 34 and particularly the 25 to 34 age groups, after which there is a steep decline. Admission of Caribbean women also peaks in the 25 to 34 age group, but this is not followed by a marked decline (Cochrane and Bal, 1989). The suicide rate of West Indian migrants is the lowest of any ethnic group in Britain, but higher than in the West Indies (Burke, 1976). Nearly 30 percent of first admissions of young West Indian male psychiatric patients received the controversial diagnosis of "cannabis psychosis" in a study at one hospital (McGovern and Cope, 1987).

The primary concern of the research in Britain is schizophrenia. The inception rate for first-contact schizophrenia of West Indians in Britain is said to be "among the highest reported in the world literature" (Harrison, 1990). It has been referred to as an "epidemic," "a major public health problem" (Glover, 1989a), and "a matter of great concern" (Littlewood and Lipsedge, 1988). Although the rate of admission for the United Kingdom as a whole has been declining, the risk for West Indians actually increased from 1965 to 1984, particularly since 1975 (Wessely, Castle, Der, and Murray, 1991). The rate for Jamaican emigrants may be higher than that for emigrants from Barbados or Trinidad and Tobago (Glover, 1989b). The second generation, contrary to expectation, has much higher rates for all disorders than the first, particularly for schizophrenia (McGovern and Cope, 1987).

One influential explanation for the high rate of schizophrenia among West Indians in Britain is that West Indians are prone to respond to stress with acute psychotic reactions, which are misdiagnosed as schizophrenia as a result of cultural differences between doctor and patient (Littlewood and Lipsedge, 1981). There seems to be some truth to this, and similar cases have been reported for Jamaican migrants in Canada (Roberts, 1990), but recent research indicates that misdiagnosis does not account for the elevated rate (Harvey, Williams, McGuffin, and Toone, 1990).

Another explanation for the elevated rate of schizophrenia is the experience of being, and growing up, black in a racist society (Burke, 1984; Littlewood and Lipsedge, 1988). A major debate has also developed around the issue of institutionalized racism in British psychiatry. Has the social control of black people been medicalized (Mercer, 1984)? West Indian patients are more likely than whites to make first contact with police, apparently because intervention by a helping agent tends to come later in the course of their illness, when they are more disturbed (Harrison, Holton, Neilson, Owens, Boot, and Cooper, 1989). West Indians in general, and young males in particular, are more likely to be admitted compulsorily and somewhat more likely to be perceived as threatening, hostile, and aggressive by health workers (Pipe, Bhat, Matthews, and Hampstead, 1991). They are more often transferred to a high security unit and treated on a locked ward (Bolton, 1984). West Indian patients are also more likely to receive major tranquilizers, electroconvulsive therapy (ECT), intramuscular medication, and to be seen by junior staff members

(Littlewood and Cross, 1980). They receive higher peak dosages and are discharged earlier too (Chen, Harrison, and Standen, 1991).

Biological explanations for the elevated rate of schizophrenia in West Indian migrants have become increasingly popular of late. They include perinatal infections such as congenital rubella, complications of pregnancy and childbirth, and low birth weight (Glover, 1989a; Harrison, 1990; Eagles, 1991; Wessely, Castle, Der, and Murray, 1991).

Emigration has had a considerable effect on life in Jamaica. Although remittances flow back to the island, many marriages, families, and kindreds have been disrupted. Separation has become a common childhood experience, as emigrating mothers generally leave their children behind, usually with maternal grandmothers. The children often follow in a few years, but they face a difficult adjustment.

Many emigrants eventually return to the island. Some do so because they became mentally ill while abroad. In 1971, every seventh readmission to Bellevue was a repatriate from the United Kingdom (Burke, 1973). This adds to the burdens of an already financially strapped and understaffed mental health system. There is, incidentally, an extremely prevalent belief in Jamaica that repatriates from Britain, but not from the United States, are more often than not "mad." Mentally ill emigrants in England are sometimes encouraged to return to their home country in the belief that they will do better there. Unfortunately, this is not usually the case in Jamaica, where they face great stigma. A study of fifty-five mentally ill repatriates from Britain to Jamaica found a poor outcome in 58 percent (Burke, 1983).

Return migration puts emigrants in "double jeopardy" (Hickling, 1991b) because they experience adjustment problems upon their return as well as abroad. People expect them to be wealthy. Successful migrants may be subjected to envy and jealousy. Unsuccessful ones may experience shame and social disgrace. The majority of repatriates in one study expressed dissatisfaction with their job situation (Taylor, 1976). In addition, children who were born or at least raised abroad often rebel upon relocation to Jamaica. The possibility that repatriation may be

pathogenic is supported by the fact that 40 percent of the repatriates seen in a private practice in psychiatry in Jamaica were first
episode patients, although they rarely presented with schizophrenia (Hickling, 1991b).

The apparently modest or "normal" rate of schizophrenia in
Jamaica needs to be tested with additional and more sophisticated
studies, in light of the clearly high rates for West Indians in Britain. It would also be extremely interesting to get comparable data
on rates of schizophrenia among Jamaicans in the United States
and Canada. These data could make a major contribution to social psychiatry and to the understanding of schizophrenia.

REFERENCES

Allen, F. A. (1985), Psychological dependency among students in a
"cross-roads" culture. *W. Ind. Med. J.*, 34:123–127.
Alleyne, E. (1984), The world view of Jamaicans. *Jamaica J.*, 17:2–8.
Barrett, L. E. (1976), Healing in a balmyard: The practice of folk healing
in Jamaica. In: *American Folk Healing*, ed. W. D. Hand. Berkeley:
University of California Press.
Beaubrun, M. H. (1966), Alcoholism and drinking practices in a Jamai-
can suburb. *Transcult. Psychiat. Res. Rev.*, 4:77–79.
Bolton, P. (1984), Management of compulsorily admitted patients to a
high security unit. *Internat. J. Soc. Psychiat.*, 30:77–84.
Brody, E. B. (1974), Psychocultural aspects of contraceptive behavior in
Jamaica. *J. Nerv. & Ment. Dis.*, 159:108–119.
Burke, A. W. (1972a), Syphilis in a Jamaican psychiatric hospital. *Brit.
J. Venereal Dis.*, 48:249–253.
——— (1972b), Physical illness in psychiatric hospital patients in Jamaica. *Brit. J. Psychiat.*, 121:321–322.
——— (1973), The consequences of unplanned repatriation. *Brit. J.
Psychiat.*, 123:109–111.
——— (1974), First admissions and planning in Jamaica. *Soc. Psychiat.*,
9:39–45.
——— (1976), Socio-cultural determinants of attempted suicide among
West Indians in Birmingham: Ethnic origin and immigrant status.
Brit. J. Psychiat., 129:261–266.
——— (1980), A cross cultural study of delinquency among West Indian
boys. *Internat. J. Soc. Psychiat.*, 26:81–87.

———— (1983), Outcome of mental illness following repatriation: A predictive study. *Internat. J. Soc. Psychiat.*, 29:3–11.

———— (1984), Racism and psychological disturbance among West Indians in Britain. *Internat. J. Soc. Psychiat.*, 30:50–68.

———— (1985), Suicide in Jamaica. *W. Ind. Med. J.*, 34:48–53.

Chen, E. Y., Harrison, G., & Standen, P. J. (1991), Management of first episode psychotic illness in Afro-Caribbean patients. *Brit. J. Psychiat.*, 158:517–522.

Cochrane, R., & Bal, S. S. (1989), Mental hospital admission rates of immigrants to England: A comparison of 1971 and 1981. *Soc. Psychiat. & Psychiat. Epidemiol.*, 24:2–11.

Cohen, Y. A. (1955), Character formation and social structure in a Jamaican community. *Psychiatry*, 18:275–296.

de Chesney, M. (1986), Jamaican family structure: The paradox of normalcy. *Family Process*, 25:293–300.

Eagles, J. M. (1991), The relationship between schizophrenia and immigration: Are there alternatives to psychosocial hypotheses? *Brit. J. Psychiat.*, 159:783–789.

Feldman, H., & Marriott, J. A. S. (1970), Diagnostic patterns and child/parent separation in children attending the Jamaican child guidance clinic. *Brit. J. Soc. Psychiat.*, 4:220–230.

Glover, G. R. (1989a), Why is there a high rate of schizophrenia in British Caribbeans? *Brit. J. Hosp. Med.*, 42:48–51.

———— (1989b), Differences in psychiatric admission patterns between Caribbeans from different islands. *Soc. Psychiat. & Psychiat. Epidemiol.*, 24:209–211.

Harrison, G. (1990), Searching for the causes of schizophrenia: The role of migrant studies. *Schizophrenia Bull.*, 16:663–671.

———— Holton, A., Neilson, D., Owens, D., Boot, D., & Cooper, J. (1989), Severe mental disorder in Afro-Caribbean patients: Some social, demographic and service factors. *Psychol. Med.*, 19:683–696.

Harvey, I., Williams, M., McGuffin, P., & Toone, B. K. (1990), The functional psychoses in Afro-Caribbeans. *Brit. J. Psychiat.*, 157:515–522.

Henriques, F. (1968), *Family and Colour in Jamaica.* London: MacGibbon & Kee.

Hickling, F. W. (1975), Psychiatric care in a general hospital unit in Jamaica. *W. Ind. Med. J.*, 24:67–75.

———— (1976), The effects of a community psychiatric service on the mental hospital population in Jamaica. *W. Ind. Med. J.*, 25:101–106.

———— (1988), Politics and the psychotherapy context. In: *Clinical Guidelines in Cross-Cultural Mental Health*, ed. L. Comas-Diaz & E. E. H. Griffith. New York: Wiley.

—— (1989), Sociodrama in the rehabilitation of chronic mentally ill patients. *Hosp. & Commun. Psychiat.*, 40:402–406.

—— (1991a), Psychiatric hospital admission rates in Jamaica, 1971 and 1988. *Brit. J. Psychiat.*, 159:817–821.

—— (1991b), Double jeopardy: Psychopathology of black mentally ill returned migrants to Jamaica. *Internat. J. Soc. Psychiat.*, 37:80–89.

—— (1992), Radio psychiatry and community mental health. *Hosp. & Commun. Psychiat.*, 43:739–741.

Jones, E. E., & Zoppel, C. L. (1979), Personality differences among blacks in Jamaica and the United States. *J. Cross-Cult. Psychol.*, 10:435–456.

Kerr, M. (1963), *Personality and Conflict in Jamaica.* London: Collins.

Littlewood, R., & Cross, S. (1980), Ethnic minorities and psychiatric services. *Sociol. Health & Illness*, 2:194–201.

—— Lipsedge, M. (1981), Some social and phenomenological characteristics of psychotic immigrants. *Psycholog. Med.*, 11:298–302.

—— —— (1988), Psychiatric illness among British Afro-Caribbeans. *Brit. Med. J.*, 296:950–951.

Marriott, J. A. S. (1973), Family background and psychiatric disorders: Experience with admissions to the University Hospital of the West Indies. *Can. Psychiatric Assn. J.*, 18:209–214.

McGovern, D., & Cope, R. V. (1987), First admission rates of first and second generation Afro-Caribbeans. *Soc. Psychiat.*, 22:139–149.

Mercer, K. (1984), Black communities' experience of psychiatric services. *Internat. J. Soc. Psychiat.*, 301:22–27.

Owens, J. (1976), *Dread: The Rastafarians of Jamaica.* Kingston: Sangster.

Phillips, A. S. (1973), *Adolescence in Jamaica.* London: Macmillan.

Pipe, R., Bhat, A., Matthews, B., & Hampstead, J. (1991), Section 136 and African/Afro-Caribbean minorities. *Internat. J. Soc. Psychiat.*, 37:14–23.

Roberts, N. (1990), Boufee delirante in Jamaican adolescent siblings. *Can. J. Psychiat.*, 35:251–253.

Royes, K. (1962), The incidence and features of psychoses in a Caribbean community. In: *Proceedings of the Third World Congress of Psychiatry*, Vol. 2. Montreal: University of Toronto Press/McGill University Press.

Taylor, E. (1976), The social adjustment of returned migrants to Jamaica. In: *Ethnicity in the Americas*, ed. F. Henry. Paris: Mouton.

Wedenoja, W. (1981), An epidemiological profile of the psychiatric patient in rural Jamaica. Unpublished report summarized in the *Transcult. Psychiat. Res. Rev.*, 19:198–201, 1982.

—— (1989), Mothering and the practice of "Balm" in Jamaica. In:

Women as Healers: Cross-Cultural Perspectives, ed. C. Shepherd McClain. New Brunswick, NJ: Rutgers University Press.

Wessely, S., Castle, D., Der, G., & Murray, R. (1991), Schizophrenia and Afro-Caribbeans: A case control study. *Brit. J. Psychiat.,* 159:795–801.

Wray, S. R., Barnaby, D. M., & McLaren, E. (1980), Hyperkinesia (minimal brain dysfunction) and other behavioural disorders in a sample of Jamaican school children. *W. Ind. Med. J.,* 29:261–272.

———— McLaren, E. (1976), Parent-child separation as a determinant of psychopathology in children: A Jamaican study. *W. Ind. Med. J.,* 25:251–259.

15.

Ancient Beliefs and Psychiatry in Mexico

Carlos Viesca Treviño and Mariblanca Ramos de Viesca

The Mexican Indians, who descended from an ancient and transcendental culture, maintain a rich cultural legacy which is transmitted from parent to child. This legacy regulates the relationship with ancestors, with their gods, and spiritual entities, reminds them of the established place of man in the cosmic order, and teaches them how to classify and treat illness. This legacy is also important in terms of social cohesion and cultural identity.

In pre-Hispanic Aztec medicine, mind and mental functions were distributed in three main vital centers, each of which had a separate soul or living spirit. These three entities are: the *tonalli*, which corresponds to the head–brain center; the *teyollia*, which corresponds to the heart; and the *ihiyotl*, which corresponds to the liver. Alterations in any one of these entities result in a variety of mental illnesses.

One illness of pre-Hispanic origin important in Mexican traditional and popular medicines is *tonalli* loss or *susto*. It was recognized early as a "traditional illness"; in recent years, anthropological literature has reported syndromes similar to *susto* all over the world (Simons and Hughes, 1985), most especially in Mindanao (Frake, 1961), and Bali (Wikan, 1989), and the special

231

significance of fright as an etiological factor is present in every different cultural context. Thus, it is possible to identify many different types of "magical fright" in various cultures rather than interpreting them as an illness.

In Mexican pre-Hispanic medicine there is a term, *Tetonal-cauatiliztli*, or fright illness, which is associated with *tonalli* loss. Later, between the late sixteenth and seventeenth centuries, *tonalli* was gradually identified with the soul as it was defined by the Spanish conquerors and evagelizers (Gruzinski, 1988). At the same time, African slaves in Mexican territory contributed the "shadow" concept, which was soon assimilated with the "European" soul concept (Aguirre Beltrán, 1963), and with the native *tonalli*, which is expressed today in some Nahuatl communities in the mountainous area North of Puebla (Cifuentes, 1990), in San Francisco Tecoxpa, and in Mexico City as the shadow soul (Sasoon, 1987).

As we stated in another paper, *susto* is not equivalent to mental illness, but sometimes it can manifest in that way (Viesca and Ruge, 1985). In fact, it doesn't correspond to any particular disease. *Susto* symptoms are most frequently general ones such as anorexia, inertia, debility, nausea, diarrhea, insomnia, nervousness, irritability, and loss of interest. Sometimes it can develop into neurotic or psychotic disorder.

A large number of *susto* patients have some depressive features. This is a logical observation if we take into account that soul loss involves a diminished functional competence, both physically and psychologically. In these cases, it is possible to obtain some therapeutic results with antidepressive treatment and psychotherapeutic management, but it will be always only a symptomatic approach. For a real cure, you need to "call" the lost soul and restore it to the body. Thus, besides a biomedical treatment, a symbolic approach is also necessary.

At times, a *susto* victim (*asustado*) develops an acute psychotic episode. This time, *susto*, as a frightening experience, will be considered as a severe stress factor in the origin of the episode which develops into illness only in high-risk people. In these cases, often asymptomatic schizophrenia is detected as a basis for the disease.

Modern folk and traditional medicines, based on pre-Hispanic beliefs, assume the pathogenic action of a certain kind of wind. Some beings may expel pathological emanations and cause illness among common people, mainly pregnant women, little babies, and adolescents. The *ihiyotl*, after death, goes out of the body and represents a real danger to others. People think also that some witches can transform themselves into whirlwinds, and in this form penetrate and possess their victims (Munch, 1983); others take a wind and use it as an invisible projectile (Sasoon, 1987). Some supernatural beings are conceived as winds and have the "virtue" of being able to cause harm. The *ehecame* (winds), as they are called in Central Mexico, are auxiliary to some major gods and may bring sickness and misfortune to sinners and people trespassing on sacred or restricted places. In some areas, like the North Gulf Coast, almost all pathogenic agents are conceived as a wind. All of them have the power to cause delusions and hallucinations.

USE OF HALLUCINOGENIC DRUGS

An exception to the rules in other countries and urban cultures, is the context within which ingestion of hallucinogenic drugs is prescribed. People may regularly eat or drink substances which induce altered states of consciousness, carrying on a tradition inherited from their ancestors. But here, these habits have a ritual significance and involve careful preparation of the group and individual, to induce the presence of socially accepted meanings in the hallucinatory experience. There are regional differences due to ecology, but the main psychotropic plants are Peyote (*Lophophora williamsii*), Ololiuhqui (*Turbina corymbosa*), and Teona-nacatl (*Psylocibe and Stropharia* Sp.), all of which contain highly active hallucinogenic alkaloids (Scultees and Hoffmann, 1979). A special pharmacological interest has been shown in psylocibine, one of the active substances in the sacred mushrooms. Psylocibine has produced psychoses during experiments. It is extremely rare to see drug addiction in Indian communities, in contrast to the relatively high number of tourists with addictive behavior. The rigorous preparation and the specific circumstances for taking a traditional hallucinatory drug, make it difficult for problems to arise, since the ritual ingestion is tightly controlled (including control of hallucinatory phenomenology) according to strict guidelines. The shaman is a qualified guide and provides socially recognized assurance (Wasson, 1957, 1980). Since pre-Hispanic times, it has been clearly understood that madness will be the punishment for those eating or drinking these drugs without preparation or without taking special measures (Hernández, 1960). Similar problems are described among Huichol Indians who become "possessed" following ingestion of a plant locally called *kieri* (*Solandra Sw. Brevicalyx*). Healers adept in the use of this plant become crazy after they stop using. In normal circumstances, possession can be clinically described as being similar to hysteria.

NERVIOS

Another popular diagnostic entity is *nervios*. The term has many meanings and people employ it in different contexts. "To be nervous" may simply mean lack of tranquility with no specific disturbance, may express anxiety, or more frequently be used to mean "to have a nervous illness" (*estar enfermo de los nervios*) and as a synonym for severe mental illness (Jenkins, 1988). In its most frequent form, *nervios* expresses distress, generally derived from social and economic pressure. *Nervios* is thought to be a "disease" of Mediterranean origin. In fact, it has been identified in Spain, Latin America, and in Greek-Canadian communities.

SPIRITUALIST MEDIUMS AND MENTAL ILLNESS

Spiritualism is a Mexican folk religion founded by Roque Rojas in 1866. It is a messianic religion which recognizes Roque Rojas as its messiah, and puts primary importance on spiritual communication. Rojas always made a clear distinction between his religion and Catholicism, Protestantism, and spiritism, fighting to develop a nationalist church. It has spread among the very poor in urban areas, and membership totals some 100,000 persons.

Aside from proper religious ceremonies, healing practices are the main spiritualist activity. Regarding illness as the product

of perturbed spirits possessing or afflicting the patient, the healing process starts with spirit identification, continues with their
expulsion (*desalojo*) from the sick body, and finishes with the education of the perturbing spirit in view of preventing a subsequent
pathogenic activity. This process is made possible by a medium
called a facilitator (Facultad), who, falling into an ecstatic trance,
is capable of receiving and translating the messages of protecting
spirits. Ethnopsychiatric studies identify different psychopathological moods in the facilitators, and it is possible to say that
mental illness from a Western perspective is common among
them. Interestingly enough, systematized delusions are perfectly
integrated with the religious world view of the medium, temple
guide, and patient. The medium sees spirits in a prescribed form,
hears voices that most of the time reassure her that she is carrying
out her healing activities correctly. Psychoses are integrated with
religious practice and acquire a religious meaning with a social
function. It is only when psychotic symptoms have immoral connotations that the problem becomes psychiatric, and only then is
psychiatric treatment sought.

MODERN PSYCHIATRY IN MEXICO

European psychiatry was introduced early in Mexico. A wide perspective of European humoral concepts arrived with the first
Spanish physicians around 1525. Some years later, the first hospitals were specially designed for the mentally ill. The earliest one,
San Hipolito Hospital, which was founded in the sixteenth century, started its work in 1567. A century later came El Divino
Salvador (Divine Saviour) Hospital exclusively used for mad
women. The existence of hospitals that admitted both general
and psychiatric patients was frequent in Colonial Mexico. In the
nineteenth century, all these hospitals, which had been managed
by friars, were modified and their direction was given to medical
doctors just a few years after the Independence War (1810–1821).
In 1910, the two main psychiatric hospitals in Mexico City, San
Hipolito and El Divino Salvador, were closed and their patients
were transferred to a new and modern building designed to be
a model institution. This new hospital was called La Castañeda

and was in operation until 1968. In other cities, the San Juan de Dios Hospitals were transformed from religious into civil hospitals, each with a psychiatric ward.

Thus, Mexico has had Western psychiatric institutions for four hundred years with professionals who followed European diagnostic practices and the more recent North American classification. Nineteenth and twentieth century sources reveal such diagnoses as mania and melancholy, lunacy or hysteroepilepsy, as well as general progressive paralysis, schizophrenia, or any other DSM-III diagnoses.

It is obvious that in Mexico, there coexist at least two ways to conceive psychiatric ailments. A Western, scientific view, specially in towns where modern medicine is regularly practiced; and a traditional indigenous view, mainly to be found in rural areas where different ethnic groups live nowadays with their traditional social structures as the underlying cultural component. The first part of this chapter dealt with an indigenous approach to mental illness. Modern psychiatry is firmly rooted and well developed in Mexico. Psychiatric diagnoses are currently used throughout the country with at least 40 percent of patients, in contrast to traditional concepts of medicine.

Epidemiological studies assert that anxiety and simple irritability are present in some 50 percent of patients seen by general practitioners, and 30 percent with depressive symptoms. In Mexico City, only 2.66 per 1000 inhabitants need psychiatric services but 8.93 percent actually utilize services (Gutiérrez and Barilar, 1986). It is interesting to observe that children are predominant in psychiatric centers in Mexico City, a situation that may be due to cultural factors—women bring children to the doctor at an early manifestation of illness, and at the same time adults find it very hard to accept psychiatric illness and treatment.

Adults, especially men, delay getting professional help until the problems have become more complicated and severe. In an epidemiological study covering the years 1973 to 1978, it was observed that the first reason for consultation in psychiatric hospitals is epilepsy, with 17.7 percent in males and 19.4 percent in females, immediately followed by schizophrenia, with an incidence of 15.4 percent, which is practically the same in both sexes (Gutiérrez and Tovar, 1984). The high rate of epilepsy observed in hospitals contrasts with a very low rate in other mental health services including general outpatient clinics (Gutiérrez and Barilar, 1986). It is necessary to consider the fact that many patients with mental illness do not go to specialized services, but receive attention from general practitioners. This situation is specially evident in alcoholism and in disturbances with somatic symptoms. Data reveal that among hospitalized patients, the number of schizophrenics is highest with 34 percent, followed by patients with epilepsy (24%) (de la Parra, Escobar, and Rubio, 1983). By contrast, drug addiction had a very low rate in 1977, only 2 percent of inpatients (de la Fuente, 1988); but in the ten years between 1976 and 1986, there was an increase in the prevalence of drug addiction among students in urban areas; use of inhalants went from 0.8 to 4.4, marijuana from 1.6 to 3.2, cocaine from 0.6 to 1.67. Heroin use is limited to cities at the northern border. A sociocultural characteristic to be emphasized is an overwhelming prevalence in inhalant use by young street people (de la Fuente, 1988). It is interesting that there has been no published study relating cultural factors to all these epidemiological tendencies. The only comments on this subject have come from general observations.

REFERENCES

Aguirre Beltrán, G. (1963), *Medicina y Magia*. México: Instituto Nacional Indigenista.

Cifuentes, E. (1990), *Herbolaria y tradiciones etnomédicas en un pueblo náhua*. México: Coordinación de la Investigación Científica, UNAM.

de la Fuente, R. (1988), Semblanza de la Salud Mental en México. *Salud Pública de México*, 30:861–871.

de la Parra, A., Escobar, O., & Rubio, S. (1983), Características psicosociales de pacientes cróicos hospitalizados. *Salud Pública de México*, 25:161–172.

Frake, C. (1961), The diagnosis of disease among the Subanum of Mindanao. *Amer. Anthropol.*, 63:113–132.

Gruzinski, S. (1988), *La colonization de l'imaginaire*. Paris: Galimard.

Gutiérrez, H., & Barilar, E. (1986), Morbilidad psiquiátrica en el primer nivel de atención de la Ciudad de Mexico. *Boletín de la Oficina Sanitaria Panamericana*, 101:648–659.

—— Tovar, H. (1984), La vigilancia epidemiológica de las enfermedades mentales. *Salud Pública de México*, 26:464–483.

Hernández, F. (1960), *Histria Natual de la Nueva España*, 2 vols. México: Universidad Nacional Autónoma de México.

Jenkins, J. (1988), Ethnopsychiatric interpretations of schizophrenic illness: The problem of *nervios* within Mexican-American Families. *Cult., Med., & Psychiat.*, 12:301–329.

Munch, G. (1983), *Etnología del Istmo Veracruzano*. México: Instituto de Investigaciones Antropológicas, UNAM.

Sasoon, Y. (1987), Espanto y mal aire. In: *Antropología y Prática Médica*. México: Facultad de Medicina, UNAM.

Scultees, E., & Hoffmann, A. (1979), *Plants of the Gods. Origins of Hallucinogenic Use*. Maidenhead, U.K.: McGraw-Hill.

Simons, C., & Hughes, C. (1985), *The Culture-bound Syndromes: Folk Illnesses and Psychiatric and Anthropological Interest*. Dardrecht: D. Reidel.

Viesca, C., & Ruge, T. (1985), Aspectos psiquiátricos y psicológicos de susto. *Anoles de Antropología* (Mexico), 22:475–492.

Wikan, U. (1989), Illness from fright or soul loss: A North Balinese culture-bound syndrome? *Cult., Med., & Psychiat.*, 131:25–50.

Wasson, G. (1957), The hallucinogenic mushrooms of Mexico: An adventure in ethnomycological exploration. *Trans. NY Acad. Sci.*, Series II, 21 (no. 4):325–339.

—— (1980), *The Wondrous Mushroom*. New York: McGraw-Hill.

16.

Uruguay: Subcultures under Apparent Cultural Uniformity

Yubarandt Bespali de Consens

The Uruguayan population is descended from European settlers: the Spanish were the primary group, but Italians and other Europeans have contributed to the diversity. There are no indigenous cultures, owing to the deplorable history of extermination of hunting tribes, about two centuries ago, soon after independence from Spain. Physical anthropologists have traced vestiges of the indigenous races in the current populations (Sanz, Mañe-Garzón, and Kolski, 1986), this in spite of the cultural myth of a definitive cultural crosscut between Amerindian and colonial cultures in Uruguay, which made Uruguayans feel "different" from other Latin Americans. Montevideo was a port of call for slave ships whose cargos were sent throughout the whole Virreinato del Perú. Today there are only a few hundred families of African origin, but they have deeply influenced Carnival musical folklore which is important in urban modern music.

Democracy, during the early part of the century, made Uruguay the *"American Switzerland,"* but in 1973 began thirteen years of military dictatorship which resulted in gross violations of human rights. Upon the disappearance of this nightmare and democracy being once more established, Uruguayans were up against sizable economic problems—Uruguay had the highest per capita debt in South America. As a result of the slump, 21 percent of households sank down to the poverty level, with their basic needs unmet. This South American region has ceased to offer a future for its young people who are emigrating in increasing numbers.

The first Asylum for twenty-eight patients was built in 1860 in Montevideo. The ceremony of opening the Manicomio Nacional took place in 1880. It is still in partial operation; the building, in the style of traditional French architecture, is a historical monument (Murguia and Soiza Larrosa, 1987).

University psychiatry began in 1908, with Professor Etchepare who was educated in Paris, and brought a long tradition with him that is still active. The French School has always dominated psychiatric theory and nosology in Uruguay. It was inspired from the sixties to the eighties, by H. Ey's work. Uruguayan authors even now make considerable use of Ey's organodynamic viewpoint (Casarotti and Gastal, 1989). Mental Health institutions have adopted the *WHO Classification* for filing purposes. The University Psychiatric Department has been a testing center for the IDC's tenth edition. The *American Diagnostic and Statistical Manual of Mental Disorders* (*DSM-III*) is often used in scientific papers, its multiaxial approach has been accepted by professionals, and is used as a reference for difficult diagnostic situations (APA, 1980). Some of its categories, which are not found in other systems, have been integrated into everyday technical language: "borderline" personality disorder has become an anglicism in Spanish.

The Psychoanalytic Association of Uruguay (founded in 1956) (Bespali de Consens, 1988), followed the Kleinian school initially, as was also true of the Argentinians. It has become popular among many of the four hundred psychiatrists and a larger number of psychologists in Uruguay. The courts used psychiatric expertise as early as 1838, and some outstanding professionals have devoted much work to forensic psychiatry. This fruitful relationship with the law has led to magistrates today sentencing a defendant to psychiatric treatment even when expert opinion has not been unanimously in favor of it.

Until recently, psychiatric care was separated from general health care. *In 1986, a community-based Mental Health plan was approved by the Ministry of Health, upon a draft made by all professionals and related groups, but government funds were not provided for it.* In the cities of the interior, patients are admitted for mental disorders to general hospitals, with less segregation than in Montevideo. *Child psychiatry* began in the forties, and specialists in this field work either in public care or in private individual consultations, with scant institutional participation. After many years of unsuccessful attempts, 1990 has witnessed the opening of a small ward at the Children's Hospital. In spite of the large number of elderly people (16% of the population), there are no special programs for their mental health.

CULTURAL ASPECTS OF MENTAL ILLNESS

Epidemiological Data

Detection of groups at risk for mental illness is mandatory in modern approaches to mental health. Some research, limited to a few specific problems, has developed during the last four decades. In 1968, a team investigating the relationship between the *mentally disturbed patient* and her or his family found a higher incidence of *mental disorders* and *alcoholism* among patients' relatives. *Alcoholism* was subject to research in the late sixties and seventies (Bespali de Consens, 1972; Ripa and Alterwain, 1969). It was estimated that in 1963, 94 liters of an alcoholic beverage were consumed per capita in the population over 15 years of age (54 liters of wine, 33 liters of beer, and 7 liters of distilled beverages). Using Jellinek's Formula (i.e., the hepatic cirrhosis death rate ratio), 1354 alcoholics with medical complications were found for every 100,000 inhabitants. The proportion of women ranged from one to every ten or twenty men according to different statistics. High figures reflect the importance of alcoholism as a neuropsychiatric complication: alcoholism appears in 30 percent of male admissions to psychiatric wards, and is the main reason for hospitalization in men. Current observation shows an increase of alcoholism in younger people, and in women.

Uruguayan society encourages people to drink at every possible opportunity: a birth, a business deal, any social occasion, courtship, and wakes. Both men and women accept drinking in males, tolerance of alcohol being part of the "machismo" ideal.

Problem drinkers are punished only in case of severe disturbance. Traffic rules do not allow blood tests for drunken drivers, and other tests are not yet available on the roads. The Penal Code considers most cases of inebriation as an attenuating circumstance. There is a large vocabulary of folkloric terms concerning drinks and drunkenness in Spanish, both written and oral. Popular folk beliefs enhance alcohol with assorted qualities: it is healthy, it is warming, it is a good nutrient, red wine cures anemia, a dose of liquor raises low blood pressure, and even what a sanitation man once told us: "One must drink to kill microbes" (Bespali di Consens, 1972).

Current research (Dajas, 1990) shows that Uruguay has the highest rate of suicide in Latin America (it increased throughout the twentieth century; it was 12.7 per 100,000 inhabitants in 1960, peaked in 1982, and slightly decreased to 8.7 per 100,000 in 1987). "A survey of the distribution of suicide according to sex and age shows a preponderance in the male at the seventh and eighth decades of life, a utilization of violent methods, and, in more than 50% of cases, it is associated with psychic disturbance. Suicide attempts show, on the other hand, a preponderance in young women (second decade) mainly due to the ingestion of psychiatric drugs" (Dajas, 1990).

From a ten-year sample of 9223 patients using private health care, social insurance, and public hospitals, Rey Tosar and Dajas (1985) found a very high percentage of depression. Unipolar depression was more predominant in the upper class (52%). They found a marked reduction of bipolar depression, with only 1 percent of melancholia. Schizophrenic patients made up almost 25 percent of the hospital diagnoses.

Between 1950 and 1960, at the University Psychiatric Ward, diagnoses were schizophrenia 11 percent, paraphrenia 1.8 percent, paranoia 0.5 percent, *bouffée délirante* or acute psychotic states 5.7 percent.

Experienced psychiatrists currently report that acute psychoses were less dramatic than they used to be twenty or thirty years ago. There has also been an increase of paranoid and schizoaffective disorders with a decrease in catatonic forms. They also noticed a general decrease of conversion symptoms in somatoform disorders.

Some mental illness appears to have been changing in frequency: anorexia-bulimia has increased during the last decade.

It is interesting to add that multiple personality disorder is perceived as locally nonexistent by many Uruguayan specialists.

CULTURE-SPECIFIC SYNDROMES

Nervios (nerves) is characterized by the following symptoms: *patient cannot sleep, is restless, bad tempered, sad, discouraged, she or he has no appetite, does not eat, and loses weight.* Half of the informants also mentioned *crying,* or *not enjoying sexual intercourse* as signs of nerves. In Uruguay, as other authors have mentioned in relation to Latinos in general, people also distinguish between *nervios* and *ataques de nervios;* this latter refers to an anxiety crisis with a strong psychomotor component. A parallelism could be made with neurotic or stress disorders.

Enloquecer (''to be driven insane'') was defined by these symptoms: *the patient babbles, acts oddly, speaks or laughs when alone, quarrels or acts aggressively, screams or cries.* Half of the surveyed people also indicated that it could *be noticeable in the patient's eyes and the ways she or he looks.* This syndrome could be roughly compared to psychotic disorders (Bespali de Consens, 1989).

Mal de ojo (evil eye) is widely known; some restrict it to child victims. The main symptom is *headache,* but also *sleeplessness, drowsiness, fever, fixed stare,* and *digestive disturbances. Mal de ojo pasado* is a severe form of *mal de ojo* which usually ends in death.

BELIEFS OF MENTAL ILLNESS AND PSYCHIATRIC TREATMENT

Popular etiology is mainly based on natural causes of mental illness, though the most significant is *psychic stress.* Other important causes are *congenital factors, toxic substances* (alcohol, drugs), and *lack of nourishment.* The only supernatural origin frequently mentioned is breaking a taboo or a moral rule (eating something evil, getting wet, or behaving improperly). Other supernatural theories of illness (sorcery, witchcraft, fate) are used much less as etiological factors in mental disorders (Bespali de Consens, 1989).

People surveyed have selected *medicines as their favorite therapeutic means for the care of the mentally ill.* They have expressed confidence in health technicians, but they reject hospitals. *Electroconvulsive therapy* (ECT) is quite widely employed with psychotic patients. A few psychiatrists claim to use it frequently, while the majority limit its use to certain cases. Both doctors and lay people use a popular euphemism, referring to ECT as the "sleep cure." *Psychotherapies,* which are currently only used in private practice, follow a variety of theoretical models: psychoanalytic, systemic family, behavioral, psychodrama, gestalt, transactional analysis, and relaxation therapies.

Herbs, *yuyos,* are known by many people as sedatives. The most popular is *Tilia europea,* prepared as a medicinal tea, or added to folk quotidian *maté* (a stimulating infusion of *Ilex Paraguayensis* drunk through a small metal tube).

Folk healers do not work with physicians in the treatment of mental illness even though they have increased in number and have contacts with all social classes. Their activities are punished by the law, but a tolerant attitude by the population is only seldom shaken by publicized accusations, in cases when an accident or a fraud has happened. Herbal or praying *curanderos* treatments are the most common ones. New religious sects (Afro-Brazilian cults, Pentecostals) deal with an increasing number of cases that require crisis management.

REFERENCES

American Psychiatric Association (1980), *Diagnostic and Statistical Manual of Mental Disorders,* 3rd ed. Washington, DC: American Psychiatric Association Press.

Bespali de Consens, Y. (1972), Some aspects of alcoholism in Uruguay. *Alcoholism,* 8:51–55.

———— (1988), Psicoanálisis en el ámbito de la Psiquiatría forense en Uruguay. Actas de ola 2as. *Jornadas de Psicoanálisis y Salud Mental,* June:63–65.

———— (1989), Conceptos populares en Salud Mental. *Rev. Psiquiatría del Uruguay,* 54:197–211.

Casarotti, H., & Gastal, F. L. (1989), *Psicosis y modelo organo-dinámico de Henri Ey*. Uruguay: Univ. Católica de Pelotas, *Educat.*

Dajas, F. (1990), Alta tasa de suicidio en Uruguay. Consideraciones a partir de un estudio epidemiológico. *Rev. Méd. Uruguay*, 6:203–215.

Damonte, A. M., & Maccio, G. A. (1989), *Uruguay: Estimaciones y proyecciones de la población urbana y rural por sexo y edad. 1975–2025.* Centro Latinoamericano de Demografía. Departmento Publ. D. G. Estad. y. Censos, Montevideo.

Murguia, D., & Soiza Larrosa, A. (1987), Desarrollo de la psiquiatría en el Uruguay. *Rev. Psiq. del Uruguay*, 52:169–179.

Rey Tosar, J. C., & Dajas, F. (1985), Algunos aspectos epidemiológicos de la depresión en nuestro ambiente. *Rev. Psiq. del Uruguay*, 50:123–138.

Ripa, J., & Alterwain, P. (1969), El Alcoholismo y su relación con el proceso salud-enfermedad. *Segundas Jornadas Urug. Psiq. Hig. Mental*, Montevideo. April.

Sanz, M., Mañé-Garzón, F., & Kolski, R. (1986), Presencia de mancha mongólica en recién nacidos de Montevideo. *Archivos de Pediatría del Uruguay*, 57:149–156.

PART V

Western Europe

17.

Social and Cultural Factors in German Psychiatry

Wolfgang Krahl

Since the beginning of the nineteenth century, the time when "modern psychiatry" evolved in Germany, there have been enormous changes in German society and culture. In the nineteenth century Germany developed from an agricultural state into an industrial one, the church lost its all-pervasive influence and was superseded by the state. (During the last twenty years, many Germans left the Catholic and Protestant churches; churches that were filled thirty years ago are today empty.) During the twentieth century alone, two World Wars originated in Germany, the monarchy was abolished, and Nazi Germany, though it existed only for twelve years, left an irradicable imprint. World War II resulted in the division of Germany, leaving two parts with completely different political and social systems, which were reunited forty years later. Today, Germany is experiencing the sometimes very painful process of reunification, a process which abolished social structures in the east before replacing them with new ones.

DEVELOPMENT OF PSYCHIATRY IN GERMANY

During the Middle Ages the mentally ill were seen as possessed by demons and devils. In 1486 the Dominican monks Heinrich

Krämer and Jakob Sprenger published their infamous book *Malleus Maleficarum* (Witches' Hammer), where they suggested that any sign of mental or physical abnormality was due to witchcraft. In the following two centuries thousands, mainly women, and many of them mentally ill, were accused of witchcraft, tortured, and executed (Ackerknecht, 1967). During the fifteenth and sixteenth centuries the citizens of prosperous German towns like Hamburg and Nuremberg would drive madmen outside their city limits or put them in Narrentürme (fool towers). The seventeenth and eighteenth centuries, the beginning of industrialization and capitalism, were no better times for the mentally ill; workhouses or Zuchthäuser were established for paupers, vagabonds, prostitutes, cripples, criminals, amoral people, politically unwanted people, and the mentally ill (Dörner, 1984).

With the beginning of the nineteenth century, psychiatry turned into science. In 1805, Johann Reil, a "Psychiker," founded the first German psychiatric journal, the *Magazin für psychische Heilkunde* and he also coined the term *psychiatry*. In those days two opposing schools existed influenced either by romanticism or natural philosophy: the "Psychiker" and the "Somatiker."

During the first half of the nineteenth century in Germany more than thirty large institutions for the insane were founded, in general outside towns. The directors of these Anstalten had a great impact on German psychiatry and some of these structures remain today.

In the second half of the nineteenth century psychiatry as taught at the university hospitals gained influence. In 1845 Wilhelm Griesinger had published his book *Pathologie und Therapie der psychischen Krankheiten* where he stated that psychological diseases are diseases of the brain. He demanded that neuropsychiatry have a scientific orientation and should abstain from making moral judgments. Most universities established departments for neuropsychiatry in the period following Griesinger. The department of psychiatry at the university of Munich was headed between 1903 and 1922 by Emil Kraepelin, whose work (1904) influenced not only German psychiatry through his nosology but DSM-III, which can be seen as a renaissance of his ideas (American Psychiatric Association, 1980).

The time between 1933 and 1945, the Third Reich, was the

darkest period in the development of German psychiatry, one that always will cast its shadow. During those days many Jewish psychiatrists and psychoanalysts had to leave countries under German control, among them, just to name a few, Sigmund Freud, his daughter Anna Freud, Karen Horney, F. Kallmann, and Melanie Klein. This was a brain drain from which German psychiatry has not yet recovered. The "Führer Decree" of 1939 resulted in the killing of more than 200,000 mental patients, not only in Germany but also in Poland and Russia. These patients were not burned by religious zealots as had happened in the Middle Ages, but were exterminated in a systematic way by physicians, psychiatrists, and other medical personnel (Lifton, 1986; Dörner, 1989). After the war, most members of the medical community reacted with denial and repression to what had happened during the Nazi regime (Schmidt, 1988). The delay of this discussion resulted in the delay of improvements for the mentally ill. Therefore the system of care remained custodial, as it had been a hundred years earlier, and no changes or reforms were made. Only in the early 1970s did the medical community start to look at what had happened more than thirty years before and this discussion is still continuing (Thom, 1990).

In 1970 the West German Parliament asked for a large-scale psychiatric inquiry that resulted in the "Psychiatrie-Enquete," which was published in 1975. It was shown that in 1974 more than two-thirds of the mentally ill were admitted to psychiatric hospitals with more than 1000 beds. At the same time West Germany had about 100,000 neuropsychiatric beds, almost 90 percent of them in institutions with more than 500 beds; only twenty-one psychiatric units in general hospitals existed at that time (Bericht über die Lage der Psychiatrie in der BRD, 1975). Though there is agreement that psychiatry should be practiced on a community oriented basis, this is changing very slowly. In 1990 there were approximately seventy large mental hospitals still in existence in West Germany, but there are also now over ninety psychiatric units in general hospitals as well as twenty-five psychiatric departments at university hospitals. Nowadays half of the acute admissions of psychiatric patients are treated in psychiatric units, the other half in large institutions. While in 1973 there were 900 neuropsychiatrists in private practice, by 1989 the number had risen to over 2500, and is still climbing (Bauer and Engfer, 1990). Until 1987 it was possible in Germany to train in neuropsychiatry, but since then a young doctor has to decide either to become a neurologist or a psychiatrist.

The reunification of East and West Germany provides an opportunity for German psychiatry. The different experiences in both parts could result in a constructive exchange of ideas and hence in the improvement of psychiatric services. It also poses threats, however, because it seems that other problems are assumed to be more important and given higher priority.

CONCEPTS AND ATTITUDES

The concept of mental illness in Germany today varies with education, social class, and the personal knowledge of a person who is suffering from a mental illness. The majority of Germans will differentiate between *Geisteskrankheit* and *Gemütskrankheit*. While *Geisteskrankheit* can be translated as insanity, *Gemütskrankheit* seems to be a very German word, the nearest translation would be mood disorder (Peters, 1989).

Geisteskrankheit is generally accepted to be a disorder in which heredity as well as organic factors play a major role. It follows its own course and can hardly be influenced by therapeutic means. It is not seen to be linked to social relationships, the economic situation, or the environment, it is something not reasonable but enigmatic. The general public thinks that if someone is suffering from insanity he is not open to reasoning at all, that he is dangerous, and that *Geisteskrankheit* (schizophrenia or psychosis) can be recognized from a person's strange clothes or staring eyes.

Gemütskrankheiten is seen as being little influenced by heredity, but by hardships in the social environment, personal relationships, and a sensitive *Gemüt* (i.e., mind, soul, feeling). The *Gemütskranke* is someone who suffers by himself and is dangerous to himself because of his gloomy thoughts. Contrary to the *Geisteskranke*, the *Gemütskranke* is seen as someone who is clear in his mind, is well-oriented, knows what he does, and his actions are understandable (Jaeckel and Wieser, 1970).

These are rather rational ideas of mental illness; however,

there are other concepts of mental illness as well. Rosin and Hammers (1979) found that one-third of the Protestant clergy and two-thirds of the Catholic clergy in Germany believe that "true" possession exists. They further believe that this phenomenon cannot be explained in psychological and psychiatric terms but that the person is possessed by the devil. This attitude on the part of the clergy has its roots in the beliefs of the general population. In some of the rural parts of Germany, a number of people still believe in supernatural causes of certain illnesses including mental illness (Rudolph, 1977; Kirfel, 1984). In addition, nowadays esoteric beliefs and practices are growing in popularity (Ruppert, 1987; Payk, 1989), but scientific psychiatry shows so far hardly any interest in these phenomena. Therefore exact data about the different ideas of the origin of mental illness are not available.

Recently, a questionnaire surveying 530 persons in Munich revealed that 54.5 percent had no or hardly any knowledge about mental illness, though 56 percent knew someone suffering from a mental illness (Lamnek and Tretter, 1991). Amazingly similar results were obtained in a comparable study in Beijing, China (Yang, 1989), showing that about half of the people questioned lack any systematic knowledge of mental disorders. Approximately half of the Germans interviewed thought that the mentally ill are aggressive and almost one-third consider them dangerous. Regarding therapy, only 40 percent thought that medication was helpful, but 11 percent were of the opinion that an operation might help. Seventy-five percent of the information about mental illness is obtained from the mass media, but most people think that mental disorders are not adequately covered.

Other studies show also that information about mental illness is quite inadequate amongst the general public. More research about attitudes, concepts, prejudices, and knowledge of mental illness is needed to develop strategies to bring a positive change; the mass media should be involved in these efforts (Korczak and Pfefferkorn, 1983; Tretter, 1985).

DEPRESSION

According to Tellenbach (1976) the "Typus Melancholicus" is characterized by orderliness, conscientiousness, meticulousness, high value achievement, conventional thinking, and dependency on conflict-free personal relationships, all values that were, at least until recently, highly valued in German society. Tellenbach calls melancholia a typical psychological disorder of Western civilization. He sees in the one-sided preponderance of high efficiency and achievement a condition for the provocation of melancholia.

To 40 percent of those questioned, depressive symptoms are the single most often named psychiatric symptom in neuropsychiatric private practice (Bochnik and Koch, 1990). The Upper Bavarian epidemiological field study, done in a rural/small town area, showed a point prevalence rate for depressive disorders (endogenous depression, depressive neurosis, depressive personality) of 11 percent for women and 4.6 percent for men (Fichter, 1990). This ratio of approximately 2 to 1 has been found in different Western cultures (Weissman and Klerman, 1977).

Across time, a change in the symptomatology of depression has been observed in Germany. Since these changes took place before the introduction of antidepressants and new psychotherapeutic interventions, the cause has to be attributed to different psychopathology mainly due to cultural and environmental factors. Lauter and Schön (1967) compared the case histories of 480 depressive patients admitted to the Psychiatric University Hospital of Munich between 1910 and 1963. They observed some important changes in psychopathology that reflect changes in German culture and society. Guilt feelings that ranked first of all the symptoms in 1910 dropped from 62 to 41 percent in 1963. Guilt feelings about religious, ethical, or sexual offenses and criminal acts all became significantly less. This is in accord with tendencies in the general population to show less involvement in religious matters and to develop more liberal views about sexuality. There is a sharp increase in guilt feelings toward partner and family. Over the past hundred years, German families have become smaller, and in the nuclear family the members are psychologically very dependent upon each other. In Germany guilt feelings toward the children are particularly strong, while in Japan where the families have also become smaller, guilt feelings toward parents are also observed (Kimura, 1965). An increase in guilt feelings regarding professional duties is reported; in 1910 only about

25 percent of the depressive patients lamented about their inability to work and about insufficiency. Half a century later this complaint was presented by approximately 75 percent of patients. The high demands of the labor market today, excessive competitiveness, and striving for high efficiency could play a role in this shift of symptomatology. Today's society is very difficult for a depressive patient. The alternative is either to be healthy and thereby fully efficient or to take on the sick role. Being depressed then means degrading oneself, which is expressed in guilt feelings regarding professional duties and feelings of insufficiency (Pfeiffer, 1984). Ideas of poverty and ruin have decreased over time, probably as a result of a much better social security system. Before the introduction of antidepressants, 25 percent of depressive patients tried to commit suicide; this number was reduced to 10 percent in 1963. But the sum of suicidal thoughts and suicidal attempts, between 40 and 50 percent, seems to remain constant over the years (Lauter and Schön, 1967).

Similar results are presented by Bron and Wetter-Parasie (1989) who investigated 301 patients between 45 and 65 years with endogenous depression, who were admitted to psychiatric hospitals between 1920 and 1982. They noticed an even sharper increase in physical and vegetative symptoms; 77 percent of the patients showed somatic complaints that had to be interpreted as depressive symptoms. While in 1920 somatization was associated with lower social class, in 1982 there was hardly any difference in somatic complaints between the social classes. This change is difficult to explain without speculation, but somatic complaints are easier for family members and society to accept than psychological complaints (Böcker, 1978). Pfeiffer (1969) compared German and Indonesian patients and found a significantly higher frequency of ideas of poverty and ruin, guilt feelings, and the feeling of professional insufficiency in the former. Somatic complaints were reported by both groups at similar rates of frequency. These results support the view that though somatization has been shown to be a predominant symptom in non-Western societies it is also very common in the West (Kleinman and Kleinman, 1985).

At the beginning of this century, suicide rates for men were around 34 per 100,000 per year and approximately 10 per 100,000 for women. During the time of economic depression and high unemployment between 1929 and 1932, the number of suicides rose to 49 per 100,000 for males. Economic hardships, despair, and hopelessness seem to have been responsible for this increase. Though there is a high unemployment rate today, suicidal rates have not increased significantly, most probably because today's better social security system works as a prophylactic. Today, suicide rates are lower than before World War II, but since 1950 there has been a slight increase. In 1987 suicidal rates were 26.7 per 100,000 for men and 11.8 per 100,000 for women, a decrease in the differences between the genders. Most probably living conditions are becoming more similar for both groups. High rates of suicide show people suffering from affective disorders, alcoholism, and schizophrenia (Häfner and Pfeifer-Kurda, 1990). Another group that shows a very high rate of suicide are men older than 65 years, especially if they are single or widowed. The social isolation, social disintegration, and often the missing family in today's German society are reasons for this phenomenon.

SCHIZOPHRENIA

In Germany the incidence of schizophrenia has apparently not changed during the last decades (Meyer, 1973; Häfner, 1985), but subtypes are different today. In the former Federal Republic of Germany incidence rates of schizophrenia are around 0.5 to 0.7 (Häfner, 1987). During his journey to South East Asia in 1904, Kraepelin observed different symptomatology in schizophrenic patients in Java than in Germany. Compared to Germany, patients in Java exhibited less catatonic symptoms, systematic delusions, as well as acoustic hallucinations, and had a better outcome for dementia praecox. Sixty years later, Pfeiffer (1971)—who had extensive clinical experience in Indonesia as well as in Germany—reported that while catatonic symptoms had lost their importance in Germany they were still common in Indonesia. Similar observations were made by other German psychiatrists who had worked in non-Western societies (Wulff, 1967; Boroffka, 1984). In general an increase of the paranoid type can be observed in the Western world, while the catatonic type is decreasing (Murphy, 1982). This change in symptomatology was observed prior to the advent of neuroleptic drugs, and it might be attributed to different social and environmental conditions which are not yet well understood. Blankenburg and Zilly (1973) compared 227 case histories of schizophrenic patients who were admitted to psychiatric hospitals between 1800 and 1890 with 246 patients admitted between 1960 to 1965. They found that there was an enormous decrease in delusions of grandeur and religious delusions. The time of heroes and monarchs is obviously over and the influence of the churches is diminishing. Sexual and homosexual delusions increased, which can be due to fewer taboos regarding sexuality. Delusions of persecution and magicomythical delusions did not change in frequency over time. Delusions with technical contents showed a marked increase, according to Murphy (1982), this is merely a reflection of change in popular thought. Delusions concerning the possession of thoughts also showed an increase. Wulff (1967) provides a challenging explanation for this. He states that in our society systematized delusions and delusions concerning the possession of thoughts are so prominent because autonomy, individual self-realization, as well as acquiring and keeping private property are highly valued and stressed, whereas a society that lacks our Western individualized ego concept, but stresses group cohesiveness, will hardly show systematized delusions or delusions concerning the possession of thoughts.

While in Germany the cumulative lifetime risk for schizophrenia is equal in both genders, there is a difference in the time of onset for the disorder. In men the first psychotic symptoms appear at a mean age of 26.6 years, four to five years earlier than in women. After the onset of the disorder, hardly any of the patients get married (Riecher, Maurer, Löffler, Fätkenheuer, an der Heiden, Munk-Jorgensen, Strömgren, and Häfner, 1991).

The Bonn study (Huber, Gross, and Schüttler, 1979) revealed some important data about the outcome of schizophrenia in Germany. Findings from this 22.4-year follow-up study with 502 schizophrenic patients showed that 22 percent of the sample had recovered, 43 percent had improved, and that 35 percent did not improve. There were no symptoms or signs at the beginning of the disease which would permit a definite prognosis of good or bad outcome. Comparable results are reported from Switzerland (Bleuler, 1972; Ciompi and Müller, 1976).

In the industrial city of Mannheim, it was shown that an uneven ecological and social distribution of schizophrenics is due to a general trend of downward mobility (Häfner and an der Heiden, 1986). This trend is enhanced since society provides little decent housing and employment opportunities for chronic schizophrenic patients (Krahl, 1991). Today's nuclear families are often not able to care for their mentally ill family members. Many of the chronic schizophrenic patients have to live in large mental hospitals or in inadequate hostels (Kunze, 1981). Though in recent years there have been efforts to provide sheltered homes and apartments as well as job opportunities for the chronic mentally ill, only in a few models has the response been adequate (Empfehlungen der Expertenkommission, 1988).

ALCOHOLISM AND DRUG ABUSE

To drink alcohol, be it beer, wine, spirits, or other alcoholic beverages, is so much accepted and expected in German society, that someone who does not drink is conspicuous. There is hardly any opportunity where no alcoholic beverages are consumed be it in public, at home, or even at work. In Bavaria beer is sometimes called "fluid bread" and many people consider it not as an alcoholic drink but as food. While in 1950 the average consumption of alcohol per person was equivalent to 3.3 liters of pure alcohol there was a steady increase over the years which peaked in 1980 with 12.7 liters and it has stayed around 12 liters per year per person since then. The consumption reached similar levels in East and in West Germany (Feuerlein, 1984; Winter, 1991). About 21 percent of the adult population are abstainers or drink rarely; 80 percent drink daily or almost daily, 14 percent of men are heavy drinkers compared to 5 percent of the women. It is estimated that today 2 to 3 percent of the German population are alcoholics; that would mean that 1.6 to 2.4 million persons in reunited Germany and their families are suffering from this disorder (Ziegler, 1984; Winter, 1991). Since 1955 a six to eightfold increase in the number of alcohol dependent persons could be observed. Alcoholism is most common in the lower social classes among men aged 25 to 45 years (Dilling, 1986; Fichter, 1990).

Unemployment is seen as one of the causes of increased alcohol consumption. Another high risk group for alcohol abuse and dependency are young men in the German army where group pressure to drink is high (Renn, 1987). In the mid-1960s it was estimated that about 10 percent of the alcoholics were women, but this number grew and today 25 to 30 percent are thought to be women (Feuerlein, 1984). Women often combine the consumption of alcohol with tranquilizers and sedatives. Alcoholic women are often single, divorced, or widowed. While German society tolerates heavy drinking in men, it despises drunkenness and loss of control in women (Stein-Hilbers, 1984). As a consequence of rising female alcoholism, each year about 1800 children are born with fetal alcohol syndrome (FAS) in West Germany (Majewski, 1987).

In the last few decades another problem has emerged: dependency on analgesics, benzodiazepines, and other anxiolytic drugs. Experts estimate the number of dependent persons to be between 300,000 and 500,000 in West Germany (Ziegler, 1984). Women are overrepresented amongst them and in treatment centers the ratio is 9 to 1 (Helas, 1982).

Compared to alcohol, the consumption of illegal drugs involves a much smaller group—it is estimated that in West Germany 80,000 people are dependent on opiates (Leune, 1990). Until the mid-1960s cannabis, opiates, and cocaine posed a minor mental health problem. Then a sudden, sharp increase in the consumption of cannabis, LSD, and opiates was observed mainly in young people. At that time the West German economy was flourishing, while simultaneously youth unrest grew, and a conflict between generations was seen (Haring, 1973). A significant number of heroin addicts came from broken homes, had bad relationships with their fathers, failed at school, and had a tendency to run away (Welz, 1987). Since the early 1980s, there seems to be a decrease of consumption of drugs among adolescents, but first-time consumers of illegal drugs are noticeably younger (Thomasius, 1991). In recent years a new, severe problem emerged in the subculture of illegal drug users. It is estimated that 20 percent of intravenous drug users are HIV positive (Drogenreport, 1991).

MIGRANTS

With the rapidly growing demand for workers in the industrial centers of West Germany during the mid-1950s, guestworkers arrived from Greece, Italy, and Spain and later from Turkey and Yugoslavia. When these labor migrants came first to Germany it was neither their intention nor the government's that they should remain permanently. It was thought that after some time they would return to their country of origin (Heilig, Buttner, and Lutz, 1990). While in 1960 there were about 280,000 guestworkers, thirty years later this number had increased to over 2 million. Many of them were joined by family members and now over 5 million foreigners are residing in West Germany, accounting for nearly 8 percent of the total population. The largest group is constituted of Turkish people, with over 1.5 million citizens. Most of them come from rural areas, are Muslims, and are still very much embedded in their own culture—a sharp contrast to German society. Most of them are employed as unskilled or semi-skilled laborers (Statistisches Jahrbuch, 1990). The general opinion that migrants always suffer from an excess of mental disorders has already been rebutted by Murphy (1982). In a case register study in the industrial city of Mannheim, it was demonstrated that the rates of psychiatric morbidity among guestworkers was significantly lower for schizophrenia, alcohol-related diseases, and organic brain syndromes than in the German population (Häfner, 1980). This outcome is partly explained by the selection prior to migration, whereby only persons who were physically and psychologically fit get a work permit. Neurotic and psychosomatic disorders showed no marked difference in both populations. There are two high risk periods for migrants: shortly after migration and after a long time in the host country (Binder and Simoes, 1978). Cranach (1976) found that foreign workers develop schizophrenialike psychosis and affective illness demanding psychiatric admission mainly during their first year of stay and he interprets this finding in terms of the specific vulnerability of these persons. When guestworkers develop mental disorders, the following are seen as typical: hypochondriacal depressive syndromes, paranoid reactions, psychosomatic conditions, especially regarding the gastrointestinal tract, sexual dysfunctions, and sleep disorders (Böker, 1975).

The "Aussiedler," a special group of migrants, are ethnic Germans who lived, sometimes for generations, in Eastern and Southeastern Europe, and tried to keep their German language and culture and who returned to Germany. Between 1950 and 1988 2 million people returned to West Germany, and with the recent political changes in Eastern Europe this number was 377,000 in 1989, and the flow is continuing (Heilig et al., 1990). Coming to Germany, they face a reverse culture shock (Hertz, 1980). Many of them have an idealized and illusory image of today's Germany and they suffer from the fact that quite a number of West Germans view them as foreigners, a situation similar to that in their former host country. Difficulties in language, housing, employment, and finances contribute to acculturation problems (Hager and Wandel, 1978). Many of the returnees complain of loneliness, isolation, anonymity, coolness, and distance of today's German society (Lanquillon, 1982). Hardly any psychiatric research has been conducted amongst this group though higher rates of depression and neurotic disorders are suspected (Häfner, 1980). While surveying admissions to a psychiatric hospital, Stöckl-Hinke (1989) found that the commonest diagnoses among returnees were alcoholism and depressive disorders with paranoid symptoms.

THE FAMILY, THE YOUNG AND THE OLD

At the beginning of this century single-person households were rarely seen in Germany, whereas today about 35 percent of the adults in West Germany live on their own. These are results of various developments: the aging of the population, delayed marriage by the young, and an increase in marriage dissolutions (by divorce, separation, death of spouse). In 1988 more Germans divorced than married (Heilig et al., 1990). This does not mean that partnership and marriage are less valued. The opposite is true, the expectations toward partnership are so high that failure becomes more probable (Nave-Herz, 1989). One of the resulting psychosocial problems of divorce is that children whose parents are separated tend to develop more conduct disorders (Lempp, 1989).

Different epidemiological studies reveal that between 12 and 21 percent of all children and adolescents in Germany show psychological problems that need professional attention (Weyerer, Castell, Bieber, Artner, and Dilling, 1988; Remschmidt and Walter, 1990). An epidemiological field study done in a small-town rural area in Upper Bavaria examined 187 girls and 171 boys aged 3 to 14 years. The individuals comprised a representative random sample drawn from the residents' register. This study gave the following 1-year prevalence rates: 15.4 percent special syndromes (ICD 307) (in particular enuresis and encopresis); 2.8 percent emotional disorders (ICD 313); 0.8 percent neuroses (ICD 300); 0.6 percent social disorder (ICD 312); the categories psychosis (ICD 299), acute stress reactions (ICD 308), personality change with brain damage (ICD 310), and hyperkinetic syndrome (ICD 314) contributed each 0.3 percent (Weyerer et al., 1988).

Suicide rates in children aged 10 to 15 years varied in the years 1968 to 1985 between 60 to 110 cases but no trend toward an increase has been observed. There seems to be a slight increase in adolescent suicide (15–20 years), about 400 to 600 suicides in this age group each year were reported for West Germany (Nissen, 1989). An increase in anorexia nervosa has been observed during the last two to three decades, supposedly related to changes in the sociocultural setting and different family dynamics (Eggers and Esch, 1988).

The prevalence of child psychiatric disorders in children of migrants has been found to be similar to that in the German population (Lempp, 1989). The only exception is enuresis which shows a high prevalence in Turkish migrants, a phenomenon that has not yet been well explained (Steinhausen, Edinsel, Fergert, Gibel, Reister, and Rentz, 1990).

As in children, the care of the old is affected by changes in family patterns. While before 1900 most of the old lived with their children, today the elderly prefer to live on their own. Today in West Germany only 12 percent of women aged 70 to 74 live with their adult children. Only 34 percent of elderly women but 81 percent of elderly men live together with their spouses. The latter is the result of the fact that women marry at a younger age to men who are older; in addition, women have a life expectancy of 77.8 years compared to 71.3 years in men (Heilig et al., 1990).

In an epidemiological field study in an urban area (Mannheim) it was shown that the prevalence of psychiatric disorders in persons older than 65 years was around 24.4 percent and that this number increases with age (Cooper and Sosna, 1983). A similar prevalence rate in the elderly was found in the Upper Bavarian epidemiological field study (Dilling, Weyerer, and Castell, 1984). Cooper and Sosna (1983) found in the population older than 65 years that 6 percent showed a severe and 5.4 percent a mild organic brain syndrome. Neuroses and personality disorders appear in 10.8 percent, while 2.2 percent suffer from functional psychosis. They report that higher frequency of organic brain syndrome is observed in lower social classes. It was also shown that living in a single-person household does not automatically mean a higher psychiatric morbidity but that social isolation and physical illness result in a high rate of psychiatric disorders. Since, in general, families cannot and do not provide the care needed for the old, institutional care becomes more and more important. In the city of Mannheim where this evaluation took place, about 5 percent of the elderly population is living in residential care (Mann, Wood, Cross, Gurland, Schieber, and Hafner, 1984).

The percentage of psychiatric disorders grows rapidly with increasing age, thus gerontopsychiatric disorders will soon outnumber the other psychiatric disorders. The decent care of these persons will be one of the great challenges in the time to come.

REFERENCES

Ackerknecht, E. (1967), *Kurze Geschichte der Psychiatrie*. Stuttgart: Enke.

American Psychiatric Association (1980), *Diagnostic and Statistical Manual of Mental Disorders*, 3rd ed. (DSM-III). Washington, D.C.: American Psychiatric Press.

Bauer, M., & Engfer, R. (1990), Entwicklung und Bewährung psychiatrischer Versorgung in der Bundesrepublik Deutschland. In: *Psychiatrie im Wandel*, ed. A. Thom & E. Wulff. Bonn: Psychiatrie-Verlag, pp. 413–429.

Bericht über die Lage der Psychiatrie in der Bundesrepublik Deutschland. Deutscher Bundestag. Drucksache 7/4200 and 4201, Bonn (1975).

Binder, J., & Simoes, M. (1978), Sozialpsychiatrie der Gastarbeiter. *Fortschr. Neurol. Psychiatr.*, 46:342–359.

Blankenburg, W., & Zilly, A. (1973), Gestaltwandel im schizophrenen Wahnerleben. In: *Gestaltwandel psychiatrischer Krankheitsbilder*, ed. J. Glatzel. Stuttgart: Schattauer.

Bleuler, M. (1972), *Die schizophrenen Geistesstörungen im Lichte langjähriger Kranken- und Familiengeschichten.* Stuttgart: Thieme.

Bochnik, H. J., & Koch, H. (1990), *Die Nervenarzt-Studie, Praxen, Kompetenzen, Patienten.* Köln: Deutscher Ärzte-Verlag.

Böcker, F. (1978), Psychosomatische Beschwerden bei endogener Depression. *Psycho*, 4:478–479.

Bodamer, J. (1953), Zur Entstehung der Psychiatrie als Wissenschaft im 19. Jahrhundert. *Fortschr. Neurol. Psychiat.*, 21:511–535.

Böker, W. (1975), Psychiatrie der Gastarbeiter. In: *Psychiatrie der Gegenwart*, Vol. 3. Berlin: Springer.

Boroffka, A. (1984), Psychiatrie in tropischen Ländern. Paper presented at the Freien Universität, Berlin, November.

Bron, B., & Wetter-Parasie, J. (1989). Erscheinungswandel der endogenen Depression im höheren Lebensalter. *Fortschr. Neurol. Psychiat.*, 57:228–237.

Ciompi, L., & Müller, C. H. (1976), *Lebensweg und Alter der Schizophrenen. Eine katamnestische Langzeitstudie bis ins Senium.* Berlin: Springer.

Cooper, B., & Sosna, U. (1983), Psychische Erkrankungen in der Altenbevölkerung. *Nervenarzt*, 54:239–249.

Cranach, M. von (1976), Psychiatric disorders among foreign workers in the Federal Republic of Germany. Paper presented at the WPA-Symposium on Transcultural Psychiatry, Kiel.

Dilling, H. (1986), Epidemiologische Aspekte der Sucht—Zur Häufigkeit des Alkoholismus. In: *Das Verhältnis der Psychiatrie zu ihren Nachbardisziplinen*, ed. H. Heimann & H. J. Gaertner. Berlin: Springer.

——— Weyerer, S., & Castell, R. (1984), *Psychische Erkrankungen in der Bevölkerung.* Stuttgart: Enke.

Dörner, K. (1984), *Bürger und Irre*, 2nd ed. Frankfurt/M: EVA.

——— (1989), Nationalsozialismus und Lebensvernichtung. In: *Der Krieg gegen die psychisch Kranken*, ed. K. Dörner. Bonn: Psychiatrie Verlag.

Drogenreport 2 (1991), AIDS im vereinten Deutschland, pp. 16–26.

Eggers, C. H., & Esch, A. (1988), Krisen und Neurosen in der Adoleszenz. In: *Psychiatrie der Gegenwart 7, Kinder- und Jugendpsychiatrie.* Berlin: Springer.

Empfehlungen der Expertenkommission der bundesregierung zur Reform der Versorgung im psychiatrischen und psychotherapeutisch/psychosomatischen Bereich auf der Grundlage des Modellprogramms Psychiatrie der Bundesregierung (1988), Herausgegeben vom Bundesminister für Jugend, Familie, Frauen und Gesundheit, Bonn.

Feuerlein, W. (1984), *Alkoholismus—Missbrauch und Abhängigkeit: Entstehung—Folgen—Therapie,* 3rd ed. Stuttgart: Thieme.

Fichter, M. (1990), *Verlauf psychischer Erkrankungen in der Bevölkerung.* Berlin: Springer.

Griesinger, W. (1845), *Pathologie und Therapie der psychischen Krankheiten.* Stuttgart: Adolf Krabbe.

Häfner, H. (1980), Psychiatrische Morbidität von Gastarbeitern in Mannheim. *Nervenarzt,* 51:672–683.

——— (1985), Sind psychische Erkrankungen häufiger geworden? *Nervenarzt,* 56:120–133.

——— (1987), Epidemiology of schizophrenia. In: *Search for the Causes of Schizophrenia,* ed H. Häfner, W. F. Gattaz, & W. Janzarik. Berlin: Springer.

——— an der Heiden, W. (1986), The contribution of European case registers to research on schizophrenia. *Schizophr. Bull.,* 12:26–50.

——— Pfeifer-Kurda, M. (1990), Das kumulative psychiatrische Fallregister Mannheim. In: *Fortschritte in der psychiatrischen Epidemiologie,* ed. M. H. Schmidt. Weinheim: VCH.

Hager, B., & Wandel, F. (1978), Probleme der soziokulturellen Integration von Spätaussiedlern. *Osteuropa,* 28:193–207.

Haring, C. (1973), Wandel im Erscheinungsbild der Sucht. In: *Gestaltwandel psychiatrischer Krankheitsbilder,* ed. J. Glatzel. Stuttgart: Schattauer.

Heilig, G., Büttner, T., & Lutz, W. (1990), Germany's population: Turbulent past, uncertain future. *Population Bull.,* 45:3–43.

Helas, I. (1982), Zahlen zum Rauschmittelmißbrauch bei Frauen —Statistische Ergebnisse aus den Suchtberatungsstellen des Diakonischen Werkes. In: *Frau and Sucht, herausgegeben von der DHS.* Hamm: Hoheneck.

Hertz, D. G. (1980), Remigration: Psychische Probleme des Rückkehrers. In: *Psychopathologie im Kulturvergleich,* ed. W. M. Pfeiffer & W. Schoene. Stuttgart: Enke.

Huber, G., Gross, G., & Schüttler, R. (1979), Verlaufs- und sozialpsychiatrische Langzeituntersuchungen an den 1945–1959 in Bonn hospitalisierten schizophrenen Kranken. Berlin: Springer.

Jaeckel, M., & Wieser, S. (1970), *Das Bild des Geisteskranken in der Öffentlichkeit.* Stuttgart: Thieme.

Kimura, B. (1965), Vergleichende Untersuchungen über depressive Erkrankungen in Japan und in Deutschland. *Fortschr. Neurol. Psychiat.,* 33:202–215.

Kirfel, B. (1984), Heilkundige in der Eifel. *Curare,* 7:239–258.

Kleinman, A., & Kleinman, J. (1985), Somatization: The interconnections in Chinese society among culture, depressive experiences, and meanings of pain. In: *Culture and Depression,* ed. A. Kleinman & B. Good. Berkeley Los Angeles: University of California Press.

Korczak, D., & Pfefferkorn, G. (1983), Psychiatrie und öffentliche Meinung. In: *Psychiatrie und Massenmedien,* ed. V. Faust & G. Hole. Stuttgart: Hippokrates.

Kraepelin, E. (1904), Vergleichende Psychiatrie. *Centralblatt für Nervenheilkunde und Psychiatrie,* 27:433–437.

Krahl, W. (1991), Rehabilitation of chronic mental patients—A comparison between Malaysia and Germany. *Proc. of the 3rd ASEAN Congress on Psychiatry and Mental Health.* Kuala Lumpur: Malaysia Psychiatric Association, pp. 308–314.

Kunze, H. (1981), *Psychiatrische Übergangseinrichtungen und Heime.* Stuttgart: Enke.

Lamnek, S., & Tretter, F. (1991), Psychisch Kranke und Psychiatrie im Meinungsbild der Münchner. *Krankenhauspsychiatrie,* 2:1–5.

Lanquillon, W. (1982), Eingliederungsschwierigkeiten—Fakten und Gründe. In: *Politische Bildung mit Spätaussiedlern.* Schriftenreihe der Bundeszentrale für politische Bildung, 184:113–143.

Lauter, H., & Schön, W. (1967), Über den Gestaltwandel der Melancholie. Archiv für Psychiatrie und Zeitschrift f.d.ges. *Neurologie,* 209:290–306.

Lempp, R. (1989), Pathogenität bestimmter Sozialfaktoren. In: *Kinder- und Jugendpsychiatrie,* ed. C. H. Eggers. Berlin, Heidelberg, New York, London, Paris, Tokyo, Hong Kong: Springer.

Leune, J. (1990), Illegale Drogen. In: *Jahrbuch Sucht 1991, Deutsche Hauptstelle gegen die Suchtgefahren.* Hamburg: Neuland.

Lifton, R. J. (1986), *The Nazi Doctors.* New York: Basic Books.

Lungershausen, E. (1973), Überlegungen zum Problem des Gestaltwandels zyklothymer Depressionen. In: *Gestaltwandel psychiatrischer Krankheitsbilder,* ed. J. Glatzel. Stuttgart: Schattauer.

Majewski, F. (1987), Teratogene Schäden durch Alkohol. In: *Psychiatrie der Gegenwart 3, Abhängigkeit und Sucht.* Berlin: Springer.

Mann, A., Wood, K., Cross, P., Gurland, B., Schieber, P., & Häfner, H. (1984), Institutional care of the elderly: A comparison of the cities of New York, London and Mannheim. *Soc. Psychiatry,* 19:97–102.

Meyer, H. H. (1973), Zum Gestaltwandel schizophrener Psychosen. In:

Gestaltwandel psychiatrischer Krankheitsbilder, ed. J. Glatzel. Stuttgart: Schattauer.

Murphy, H. B. M. (1982), *Comparative Psychiatry: The International and Intercultural Distribution of Mental Illness*. Berlin: Springer.

Nave-Herz, R. (1989), Zeitgeschichtlicher Bedeutungswandel von Ehe und Familie in der Bundesrepublik Deutschland. In: *Nave-Herz, Handbuch der Familien- und Jugendforschung*, ed. M. Makefka. Neuwied Frankfurt: Luchterhand.

Nissen, G. (1989), Suizidversuche und Suizide. In: *Kinder- und Jugendpsychiatrie*, ed. C. H. Eggers. Berlin: Springer.

Payk, T. R. (1989), Von der Parapsychologie zur Parapsychotherapie. *Fundamenta Psychiatrica*, 3:165–168.

Peters, U. H. (1989), Emotionspsychopathologie: Zur Problemgeschichte eines Widerspruchs. In: *Schizoaffektive Psychosen Diagnose, Therapie und Prophylaxe*, ed. A. Marneros. Berlin: Springer.

Pfeiffer, W. M. (1969), Die Symptomatik der Depression in transkultureller Sicht. In: *Das depressive Syndrom*, ed. H. Hippius & H. Selbach. München. Urban und Schwarzenberg

——— (1971), *Transkulturelle Psychiatrie*. Stuttgart: Thieme.

——— (1984), Transkulturelle Aspekte der Depression. *Nervenheilkunde*, 3:14–17.

Räder, K. K., Krampen, G., & Sultan, A. S. (1990), Kontrollüberzeugungen Depressiver im transkulturellen Vergleich. *Fortschr. Neurol. Psychiat.*, 58:207–214.

Remschmidt, H., & Walter, R. (1990), Psychische Auffälligkeiten bei Schulkindern. *Z. Kinder-Jugendpsychiat.*, 18:121–132.

Renn, H. (1987), Prävention, Organisatorische und evaluative Aspekte. In: *Psychiatrie der Gegenwart 3, Abhängigkeit und Sucht*. Berlin: Springer.

Riecher, A., Maurer, K., Löffler, W., Fätkenheuer, B., an der Heiden, W., Munk-Jorgensen, P., Strömgren, E., & Häfner, H. (1991), Gender differences in age and onset and course of schizophrenic disorders. A contribution to the understanding of the disease? In: *Search for the Causes of Schizophrenia*, Vol. 2, ed. H. Häfner & W. F. Gattaz. Berlin: Springer.

Rosin, U., & Hammers, A. J. (1979), Parapsychologie, Okkultismus, Teufelsglauben, Besessenheit, Exorzismus und Wunder. In *Die Psychologie des 20. Jahrhunderts*, ed. G. Condrau. Zürich: Kindler.

Rudolph, E. (1977), *Die geheimnisvollen Ärzte. Von Gesundbetern und Spruchheilern*. Olten und Freiburg im Breisgau: Walter.

Ruppert, H. J. (1987), Neues Denken auf alten Wegen: New Age und Esoterik. In: *Die Rückkehr der Zauberer*, ed. H. J. Hemminger. Reinbek bei Hamburg: Rowohlt.

Schmidt, G. (1988), Das unerwünschte Buch. In: *Aktuelle Kernfragen in der Psychiatrie*, ed. F. Bîcker & W. Weig. Berlin: Springer.

Statistisches Jahrbuch (1990), *für die Bundesrepublik Deutschland*. Stuttgart: Metzler-Poeschel.

Steinhausen, H. C., Edinsel, E., Fergert, J. M., Gîbel, D., Reister, E., & Rentz, A. (1990), Child psychiatric disorders and family dysfunction in migrant workers' and military families. *Eur. Arch. Psychiatr. Neurol. Sci.*, 239:257–262.

Stein-Hilbers, M. (1984), Drogen im Leben von Frauen. In: *Band 26 der Schriftenreihe zum Problem der Suchtgefahren; herausgegeben von der Hauptstelle gegen die Suchtgefahren*. Hamm: Hoheneck.

Stöckl-Hinke, M. (1989), Mental health problems of "Aussiedler" from Eastern Europe. In: *Psychiatry Today. VIII World Congress of Psychiatry, Abstracts. Excerpta Medica International Congress Series 899*. Amsterdam, Oxford, New York.

Tellenbach, H. (1976), *Melancholie*, 3rd ed. Berlin: Springer.

Thom, A. (1990), Ethische Werte und moralische Normen sozialpsychiatrischen Handelns. In: *Psychiatrie im Wandel*, ed. A. Thom & E. Wulff. Bonn: Psychiatrie-Verlag.

Thomasius, R. (1991), Drogenkonsum und AbhÑngigkeit bei Kindern und Jugendlichen. Ein Überblick zum Forschungsstand. *Sucht*, 37:4–19.

Tretter, F. (1985), Verbindungswege zwischen psychisch Kranken und Offentlichkeit. *Deutsches érzteblatt*, 24:1835–1843.

Weissman, M. M., & Klerman, G. L. (1977), Sex differences and the epidemiology of depression. *Arch. Gen. Psychiatry*, 34:98–111.

Welz, R. (1987), Epidemiologie des Drogenmi·brauchs. In: *Psychiatrie der Gegenwart 3, Abhängigkeit und Sucht*. Berlin: Springer.

Weyerer, S., Castell, R., Bieber, A., Artner, K., & Dilling, H. (1988), Prevalence and treatment of psychiatric disorders in 3 to 14-year-old children: Results of a representative study in the small town rural region of Traunstein, Upper Bavaria. *Acta Psychiatrica Scand.*, 77:290–296.

Winter, E. (1991), Alkoholismus im Sozialismus der Deutschen Demokratischen Republik—Versuch eines Rückblickes. *Sucht*, 37:71–85.

Wulff, E. (1967), Psychiatrischer Bericht aus Vietnam. In: *Beiträge zur vergleichenden Psychiatrie*, Vol. 1, ed. N. Petrilowitsch. Basel: Karger.

Yang, H. (1989), Attitudes towards psychosis and psychotic patients in Beijing. *Internat. J. Soc. Psychiatry*, 35:181–187.

Ziegler, H. (1984), Sucht und Gesellschaft—Zur Situation in der Bundesrepublik Deutschland. In: *Band 26 der Schriftenreihe zum Problem der Suchtgefahren; herausgegeben von der Hauptstelle gegen die Suchtgefahren*. Hamm: Hoheneck.

18.

Modernization and Mental Illness in Greenland

Inge Lynge

The aboriginal people of precolonial Greenland were primarily Inuit (Eskimos). Most of their ancestors migrated from the Western Arctic about 1000 years ago, though the present population in the polar gateway, Thule, came as late as the eighteenth century. In East Greenland the Inuit may have mixed with an older population of the Dorset people. The language is Greenlandic, an *Inupiaq* (Alaskan Inuit) language with three main dialects: West, North, and East Greenlandic. The contemporary native Greenlandic population is mixed with Europeans. In West Greenland the ratio of Greenlandic to European genes is presently estimated to be 3 to 1, or 2 to 1 (Harvald, 1989). The admixture in North and East Greenland began much later and is much less; however, recent data are lacking on this.

The colonization of Greenland took place in three stages: (1) In Western Greenland the first Danish trade and mission station was established in 1721, and most of the sparse population was Christianized before the end of the century. (2) In Ammassalik, East Greenland, a rather isolated declining tribe was discovered in 1884. There had already been some migration to colonized West Greenland from the southern part of the east coast, and during the following years many Ammassalik Eskimos also moved south and west to take advantage of possibilities for trade. This migration was stopped and reversed ten years later, when a Danish/West Greenlandic trade and missionary station was established in Ammassalik. In 1923 all East Greenlanders were Christianized. (3) In Thule, North Greenland, a missionary station staffed by West Greenlanders was established in 1909 and a trading station in 1910. In the previous 20 years there had been contacts with whalers and explorers, first and foremost Robert Peary, who on many expeditions between 1892 and 1909 charted part of the area and searched for the geographic North Pole. He brought guns, domestic utensils, knives, and wood for sledgerunners, but the supplies were very unstable, thus endangering the Thule people who had become accustomed to the modern goods. On request from the local population the Danish explorer Knud Rasmussen founded the above-mentioned private trading station, after repeated appeals to the Danish government had failed.

In traditional Inuit society all illnesses were regarded as being caused by transmigration of souls. A soul could leave the physical body or a foreign soul could occupy it. The *angakkoq* (shaman) communicated with the spiritual world, found out what had gone wrong and gave prescriptions for the restoration of order. Sometimes, a transmigration might be diagnosed as the result of violation of a taboo, or in other cases as a result of sorcery. In the first case recovery was conditional on a complete confession. An *ilisiitsok* (witch or sorcerer) had supernatural power like the *angakkoq*, but unlike the latter the *ilisiitsok* operated in secret and destructively. Especially in the Ammassalik area *ilisiitsut* were very much feared, and people who behaved in an odd manner or lived in social isolation were often suspected of sorcery. Delirium was looked upon with great fear because it was suspected that the delirious person was a witch. Dangerously insane persons were abandoned, tied up, or sometimes killed. Glahn, a Danish missionary in West Greenland in the 1760s, notes: "Mad people are removed (from the house) or killed, not from cruelty, more from fear" (Glahn, 1921).

Information about the occurrence of mental illness in the precolonial and newly colonized societies in Greenland is scanty and rather casual. When Peary was a regular visitor to Thule he saw many cases of a dissociative-type reaction called *pibloktoq* or arctic hysteria (Brill, 1913). In Thule some occasions were especially known for triggering *pibloktoq*, for instance, being on Peary's ship in open sea and out of sight of land. In 1915, 16 out of the 216 lnuit in Thule district had frequent attacks of *pibloktoq* (Freuchen, 1915), but nowadays the syndrome is never reported. (For a more extensive treatment see Foulks, 1972).

While the art of shamanism was highly developed in East Greenland and life was imbued with fear of witches and evil spirits, life at that time was far more relaxed in Thule, North Greenland. Shamans had less power and fewer techniques than in East Greenland. Because of the relatively wealthy life there was not the same need for invocation of supernatural forces, and people had forgotten the art of their forefathers.

THE DEVELOPMENT OF MODERN PSYCHIATRY IN GREENLAND

In the late nineteenth century the Danish government developed a local health service, which eventually took responsibility for most disturbed patients. Yet in isolated areas there was no alternative in some cases to the traditional ways of managing dangerous situations. With the introduction of the Danish health service, European ideas about illness and diagnosis were imported. There has never been an attempt to combine traditional and modern ideas. Inuit concepts of illness were too intertwined with the religious ideas that were disparaged by practitioners of the new religion. Now people have moved too far away from Inuit traditions to make a rapprochement meaningful. In 1950 a large-scale and pervasive program of modernization was started in Greenland. Improvement of the health service was given high priority, and patients, including some who were mentally ill, were referred in increasing numbers to hospitals in Denmark.

Greenland now has 54,000 inhabitants, of whom 45,000 are native Greenlanders, living in 126 towns or villages, along a coast more than 4000 kilometers long. The general health service is organized into sixteen districts, each with a chief medical officer and a small district hospital. In the capital, Nuuk/Godthåb, a

TABLE 18.1
Psychiatric Admissions Per Year 1984–1988

Institutions	Average Number
In Greenland	
District hospitals	500
Queen Ingrid's Hospital / Psychiatr. Dept.	190
In Denmark	
Mental Hospitals	50
High Security Ward	3

Sources: Greenland Health Service and Institute of Psychiatric Demography, Århus, Denmark.
From I. Lynge (1991).

town of 13,000 inhabitants, Queen Ingrid's Hospital serves as district hospital and at the same time as central hospital for the whole country. The first psychiatric consultant at Queen Ingrid's Hospital was appointed twenty years ago, and in 1980 a psychiatric ward with twenty-five beds was established. This ward is not adapted to the long-term residence of severely disturbed patients. Patients in need of facilities not available in Nuuk are still referred to a Danish mental hospital. The Health Service, which up till now has been a Danish governmental responsibility, was taken over by the Greenlandic Home Rule government in January 1992.

THE ORGANIZATION OF PSYCHIATRIC SERVICES TODAY

Psychiatric treatment and care is offered on four levels: (1) The local primary health service, including district hospitals, with some supervision from the psychiatric service in Nuuk; (2) the psychiatric in- and outpatient service in Nuuk; (3) a mental hospital in Denmark; (4) a high-security ward in Denmark.

Table 18.1 indicates admission figures, and Table 18.2 beds in use in the four types of institutions. The delivery of psychiatric service to a population that is widespread and undergoing tremendous social changes is a great challenge. Reforms aiming at more emphasis on caretaking in the local community are planned. A precondition for successful transfer of the "heaviest" part of hospital treatment to Greenland is a well-trained staff, familiar with the Greenlandic language and ways of life. Many

TABLE 18.2
Beds in Use for Psychiatric Inpatients 1984–1988

Institutions	Average Number
In Greenland:	
District Hospitals	11
Queen Ingrid's Hospital/Psychiatr. Dept.	20
In Denmark:	
Mental Hospitals	24
High Security Ward	6

Sources: Greenland Health Service and Institute of Psychiatric Demography, Århus, Denmark.
From I. Lynge (1991).

norms and values, for instance, traditional ways of handling conflicts, are still at work even though their consequences are quite
different in today's pluralistic society. To take care of the most
seriously ill patients in Greenland in all phases of their illness will
also demand special mental resources in order to contain and
confront the overwhelming emotions that are often exposed by
these patients. The traditional strategies of noninterference or
expulsion are no longer adequate. The psychiatric service should,
however, be careful not to push but to support necessary developments. A main task is the encouragement and education of more
native Greenlanders to join the staff.

EPIDEMIOLOGY OF MENTAL ILLNESS

Our knowledge of the epidemiology of mental illness in Greenland is derived mainly from health service statistics and is insuffi-
cient. The World Health Organization's (WHO's) international
classification (ICD-8) is used, and the common diagnoses of organic and functional psychoses, neuroses and personality disorders are applied without special difficulties. The figures for all
admissions (Table 18.3) suggest certain differences between the
sexes: far more admissions for schizophrenia among men and
more for manic–depressive psychosis among women. No cases of
eating disorders such as bulimia and anorexia nervosa have been
met with. Puerperal psychoses seem to be uncommon. The preponderance of male schizophrenia is confirmed in an ongoing

TABLE 18.3

**All Admissions in the Five Years 1984–1988 to Psychiatric Institutions
in Greenland and Denmark of Patients from Greenland**

Diagnosis	Male	Female
Schizophrenia	161	47
Manic-Depressive Psychoses	35	66
Organic Psychosis	15	12
Reactive Psychosis	64	75
Not Classifiable Psychosis	25	21
All Psychoses	300	221
Neuroses	18	68
Personality Disorder	75	77
Alcoholism	120	112
Other	82	109
Neurotic States	295	366
All Admissions	595	587
Yearly Admissions per 1000 inhab>/15 years old	5.3	6.4

Source: Institute of Psychiatric Demography, Århus, Denmark.

(not yet published) follow-up study of first-admissions, which has found a yearly incidence among males of 33.7 and among females 15.6 per 100,000 above 15 years of age. The rates of inpatients, divided by age groups, from Greenland in psychiatric institutions in Greenland and Denmark (district hospitals not included) are seen in Table 18.4 (Lynge, 1991). The corresponding figures for inpatients from all Denmark is also shown. Compared to Denmark, more young and fewer older people from Greenland are psychiatric inpatients. Most are males and about 25 percent are forensic cases, which explains the rather heavy use of the high security ward indicated in Table 18.2.

CULTURE-SPECIFIC SYNDROMES AND CHANGES THEREIN, FOLLOWING SOCIAL AND CULTURAL CHANGES

Today the term *pibloktoq* (mentioned in the introduction) is an obsolete term for humans in West Greenland. It has become a derogatory term for a mad dog. In former days when an individual

TABLE 18.4
Prevalence of Psychiatric Inpatients

Age	Greenland* per 10,000	Denmark** per 10,000
15–24	10.2	6.2
25–44	20.2	13.1
45–64	13.7	18.2
65–	8.4	47.5

* Greenland: Average of 5 cross-sectional surveys 1984–1988.
** Denmark: Cross-sectional survey on February 27, 1985.
Source: Institute of Psychiatric Demography, Århus, Denmark.
From I. Lynge (1991).

permanently left society in anger to live alone, tradition said that he was transformed into a ghost, a *qivittoq*. Even today the old fear of *qivittut* can lurk, when people disappear without leaving traces (as in some fatal accidents at sea). Thus a woman in deep depression "confessed" that she had supported a *qivittoq* with food. The idea of *qivittut* was pervasive among West Greenlandic Inuit and might have served as a strong warning against separation. In West Greenland there seem to have been an increasing number of runaways in the colonial period.

Whereas *pibloktoq* and *qivittoq* are feared and repellent conditions, another culture-specific syndrome is apparently accepted without connotations of shame: *nangiarneq* (anxiety in kayaks and at the edge of abysses). *Nangiarneq* is a phobic state that was known (and named) in West Greenland before colonization, but which may have been rather infrequent in those days. The first missionaries and traders do not mention it as a problem. At the end of the nineteenth century, however, it had developed into a widespread disorder, afflicting 11 to 15 percent of active hunters in the districts of West Greenland. Bertelsen (1940) gives a very detailed account and based on that, Gussow (1963) indicates the similarity of the kayak anxiety with the anxiety that overcomes jet pilots, who are also alone under conditions in which sensory inputs are very few. Gussow sees kayak anxiety as an indication of a general Eskimo type of response and adaptation to stress, namely withdrawal. A common element of intentional social withdrawal is found in kayak anxiety, going *qivittoq* and suicide, whereas in *pibloktoq* the withdrawal is unconscious, taking the mind on a trip for a time and forgetting. It was suggested that when anxiety could not be handled with support from the group and when anger could not be expressed openly, there were few alternatives to withdrawal. The cultural and religious blank space, which was left by the collapse of the pagan defenses against anxiety (rule-governed behavior, use of amulets, etc.) might explain the increase in *qivittoq* behavior, *pibloktoq*, and first and foremost *nangi-arneq*. As for suicide, the utmost consequence of withdrawal, the course has been otherwise: In traditional society suicide was accepted, could even be approved of in certain circumstances, for example, in the case of old age, illness, or other conditions that made the person a burden to society. But when the Christian view was adopted, that life and death belong to God, suicide became a sin. So in the colonial era, the suicide rate was very low (3 to 4 per 100,000 per year) (Bertelsen, 1935). But in the last twenty to thirty years of rapid social change, suicide rates have increased immensely, especially among young men, who now have rates up to 500 to 600 per 100,000. The highest rates are found in East and North Greenland and in the capital Nuuk (Bjerregaard, 1991), that is, in the areas that were colonized first and latest (Lynge, 1985; Thorslund, 1990). When settlement types are compared, the picture is quite complex, but there are great differences between districts. A controlled study in Nuuk found that suicidal acts were correlated with emotional conflicts with close relations, and with disharmonious parental homes, characterized by alcohol abuse. Suicide victims themselves often abused alcohol (Grove and Lynge, 1979). Violence and homicide have also increased dramatically and again alcohol is implicated.

In a field study in Umanak in 1949 including 1003 persons 6 years old or more, Ehrstrøm saw no psychoses, but neuroses, mainly of the hysteric or phobic type, were not infrequent. Psychophysiological disorders were rare among those who were living in a traditional manner but were rather common among those Greenlanders who lived and worked in the colony, in contact with the mode of life and thought of Western civilization. Various reasons for these findings were discussed, for instance the fact that a certain verbal ability is obligatory in psychosomatic cases. Thus partially trained persons, who have a greater capacity to express themselves in words, are in a tautological way more apt to show psychosomatic disturbances. Ehrstrøm also found that contact with Europeans had created a feeling of inferiority, especially on the part of the population that lived nearest to Europeans (Ehrstrøm, 1951). A similar finding is reported from Alaska, where a survey of treated mental disorders in Native Alaskans in 1968 indicated frequent psychophysiological disorders among Southeast Alaskan Indians, who also lived in larger urban areas in close contact with the white world (Foulks, 1972).

SEX DIFFERENCES IN TRADITIONAL SOCIETY, AS WELL AS THE EFFECTS OF RECENT CHANGES IN SEX ROLES ON MENTAL ILLNESS

In traditional Greenlandic society the roles of the sexes were very well defined. Skilled hunters had high status and women were totally dependent on them as providers. But hunters also depended on efficient wives, and a well-balanced relationship between husband and wife was possible. Male children were brought up as future providers. Traditional upbringing with its deep concern for the process of socialization was molded for life in the homogeneous small-group society, where people grew into their preformed adult roles (Briggs, 1970, 1990). In a modern pluralistic society the roles are not laid down in the same way, but are created over a lifetime. Whereas in the traditional society the identity was deeply rooted in the group, individualism is now growing, and questions about personal identity become important.

In modern Greenlandic society there is still a tendency to adore the male child, but as he grows up, his status is reduced. Female emancipation has been quite successful. Society has become very complicated and in need of highly educated professionals, far more than the society itself can produce in spite of the advanced educational programs that are now available. Better jobs are still in Danish hands, often those of single males. Thus the situation is highly stressful, especially for young Greenlandic men.

FUTURE DIRECTIONS OF PSYCHIATRIC RESEARCH

Mental health problems cause much pain in contemporary Greenland. In the process of modernization the gap between those who can take advantage of the new challenges and those who fail to do so is increasing. High alcohol consumption, high rates of male suicide and homicide, violence, and sexual abuse are strong indicators of societal distress. But also more strictly psychiatric phenomena such as the rather high rates of hospitalized schizophrenia, especially among men, claim our attention. Greenland has a well-established national register of demography, and in the small local communities there is a high degree of personal knowledge, so the preconditions for basic psychiatric research on incidence, forms, and course of mental illness in various areas and among various groups are fair. The different socioeconomic conditions in the various districts and their varying histories of acculturation make fruitful soil for sociopsychological as well as biological psychiatric research.

SUMMARY

There are many indicators that mental illness is a major health problem in today's Greenland. The colonization and christianization of West Greenland in the eighteenth century and East and North Greenland in the beginning of this century initially alleviated the poverty and kept the family structure and the small-group society rather stable. But from different causes the traditional way of life gradually broke down. Climatic changes made the seal vanish and it was replaced by the cod. Impoverishment and increasing ill-health, above all high rates of tuberculosis, followed. After the Second World War a large-scale program of modernization was developed with the ultimate aim of building a fishing industry and a self-supporting modern economy. In the wake of the cash economy, family and societal structure has disintegrated with serious consequences, especially for the young men, who today have soaring rates of suicide, homicide, and alcohol problems. Psychiatric morbidity is high, and the Greenlandic

Home Rule Government, which recently has taken over responsibility for the health service, is faced with a huge task, demanding not only financial support, but maybe first of all an improvement of the general public's awareness of the field of mental hygiene.

REFERENCES

Bertelsen, A. (1935), Grønlands medicinsk Statistik og Nosografi. *Meddelelser om Grønland*, Reitzel, København, 117:58–65. English Summary.

———— (1940), Grønlands Medicinsk Statistik og Nosografi. *Meddelelser om Grønland*, Reitzel, København, 117:181–190. English Summary.

Bjerregaard, P. (1991), Disease pattern in Greenland. *Arctic Med. Res.*, 4:40–41.

Briggs, J. (1970), *Never in Anger*. Cambridge, MA: Harvard University Press.

———— (1990), Playwork as a tool in the socialization of an Inuit child. *Arctic Med. Res.*, 49:34–38.

Brill, A. A. (1913), Pibloktoq or hysteria among Peary's Eskimos. *J. Nerv. & Mental Disease*, 40:514–520.

Ehrstrøm, M. C. (1951), Medical investigation in North Greenland 1948–49. *Acta Psychiat. Scand.*, 4:254–264.

Foulks, E. F. (1972), The arctic hysterias of the North American Eskimo. In: *Anthropological Studies* #10, ed. D. H. Maybury-Lewis. Washington DC: American Anthropological Association.

Freuchen, P. (1915), Om Sundhedstilstanden blandt Polareskimoerne (On the condition of health among the Polar Eskimoes) (in Danish) Ugeskr laeger: 1089.

Glahn, H. C. (1921), *Missionær i Grønland Henric Christopher Glahns dagbøger for årene 1763–64, 1766–67, or 1767–68* (The Diaries of Missionary in Greenland: Henric Christopher Glahn). Det grønlandske selskabs skrifter. In: *GEC Gad København*, ed. H. Ostermann. Copenhagen: Greenlandic Society, GEC Gad.

Grove, O., & Lynge, I. (1979), Suicide and attempted suicide in Greenland. A controlled study in Nuuk. *Acta Psychiat. Scand.*, 60:375–391.

Gussow, Z. (1963), A preliminary report of kayak-angst among the Eskimos of West Greenland: A study in sensory deprivation. *Internat. J. Soc. Psychol.*, 9:18–26.

Harvald, B. (1989), Epidemiology of Greenland. *Arctic Med. Res.*, 48:171–174.

Lynge, I. (1985), Suicide in Greenland. *Arctic Med. Res.*, 40:53–60.

————— (1991), Mental health problems and services in Greenland. In: *Proceedings of the Eighth International Congress on Circumpolar Health,* ed. B. D. Postl. Canada: University of Manitoba Press.

Thorslund, J. (1990), Inuit suicides in Greenland. *Arctic Med. Res.*, 49:25–33.

19.

Culture and Mental Illness in the Iberian Peninsula

A. Seva and A. Fernandez-Doctor

Spain and Portugal are in a unique cultural situation, forming a bridge between the Southern European countries and those South American countries which were formerly their colonies. Thus, there are certain similarities between some psychological and psychopathological signs and symptoms in both Iberians and Ibero-Americans, which are also similar to those found among the other European Mediterranean races.

Spain's contribution to the development of psychiatry has been considerable, particularly regarding the treatment of the mentally ill. Muslim influence in the Peninsula was of great importance, and their methods for the treatment of mad people can be seen as far back as 1367 when Mohamed V founded the first psychiatric hospital in Granada (Spain). Shortly afterwards, in 1409, King Martin the Humane established the first Christian hospital in Valencia (Spain) mainly due to the efforts of Father Gilbert Jofré who belonged to the Order of Our Lady of Mercy. In 1425 in Saragosse (Spain) a general hospital was founded, which included a psychiatric department. This was the Royal and General Hospital of Our Lady of Grace, whose care and treatment, and above all, the occupational therapies, influenced Philip Pinel's reorganization of French psychiatry following the French Revolution.

Early in the fifteenth century, several psychiatric hospitals were set up in the Peninsula and various countries in America, along humanitarian lines. At about that time, the great mystic and humanitarian, St. John Of God (1495–1550), who was born in Portugal, was inspired to found hospitals in Spain, Germany, and France. In Portugal, however, psychiatric services were established at a later date, and in 1539, mentally ill patients were already being treated in Todos Los Santos Hospital in Lisbon. Scientific psychiatry appeared in Portugal in 1883, with the setting up of the Asilo de Alienados Conde Ferreira in Oporto (Fernandes de Fonseca, 1984).

At present, Spain has some 40,000 psychiatric beds, of which about 55 percent come under regional and provincial government, and 27 percent belong to the Catholic Church, 12 percent are private, 5 percent come under the Ministry of Health, and 0.5 percent under the Ministry of Justice. Only 3,000 beds are to be found in general hospitals and the rest are in large psychiatric hospitals, about half of which were built nearly 100 years ago.

The ratio of beds per 1000 inhabitants is 1.26 but their utilization is low as the ratio of patients per bed over 12 months is 1.29 and the ratio of personnel to bed is 0.3 over the whole country, dropping to 0.16 for hospitals run by the county councils and religious orders. Standards are higher in the psychiatric departments of general hospitals, with 7.7 patients per bed and year.

The new Health Law, which included psychiatric reform, came into force in the 1980s in the various Spanish regions. The main idea behind this law was to decentralize psychiatric care by means of regional mental health centers.

Furthermore, the setting up of acute psychiatric beds in general hospitals is encouraged, and at the same time the number of beds for chronic patients in the old psychiatric hospitals has been reduced. Creation of day hospitals and centers is also encouraged, together with supported housing, and at the same time an attempt is being made to integrate psychiatric attention and care within the area of general medicine. Even today there is a great deal of resistance to this reform; there are also economic difficulties in implementing changes.

Beginning in the 1960s Portugal began to see a change in the type of patient care previously available. Until then the greater part of care was centered in the Julio de Matos hospital in Lisbon, in the Sobral Cido hospital in Coimbra, and in the Magalhaes Lemos hospital in Oporto. The setting up of the Instituto de Asistencia Psiquiatrica following the new Law of July 25, 1958, meant a reactivation of psychiatric care through the creation of dispensaries and mobile psychiatric terms. It was not until the 1974 Revolution, however, that an attempt was made to integrate all psychiatric care within the community. At present, as pointed out by Fernandes da Fonseca (1984), the demand for psychiatric consultations has increased to such an extent that one quarter of the population of Portugal makes use of such services. The total coverage of psychiatric care by social security, the great increase in stressful situations, and the increased life span are the factors contributing to this new situation.

EPIDEMIOLOGY OF MENTAL ILLNESS AND SOCIOCULTURAL CHANGES

The first community survey in the Peninsula was probably that carried out on the island of Formentera, the most notable features being the frequency of alcoholism in men and of neuroses in women. Epidemiological investigations on alcoholism are the most frequent, due to the grave problem this represents in our society.

The Iberian countries have traditionally been noted for emigration, first to Latin America, Africa, and Asia, and then, during the 1970s, to central and northern Europe. Furthermore, it was during this period that an intense internal migration took place from rural to urban areas. If we add to this the importance of the tourist industry, which brings millions of foreigners each year to the Peninsula, it is understandable how traditional cultural norms have changed radically. We have seen this in our studies carried out in Castilla (Seva and Civeira, 1982) and in the town of Saragosse (Seva, 1983). Great changes have been detected in family size and structure, and at the same time a breakdown in traditional ways of solving conflicts. We very frequently find depressive and anxious disorders among housewives who are working in unskilled jobs and who have a low educational level. They experience difficulties in adaptation after migrating to towns, and some have suffered affective deprivation in childhood.

Epidemiological studies carried out in rural areas show excessive psychiatric pathology when isolation and consanguinity increase. In Galicia, various authors such as Diaz-Fernandez and Gestal-Otero (1987) studied the prevalence of some disorders in rural areas, and found high rates of mental deficiency in those mountain areas which were most isolated geographically and where there was a high degree of inbreeding. Within an urban population such as Saragosse (Seva, 1990) the following psychiatric pathology had already been detected by means of a two-phase investigation (General Health questionnaire and Clinical Interview Schedule) carried out under the Samar Project-89: dysthymic disorders 2.1 percent; alcoholism 1.9 percent, anxiety disorders 1.95 percent, disorders of adaptation 1.16 percent; depressive disorders 1.1 percent; personality disorders 0.9 percent; dementia 0.6 percent; schizophrenia 0.2 percent; mental retardation 0.2 percent. General psychiatric morbidity showed an overall prevalence of 11.8 percent, which is seen to be slightly lower than that found in the rural environment of Cinco Villas using the same methodology.

Internal migration, especially from Andalucia to Cataluña, was studied from a transcultural point of view by Rojo (1960). Using an analysis of local myths and legends, Rojo found the Granadians to be imbued with a sense of mystery and magical modes of thinking related to important Arab influences occurring up to the late fifteenth century, which is not found among the more realistic Catalonians, and this was reflected in their respective psychopathologies (there were more themes of magical influence and bewitchment states in the symptoms of Granadians).

Rendueles-Olmedo and Franco-Vicario (1976) also studied the appearance of psychotic episodes among rural emigrants going from Andalucia to Catalonia. These began with digestive disorders, followed by psychomotor agitation, anxiety, depersonalization, and an incapacity to differentiate between reality and fantasy. These clinical pictures are thought to be produced by a hypersensitivity to the new cultural conditions together with great difficulty in adapting to them. These cases showed a complete cure with treatment or on return to the south.

Rojas and Rojo (1962) pointed out that Spanish emigrants to Germany, by comparison with other migrant groups, were particularly prone to delusions regarding poison and sexual infidelity. They discussed in passing the cultural basis for these delusions, commenting that in Germany, rural Spanish migrants are confronted by striking cultural contrasts in social and dietary habits and greatly increased sexual freedom. As with other emigrants, they note that repatriation was the best medicine for such patients.

In Spain, the possibilities of carrying out comparative ethnic or religious studies were minimal as there were no racial or religious divergences of any importance in our territory. Only the gypsy population has been the object of occasional analysis and studies by means of the Rorschach test (Morales, Sanchez, Serrat, Civeira, and Jauregui, 1981) and form the most practical angle of attempting to assess the effect of the marginal economic status of the group and the irregular education on the mental health of children (Civeira, 1981). Belief in the evil eye as a cause of illness persists especially among gypsies and rural populations.

One of the most relevant phenomena of change in psychiatric diagnoses in the Spanish cultural environment is that neuroses have decreased in favor of depressive syndromes. To this should be added the changes encountered in the consumption of alcohol, which has changed from being almost exclusively drunk on a daily basis, as is usually in Mediterranean countries, to an excessive intake at the weekends, thus following the pattern of Anglo-Saxon and Northern European countries. Women also have greatly increased their alcohol intake, thus causing an increase in female alcoholism beginning in the 1960s. In Portugal, Ferreira (1976) dealt with these alcohol related problems some years ago. In hospitalizations, the percentage of patients with schizophrenia and organic dementia is declining and that of alcoholics is rising.

Sexual differences are steadily decreasing in our cultural environment and this is accompanied by similarity of psychopathological experiences which some years ago were peculiar to men or women. This occurred in the case of alcoholism, which affects 9 percent of the population, and at present the proportion of female to male alcoholism has changed from 1:9 in 1954 to 1:4

in 1976 (Alonso-Fernandez, 1976). Seva and Sarasola (1991) detected an excessively high ratio of male/female consumption of 28 to 1 in the rural area of Cinco Villas which, curiously enough, becomes 7 to 1 on weekends, thus demonstrating that women show an extraordinary increase in their alcohol intake at the weekend.

Regarding suicide and attempted suicide, an important change has again been seen, so that, as pointed out by Castro and Martins (1987) since 1977, in Portugal, the rates have risen for all age groups of those still professionally active. On the other hand, suicide attempts and anorexia nervosa, which were almost exclusively found in women, are now also found in men.

The increasing number of women in psychiatric epidemiological studies with anxiety and depressive disorders, is balanced by including alcoholism, where the number of men is greater. And this would be even greater if we included the hospitalized psychiatric population and those carrying out delinquent acts as a consequence of their psychiatric illness, where the number of men is found to be higher.

In Spain, dedication to child psychiatric problems goes right back to the beginning of this century, with the main interest being centered on psychometric studies in schools. Moreover, child psychiatry developed much more under the influence of psychiatry than under the influence of pediatrics. Protection of mentally retarded children, which reached its culmination in the 1960s, took up a great part of public and private activity. Child psychiatry does not exist as an independent specialty in Spain, however, though there are many psychiatrists, psychologists, and pediatricians who are active in this field, where the most common problems are "school failure," lack of adaptation in school and family, drug addictions, and anorexia.

In some areas, such as those studied by Oliveras (1989) in Alicante Province (Alto Vinalopó), the idea of the "evil eye" is accepted by 30 percent of the population, and obviously the "healers" or "bonesetters or quacks" are those asked to treat these patients. Furthermore, Oliveras showed, in his investigation, that a quarter of the patients attending a mental health center in this area had visited a "healer" in the first phase of their illness, and 8.6 percent continued to visit them.

PROGNOSIS AND THE EFFECTS OF PSYCHIATRIC TREATMENT

The prognosis of mental illness in the Iberian Peninsula has improved enormously over the last thirty years, thanks to the new psychopharmacological treatments and also to the psychiatric care network. As earlier doctors, and more recently Ruiz-Ripoll (1990) pointed out, however, the "new chronics" constitute a serious problem in spite of the many preventive measures which are underway.

Moreover, the poorly coordinated "psychiatric reform" which was put into practice in the 1980s, based on the idea of closing psychiatric hospitals without setting up other methods of care and attention (day centers, day hospitals, therapeutic apartments, psychiatric units in general hospitals, rehabilitation centers, ctc.), has created situations which are extremely difficult for some patients and their families, who find themselves suddenly forced to adapt to the new situation, with little or no economic, therapeutic, or rehabilitative support.

Therapy for the mentally ill is based on psychopharmacological treatments, whereas psychotherapy takes a very secondary place and is mainly within the framework of private medicine. The actual dosage of neuroleptics, tranquilizers, or antidepressants utilized in each case, and likewise the secondary effects are similar to those encountered in other European countries. We have been unable to find any significant differences in any of the international multicenter psychopharmacological investigations in which Spain participated together with other hospitals in Western Europe.

REFERENCES

Alonso-Fernandez, F. (1976), *Fundamentos de la Psiquiatria actual.* Madrid: Paz Montalvo.

Castro, E. F. de, & Martins, I. (1987), The role of female autonomy in suicide among Portuguese women. *Acta Psychiat. Scand.*, 75:337–343.

Civeira, J. M. (1981), Experiencia de investigacion sanitaria psiquiatrica en una poblacion marginada ne niños gitanos. *Comunicación Psiquiatrica*, 8:175–185.

Diaz-Fernandez, F., & Gestal-Otero, J. J. (1987), The influence of habitat on the prevalence of mental handicap. *Internat. J. Epidemiol.*, 16/1:52–56.

Fernandes da Fonseca, A. (1984), Evolución de la salud mental en Portugal. *Rev. Depto. Psiqu. Fac. Med. Barcelona*, 11:373–382.

Ferreira, A. G. (1976), Alcoholism in Portugal. *Internat. J. Ment. Health*, 5:63–73.

Morales, C., Sanchez, A., Serrat, D., Civeira, J. M., & Jauregui, J. (1981), Un estudio de población gitana a traves del test de Rorschach. *Comunicación Psiquiatrica*, 8:41–51.

Oliveras, M. A. (1989), Los modelos y la conducta de enfermedad en la poblacion psiquiatrica de la comarca del Alto Vinalopo. Doctoral dissertation. University of Alicante.

Rendueles-Olmedo, G., & Franco-Vicario, J. M. (1976), Episodes of transient delirium in Andalusian immigrants to Cataluna. *Rev. Psiq. y Psic. de Eur. y Amer. Lat.*, 12/6:365–374.

Rojas, L., & Rojo, M. (1962), Sindromes mas frecuentes observados en los emigrantes. Actas del VII Congreso de Neuropsiquiatria. Pamplona, Departamento de Psiquiatria. Typescript.

Rojo, M. (1960), Estudio de los estratos socitimicos catalan y granadino por el metodo de las leyendas. Paper presented at Libro de Actas del VII Congreso Nacional de Neuropsiquiatria. Barcelona, Departamento Universitario de Psiquiatria.

Ruiz-Ripoll, I. (1990), New chronics. *Brit. J. Psychiat.*, 156:447–448. (Special Issue: Cross-cultural psychiatry.)

Seva, A. (1983), El alma del asfalto. La salud mental en la población urbana de Zaragoza. Zaragoza, Excmo. Ayuntamiento y Universidad de Zaragoza.

———— (1990), La Salud mental de los aragoneses y su asistencia. Paper presented at the Real Academia de Medicina (Distrito de Zaragoza). Zaragoza, Real Academia de Medicina de Zaragoza.

———— Civeira, J. M. (1982), Analisis higienico sanitario de la salud mental de Soria. Soria, Excma. Diputación Provincial.

———— Sarasola, A. (1992), Epidemiologia psiquiatrica en la comarca rural de las Cinco Villas de Zaragoza (Proyecto SAMAR-89). Zaragoza, Diputación General de Aragon. Colección El Cierzo.

PART VI

Eastern Europe

20.

Culture, Politics, and Mental Illness in the Czech and Slovak Republics

Ctirad Skoda

There is a long history of mental health care and education in the former Czechoslovakia (CSFR). In 1886, Czech psychiatry started its scientific and pedagogical development in the newly founded Psychiatric Department of the Czech University School of Medicine in Prague. From the beginning, psychiatry and neurology developed independently. Until the end of World War I the territories of both republics were parts of the Austro-Hungarian Empire. The Czech lands belonged to industrial Austria and Slovakia to feudal Hungary. Mental health care was mostly to be found in inpatient treatment facilities. Those in the Czech region were built according to the Austrian model (large mental asylums located primarily outside of larger towns or in the country), whereas in Slovakia they followed the historical trend of Hungary to form psychiatric departments as integral parts of general hospitals which served administrative areas. Most of these psychiatric beds were concentrated around the Hungarian capital of Budapest. The end of World War I brought the separation of Slovakia

All figures in this chapter are based on data published in UZIS yearbooks or archived there as computer printouts.

Acknowledgment is due to Eva Dragomirecka, Ph.D., for all her stimulating technical help in manuscript preparation.

291

from Hungarian rule and the few remaining Slovak psychiatric asylums were damaged or destroyed during World War II. As a result of these separate histories, the Czech and Slovak republics have shown substantial differences in the structure of their inpatient psychiatric facilities. These differences are reflected in the proportions of psychiatric beds located in general hospitals and the number of beds per 100,000 inhabitants (see Table 20.1). After World War II, especially during the 1960s and 1970s, there was a general increase in the availability of outpatient psychiatric services (Table 20.1).

The concepts used in classification, treatment, and rehabilitation of mental disorders were those of the German and Swiss psychopathology schools, and the French rehabilitation and resocialization models. These concepts prevailed until the past three decades, when the influence of the Leningrad and Moscow schools of psychiatry were accepted and incorporated into the practice of Czech and Slovak psychiatry. Ten-yearly revisions of ICD (WHO) were widely used, complemented by the rising interest in DSM-III and DSM-III-R (APA, 1980, 1987) in recent years as diagnostic tools.

SOME EPIDEMIOLOGICAL DIFFERENCES

Mental Morbidity and Mental Health Care Consumption

The main problems faced by CSFR psychiatry in recent decades were the same as those declared by the European WHO Office in Copenhagen as problems all European WHO member states have to face. These problems include the aging of the population and an associated rise in risk of mental disturbance with age, an epidemiclike rise in alcohol dependence and abuse, abuse of other psychoactive substances, the hidden psychiatric morbidity in general practice and primary care, need of internationally comparable psychiatric information systems.

These are especially evident from the time series of average daily sick leave from work per 1000 insured employed inhabitants (Fig. 20.1). These series are based on the examination of a 20

Figure 20.1 Average Daily Sick Leave Per 1000 Insured
(ICD 290 to 318 Diagnostic Subgroups)

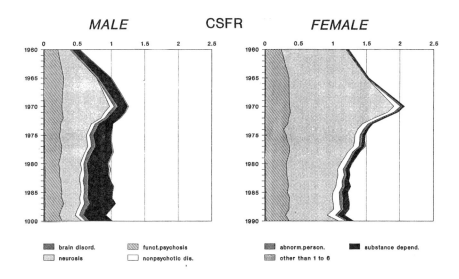

From 1989, agriculture cooperatives are included
Source: Sick Leave Yearbook, UZIS Prague and Bratislava

percent sample of all administrative forms which declared patients incapable for work during the calendar year. These forms
include the ICD diagnosis and must be signed by a physician.
Analysis of these statistical data shows that average daily sick leave
(ADSL) due to neurosis has decreased in both genders since
1970. In males, however, this decrease is outweighed by a conspicuous ADSL rise in substance abuse, dependence, and their psychotic complications. In the last three years these diagnostic
categories accounted for approximately one-third of the total pay-
ments of sick leave compensation for employed and insured males
in the CSFR, an alarming development indeed.

In all age groups a conspicuous rise in the proportion of first-
time inpatient treatment for substance dependence and abuse in
males (about +100%) and females (about +800%) is evident in
the 1963 to 1988 period, and in the 60+ age group a rise in brain
disorder incidence of hospitalization (Table 20.1). All this is in

TABLE 20.1
Various Descriptors of the Availability and Consumption of Mental Health Services in Czech (CR) and Slovak (SR) National Republics and in CSFR

All rates given per 100,000 inhabitants; the differences given in % of 1960 value	CR			SR			CSFR		
	60	89	dif	60	89	dif	60	89	dif
Psychiatric Beds									
total	155.5	146.9	−5.3	90.0	86.9	−3.4	133.4	126.1	−5.5
In mental hospitals	146.3	130.2	−11.0	49.2	58.0	+17.9	117.9	105.9	−10.2
In psychiat. depts of general hospitals	9.2	16.7	+81.5	30.8	27.5	−10.7	15.5	20.3	+31.0
% of total in psychiatric depts. of general hospitals	5.9	11.3	+91.5	38.5	32.2	−16.4	11.6	16.1	+38.8
Psychiatrists									
Serving all beds	2.8	4.8	+71.4	1.8	3.6	+100.0	2.5	4.4	+76.0
beds in general hospitals	2.5	3.7	+48.0	.7	1.8	+157.1	2.0	3.1	+55.0
beds in psychiatric depts. of general hospitals	.4	1.1	+175.0	1.1	1.8	+63.3	.6	1.4	+133.3
In outpatient psychiatric services	.87	3.88	+346.0	.54	3.47	+542.6	.78	3.74	379.5
In outpatient antiaddicts services	.03	.18	+500.0	.01	.39	+3800.0	.15	.45	+200.0
Total in health care service	3.20	8.87	+177.2	2.33	7.27	+212.1	3.32	8.33	+150.9

Inpatient Treatment Incidence per 100,000 civilian population	CR			SR			100*SR/CR (%)[1]	
Male	1960	1988	dif[1]	1960	1988	dif[1]	1960	1988
Age Group 15–29								
Brain syndrome	11.9	2.4	−79.7	8.9	4.6	−48.2	75.3	190.9
Functional psychosis	30.2	25.1	−16.9	30.4	33.2	+9.3	100.6	132.3
Neurosis and other nonpsychotic disorder	67.7	79.5	+17.4	38.0	58.0	+52.4	56.2	73.0
Substance abuse, dependence and their psychotic complications	41.0	70.3	+71.6	35.3	87.2	+147.3	86.0	124.0
All mental disorders	211.0	240.6	+14.0	155.1	232.0	+49.6	73.5	96.4
Age Group 30–59								
Brain syndrome	22.0	11.4	−47.9	13.5	12.9	−5.0	61.8	112.7
Functional psychosis	42.0	24.3	−42.0	47.3	40.1	−15.4	112.9	169.9
Neurosis and other nonpsychotic disorder	83.1	49.0	−41.0	68.9	43.8	−36.4	83.0	89.5

TABLE 20.1 (continued)

Substance abuse, dependence and their psychotic complications	71.1	116.0	+63.2	110.4	255.4	+131.0	155.4	220.2
All mental disorders	248.2	228.0	−8.1	270.5	372.0	+37.5	109.0	163.1
Age Group 60+								
Brain syndrome	135.2	198.4	+46.7	57.1	140.5	+146.1	42.2	70.8
Functional psychosis	28.3	20.7	+26.7	33.0	33.2	+0.5	116.6	159.9
Neurosis and other nonpsychotic disorder	26.8	32.4	+20.9	20.1	31.6	+57.4	75.0	97.7
Substance abuse, dependence and their psychotic complications	11.9	18.0	+51.7	13.4	53.8	+302.2	112.9	299.4
All mental disorders	214.5	290.7	+35.5	139.2	262.5	+88.6	64.9	90.3
Female								
Age Group 15–29								
Brain syndrome	7.1	3.0	−57.3	4.3	2.6	−40.4	61.2	85.4
Functional psychosis	32.0	34.9	+12.3	32.2	39.5	+22.4	100.7	113.2
Neurosis and other nonpsychotic disorder	98.2	80.1	−18.0	68.4	63.1	−7.8	69.6	78.3
Substance abuse, dependence and their psychotic complications	2.0	11.5	+484.8	2.4	10.9	+356.0	121.2	94.5
All mental disorders	173.4	160.2	−7.1	138.2	135.1	−2.3	79.7	84.3
Age Group 30–59								
Brain syndrome	13.7	6.2	−54.5	9.6	6.9	−28.2	70.5	111.3
Functional psychosis	55.6	43.7	−21.3	56.5	58.4	+3.5	101.5	133.6
Neurosis and other nonpsychotic disorder	103.8	74.1	−28.6	102.0	76.2	−25.3	98.3	102.8
Substance abuse, dependence and their psychotic complications	3.4	27.4	+706.3	6.0	49.8	+732.0	176.0	181.5
All mental disorders	191.3	169.6	−11.3	191.4	205.2	+7.3	100.0	121.0
Age Group 60+								
Brain syndrome	135.7	230.3	+69.6	40.6	134.0	+230.5	29.9	58.2
Functional psychosis	40.0	43.6	+9.2	30.0	57.4	+91.4	75.0	131.5
Neurosis and other nonpsychotic disorder	31.5	44.0	+39.8	22.2	40.2	+80.6	70.6	91.2
Substance abuse, dependence and their psychotic complications	0.5	3.8	+754.9	1.4	8.7	+519.5	315.0	228.2
All mental disorders	213.6	338.6	+58.5	99.1	246.8	+149.0	46.4	72.9

[1] All differences and percentages are calculated from unrounded values.

agreement with the already mentioned European WHO Regional Office in Copenhagen report. Alcohol abuse, however, presents a much greater problem in the CSFR than other substance abuse.

Some of the differences in availability of mental health care services in both national republics have already been demonstrated. The population in the Czech Republic is about twice that of the Slovak Republic. Both nationalities feel themselves historically and culturally different, but the Czech and Slovak languages are very similar and the people do understand each other without any difficulty, especially through the influence of TV programs. In the Slovak Republic there is a strong Catholic majority. In the Czech Republic the historical influence of the protestant movement (Johannes Hus and the Hussite's wars) is evident, though religion was an item omitted from official statistics during the past forty years when atheism was the official doctrine and religious activities were persecuted by the Communist Party leadership and administration.

In 1945 most of the German minority in the Czech Republic was transferred back to Germany. In the Slovak Republic a strong Hungarian minority still exists, concentrated along the Hungarian frontier. Gypsies form an ethnic group dispersed throughout the whole region of the Czech and Slovak republics, with increasing concentrations to the East. Unfortunately, during the last forty years they were not the subject of the all-state Psychiatric Information System (PIS).

Suicidal Behavior in Czech and Slovak Republics

Long-term time series of suicide rates exist in past Czechoslovak statistical yearbooks. Ruzicka (1968) has summarized and analyzed them in a monograph. One of his tables shows fatal suicide rates covering the time span 1895 to 1964 in five-year periods for the Bohemian regions. A decrease in suicide rates during World War I is clearly evident. It cannot, however, be excluded, that the second marked decrease from 1950 is partly due to the transfer of the large German minority back to Germany in 1945, as this minority was known to have the highest suicide rates in Czechoslovakia. For Slovak regions only rates after the formation of Czechoslovakia in 1918 are available. Since 1963 elaborate statistical yearbooks have been published about various aspects of suicidal behavior in both national republics. Figure 20.2 summarizes a few of the global findings. Fatal suicide rates were traditionally higher in males than females and higher in the Czech than the Slovak Republic. In the last figure the Czech 1938 to 1945 values demonstrate the known decrease of fatal suicide during times of social turmoil. A similar but not profound decrease is evident in the 1967 to 1969 interval in Czech males, followed by a peak in 1970 after which a steady decrease occurs. In Czech females a slight and steady decrease takes place throughout the whole period except the peak in 1945. Fatal suicide rates in Slovak females are lowest and steady. Conversely the rates of Slovak males show a steady increase until 1980 when they reached the values of Czech men. After 1980 they followed the descending trend which in Czech males started in 1970.

In contrast to fatal suicides, suicidal attempt rates were traditionally higher in females than in males, and here again higher in CR than in SR. The analysis of the age group profiles of suicide rates shows that the highest incidence of fatal suicide occurs in the 70+ age group, whereas in suicidal attempts the rates are highest in the 15 to 19 age group. The 1979 to 1989 comparison presents a massive reduction in the incidence of suicide attempts and fatal suicides for all subgroups, regardless of gender or geography, except for fatal suicide rates in Slovak women which represent low and stable profiles.

Macrosocial Stress of Prague Spring and Its Defeat by Warsaw Pact Forces

In 1969 two volumes of research results (Černý, Vrba, and Černá, 1969; Vrba and Černý, 1969) examined macrosocial stress (MS) defined as a "situation when large population groups are exposed to massive stress load." Such a situation took place in the Czech Republic during 1968 and 1969, when the period of generally shared trust in favorable change of political orientation was replaced by disappointment and helplessness induced by the occupation by Warsaw Pact forces led by the Soviets on August 21, 1968. This unique "natural experiment" was utilized in several

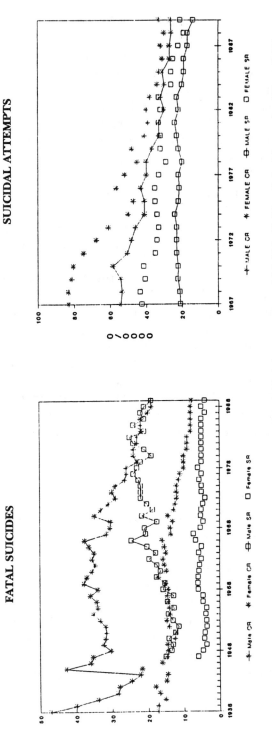

Figure 20.2 Time Series of Fatal Suicides and Suicidal Attempts per 100,000 Civilian Inhabitants in CR and SR

designs that studied the impact of MS on various aspects of mental health and illness.

One such aspect studied was the suicide rates. It has already been stated that in the geographic area of the present Czech Republic, an important decrease was observed in suicide rates during World Wars I and II. From 1910 to 1914, 29.7 persons died by suicide per 100,000 population (= o/oooo); in 1917 the greatest decrease was observed with only 14.4 o/oooo realized suicides. During 1935 to 1937 the rates were 33.6, o/oooo, followed by a decrease during the war years with minimum rate in 1944 equal to 18.2 o/oooo. Similar changes were observed in Italy, France, in occupied Netherlands, and neutral Sweden. On the other hand there was an increase of suicide rates in neutral Switzerland, occupied Denmark, and Norway (Ruzicka, 1968). According to some authors there were low suicide rates in concentration camps. The Cerny study calculated the expected monthly suicide rates from the 1964 to 1967 data. In 1968 the observed realized suicide rates in males were significantly lower than expected from May to October with a minimum in July; in females lower rates were observed in September and October. Observed 1968 suicidal attempts' rates in males were significantly lower only in July and October, in females in August only. Further analysis revealed that the age group 20 to 39 was most responsible for the change in expected monthly values along with the rising trend in realized and attempted suicide rates between 1964 and 1967. The authors (Cerny et al., 1969) explain this by the changes in attitudes following the resignation of general Communist Party secretary and president Novotny and the election of Alexander Dubcek. There was a sudden rise of interest in political issues and active involvement of the population, and particularly of males in social and political affairs after a long period of passivity and resignation.

The second of the designs was a survey of forty scientific workers aged 27 to 58, twenty-seven male and thirteen females: by standardized interview in the presence of two observers, changes were compared for three time intervals (I.—Jan. 1 to Aug. 20, 1968; II.—Aug. 21 to Sept. 21, 1968; III.—Sept. 21, 1968 to start of April 1969) of motivation to work, work output, mental efficiency, and emotional and neurotic problems respectively.

The most conspicuous findings were those of emotional states. In period I, better than usual results were found both individually and when compared with general norm. In period II a negative emotional state of mind was reported by all participants in the experiment with prolongation of these findings into period III. This trend was present in the mental efficiency and work output as well.

The authors emphasize that though there was an increase in neurasthenic symptoms (one-fifth during I, two-thirds in II, and over half of the volunteers in period III) more significant impacts were found in the overall mental state of all subjects which resulted in the worsening of work output and lowering of work motivation (Cerny et al., 1969).

The third design measured depressive symptomatology by means of the Zung self-rating scale from June to October 1968 in 120 subjects examined before and after August 21. The insignificant decrease of symptomatology after August 21 in the whole sample and the significant increase in individuals younger than 40, compared with the 40 years and older group, was explained by the tendency of men to experience sthenic reactions when living under menacing conditions (Vrba and Černý, 1969).

A similar comparison was conducted in 100 admissions to the Charles University School of Medicine, Department of Psychiatry between August 7 and September 24, 1968. An original scale rating the level of emotional harmony and standardized interviews were utilized. About half of the sample was influenced by MS, mostly as worsening of symptoms in the inpatient treated subjects or as a release of a new episode in those admitted later on. In agreement with world literature the authors found little influence of MS on the course of schizophrenia. This was confirmed by results of MS influence on treated outpatients living in central City Prague—1 district. When the periods August 1 to September 30 of 1967 and 1968 were compared, it was found that schizophrenics were the least and depressive phases of affective disorders the most influenced. In 1968 marked reduction in contacts of patients aged less than 20 years could be stated and an increase of contacts in age groups between 31 and 39.

In the analyzed MS period, twenty-nine cases of specific suicidal behavior, self-burning, took place in the first half of 1969, a very unusual behavior in a European culture. From very detailed analysis of all cases by Cerny (1969), it is evident that the first event (J.P.) was not intended as suicide; it was a clear political protest, the unusual form of which was expected to evoke the highest possible public reaction. Similar conclusions were drawn from two other impersonally motivated events (J.Z. and E.P.), evoked by a political situation in individuals free of psychopathology. According to the author, the remaining twenty-six events were under the suggestive influence of the first widely published and discussed event with intent to give to the suicidal attempt impersonal features or increase the threat to the social environment.

The public burial ceremony of J.P., the student from the Charles University School of Philosophy, the first of the three live self-immolations, became a quiet demonstration by thousands of citizens against the August occupation. For twenty-two years every possible action was attempted to expel this event from the nation's memory, but the attempts were in vain. In January 1988 the brutal police action against people ready to lay flowers at the place where J.P. performed his act of self-immolation was one of the events that started the velvet November revolution.

REFERENCES

American Psychiatric Association (1980), *Diagnostic and Statistical Manual of Mental Disorders*, 3rd ed. (DSM-III). Washington, DC: American Psychiatric Press.

———— (1987), *Diagnostic and Statistical Manual of Mental Disorders*, 3rd ed. rev. (DSM-III-R). Washington, DC: American Psychiatric Press.

Černý, M., Vrba, V., & Černý, H. (1969), Macrosocial stress I. Final report of Research task Z-21-41. (In Czech.) Research Unit, Psychiatric Dept. of Charles University School of Medicine. Prague.

Ruzicka, L. (1968), Suicide in Czechoslovakia from the point of view of demography and sociology. (In Czech.) Prague: Academia.

UZIS: Health statistics of CSFR. Suicides 1964–1992. In Czech—contains detailed analysis of 1963–1991 data. Institute of Health Information and Statistics, Prague 1964–1992.

UZIS: Health statistics of CSFR. Mental Health Care 1960–1991. In Czech—contains detailed analysis of 1960–1991 data. Institute of Health Information and Statistics, Prague 1960–1991.

UZIS: CSFR Health Care 1960–1990. In Czech—contains detailed analysis of 1960–1990–1 data. Institute of Health Information and Statistics, Prague 1960–1990.

Vrba, V. & Černý, M. (1969), Macrosocial stress II. Final report DU Z-21-41. (In Czech.) Research Unit, Psychiatric Dept. of Charles University School of Medicine, Prague.

21.

Hungarian Culture and Mental Illness

Béla Buda and János Füredi

Marxist ideology was unfriendly toward sociology and cultural anthropology. It only tolerated scientific disciplines and allowed their existence in a rather restricted form. Thus there were no proper scientific investigations of culture and cultural processes in the country during the Communist era. There are only qualitative data, limited observations, anecdotal evidence, and a few studies which have dealt with the relationship between culture and psychopathology in Hungary. Interestingly, on the other hand, there is a strong belief among professionals that many manifestations of mental illness and deviant behavior are deeply influenced by some cultural characteristics of the population and the Hungarian mentality.

THE HISTORY

Traditionally, the country was stratified and differentiated in many dimensions. Before World War I, as part of the Austro-Hungarian Empire, the country was a multinational entity, with large segments of Slovaks, Romanians, Serbians, Rutenians, with many scattered German groups, Gypsies, and Jews who came from Russia and Poland in a constant flux, fleeing discriminatory laws and pogroms (the Austro-Hungarian Empire had a liberal immigration and settlement policy). In 1920 the Trianon Treaty dissolved the Empire, dividing it into many countries. Hungary became a small country with a relatively homogeneous population, while many millions of ethnic Hungarians remained in the new neighboring states. The forced partition of the historical Hungarian territory was a terrible blow to the national identity of the country. It was the main reason why the country entered the Second World War. Because of the present discrimination and suppression of Hungarians in these new states, it is still an acute problem of national self-esteem.

Hungary's culture was determined in the last century largely by the *ethnic subcultures* and by subcultures of social classes and strata. Ethnic Germans were diligent, disciplined, willing to learn handicrafts and trades, and thus, the German population was the main labor force in the initial industrialization of the country. Slovaks and Romanians were mainly migrant and unskilled workers. Jews dominated commerce, banking, and the entrepreneurial sphere.

Religion has always had a great impact on the country. The Catholic church had the largest membership in all Hungary, after a forced reconversion of the Protestant population during the seventeenth and eighteenth centuries. Protestantism has had such strong roots, however, that remnants of the Protestant mentality can be discovered also in predominantly Catholic regions. An example of this is suicide. Suicide rates, in contrast to the Western European countries, did not (and do not) show great differences between Catholic and Protestant regions, and tolerant attitudes toward suicide are the same in the different religious groups. The Protestant ethic is characteristic of the Hungarian peasant population, which is hard-working and future oriented and always prone to delay of gratifications, if work or future investment requires it. In the old Hungary, church-going played a great role in social integration. Priests had high moral authority and were officially recognized as agents of social order, especially in villages.

Since Hungary was an agricultural country, the largest part of the population consisted of peasants living in small villages and in the Eastern territories of the country, on the so-called

Hungarian lowlands. Many lived (and hundreds of thousands still live) in hamlets scattered throughout large areas, on average 1 to 2 kilometers apart. The original *peasant culture* was a rather rigid one which placed great stress on traditional distribution of work, on traditional sex roles, on paternalism, and on dependency of children on paternal authority. Rules and norms were enforced strictly, deviation was not tolerated and was treated with rejection and ostracism. Since exclusion from the traditional community was a severe punishment, many considered suicide. *Suicide* in Hungary still includes this element. There is a strong pressure within families, kinship, and communities on persons rejected (because of behavioral offenses, rule-breaking, or social failure) to kill themselves. In the old Hungary there were also patterned responses. Girls who got pregnant out of wedlock used to jump into pits, servants from the country who got into conflicts in towns poisoned themselves with phosphorus obtained from safety matches. After matches were made phosphorus-free, servants began to drink natron lye found in households in large quantity. Men who failed in business or social life jumped from bridges and high places. Soldiers shot themselves. Old men who were ill or had become intolerable drunkards hung themselves. There are still influences of these traditions. Hanging is still the main method of suicide for old rural people and the "popularity" of this method, which is slowly being superseded by the equally lethal method of swallowing pesticides and taking medication contributes to the high rate of suicidal deaths in Hungary.

Interestingly there are characteristic regional differences in suicide rates within the territory, the patterns of which have been relatively constant over the last 100 to 120 years. Suicides are much more frequent in the southern and southeastern counties of Hungary (Bács-Kiskun, Csongrád) while to the west and north the suicide rates decrease. In the mid-eighties the country's suicide rate was about 45 per 100,000, in the above-mentioned high-rate counties it was 65 to 67, while in the western regions it was 20 to 25. There are slight changes in the rates of the counties (i.e., larger administrative districts which have traditional borders defined centuries ago), thus while some counties change place in the frequency list, regions preserve their position. This is considered by experts as a sign of cultural determination of suicidal behavior. Regional cultures really favor the southern parts of the country where there are withdrawal tendencies, escapism, suicidal responses, and a marked trend in the population to accept and approve suicides as brave acts of protest and defiance against fate or oppression. Hanging is the traditional method of self-destruction in these regions, especially for men; but in comparison to other countries a very high proportion of women also utilize this almost inevitably fatal method.

The original peasant culture acted to inhibit aggression. Many historians believe that this is a consequence of the fact that the country survived the last five centuries under constant foreign occupation and repressive political regimes. Retreating forms of deviant behavior were allowed instead of aggression. For example, the homicide rate has been traditionally low in the country, while self-destructive behavior patterns have been tolerated or even cultivated, such as suicide, heavy drinking, risk-taking tendencies in desperate situations, and fatalistic attitudes toward danger. Mental illnesses were partly tolerated and partly used as a scapegoat by the community. Not only did each village have its "fools" but there was a long tradition in royal courts and aristocratic houses of having a fool who was used for amusement or even sometimes for political purposes.

Inhibition manifests itself also in the escapist abuse of alcohol which is a traditional way of coping with stress. It also has to do with the fact that the country is a traditional center of wine production. Alcohol consumption is very high in the country, although the peak quantity of 13 liters of absolute alcohol per capita has decreased slightly in the last few years to 11.5 liters. Spirit consumption is constantly rising, however, and now exceeds 8 liters, an alarmingly dangerous trend which is reflected in the rapidly increasing rate of cirrhosis of the liver, a twentyfold increase in the past twenty-five years! The distribution of alcohol consumption and alcoholism rates are not known exactly, but data on the rate of delirium tremens parallel the rate of suicide in the counties (with some irregularities, since in one of the low suicide rate counties there is a high rate from complications of alcoholism).

NATIONAL CHARACTERISTICS

Hard work and obedience, and reactions to repression and traumas concerning feelings of national identity, seriousness, and sadness are all considered characteristics of the Hungarian "soul."
Folk songs and fairy tales have had predominantly sad themes
and in almost all neighboring countries, there are proverbs and
sayings expressing observations concerning Hungarian sadness
("you are sad like a Hungarian . . ."). There are anecdotes of
traveling or emigrant Hungarians whose ethnic origin has been
repeatedly identified because of their "sad" behavior. This sadness is believed to play a role in the high rate of suicide in the
country (actually the country has the highest recorded rate in the
world, fluctuating between 43 and 45 per 100,000, and the rate
has stayed very high during the past two centuries, according
to existing statistics). Today psychiatrists tend to interpret these
observations as signs of greater proneness to depression in the
Hungarian population (Zonda, Rihmer, and Lester, 1992).
Chronic and characterological manifestations of the depressive
spectrum, described by modern researchers, such as Akiskal
(1985), support such interpretations. There are speculations
(based on some epidemiological data) among psychiatrists that
depression is underdiagnosed even now after decades of strong
campaigning by pharmaceutical companies. Cultural standards of
depressionlike behavior might be the main cause of the increased
suicide rates in the country, and may play a role in widespread
alcohol abuse and alcoholism.

If the view is held that depression is more common in Hungary than in other countries (an assertion which has not been
tested by any comparative investigation) there are many explanations. Increased genetic vulnerability of the Hungarian population can be mentioned (though still not proved) as well as the
role of a depressive culture. Suicide and alcoholism rates (the
latter being measured by the incidence and prevalence of serious
complications of abusive drinking, such as alcoholic psychoses,
delirium tremens, etc.) vary in the country between different regions along the pattern discussed previously. Their distribution
patterns are remarkably consistent and have changed very little.
This is a well-established statistical and epidemiological fact, that

yields itself to a cultural explanation, pointing to the role of regional subcultures (norms of behavior, reaction patterns to stresses, socialization mechanisms, tension release, customs, etc.). Cultural research is lacking in this area. There is much speculation concerning the effects of historical development, ethnic and religious composition, economic and social development, of the given regions. Hungary has always had a rather rigid district or county structure and public administration and this structure has historically also reinforced the existing characteristics of the region and contributed to the development of a *regional identity*. The cultural explanation relies on observations concerning the strong pressure on the children to achieve, the high frequency of a perfectionist, ambitious, hard-striving, competitive character structure within the population. This structure predisposes one to exhaustion, as well as making one vulnerable in terms of self-esteem even in instances of minor frustration and failure. This hypothesis can be corroborated also by some observations: that helping and supporting behavior patterns are not developed in the country. This is true also in historical retrospective. The only source of support in old Hungary was the large family and kinship, but this has disintegrated through migration, urbanization, and industrialization which have been taking place during the last decades at an accelerated pace. Only a few communities have the resources and traditions to provide organized support in times of crisis for individuals or families, and the Communist regime suppressed even these community supports since they were regarded as being dangerous to a totalitarian control system.

Some consider the Hungarian language to be poor in expressing feelings and relationships, and thereby contributing to difficulties in meaningful emotional communication during conflicts and crises, presenting adequate problem solution, and tension relief. The poor communication in interpersonal relations and family life is pointed out by psychotherapists and is believed to be an important factor also in suicide, divorce, and the neurotic reactions of the Hungarian population.

CULTURE AND NEUROSIS

Subjective acceptance of neurotic symptoms and complaints is high in Hungary, corresponding to environmental willingness to accept neurotic persons, if somewhat devaluing them and putting them at a disadvantage in everyday competitions (e.g., in the workplace, in organizations, etc.). There is a change taking place now in this respect in the country, especially in the capital and the larger towns. This change is due to the prevalence of Western standards of self-image and social performance that are spreading and are causing higher ambitions.

In general, the opinion of experts about the relationship of culture and neurosis in Hungary tends to be that public life is dominated now by people who either themselves were formerly peasants, and became workers in industry and public services after moving to large towns, or are children of such people. There are data from the 1950s and 1960s that show more than 50 percent of the Hungarian population changed its place of residence and occupation, almost all of them left villages and peasant life and went to towns as workers. A similar large transformation of society took 100 to 150 years in England and France. Women were motivated to enter the labor force, though sometimes constrained from doing so. These rapid changes disrupted both patterns of family relationships and individual schemes of orientation and coping. The stress of societal transformation became an important factor in neurosis, in the increase of suicide and alcoholism (later in other forms of substance abuse).

It can therefore be said that the original peasant subjective culture was not able to assist or to serve people in this rapid process of *social transformation*. They could not cope with the many adaptational and relational problems and failures. Since the Communist regime persecuted the aristocracy and the thin stratum of bourgeois living in towns (the prewar population of Hungarian cities consisted mostly of urbanized peasants), there were no behavior models for a civic urban life-style and therefore cultural change could not be handled by following existing models. Later, this situation may explain how Western models of behavior and personal values (e.g., consumerism, "sexual revolution," fashions, etc.) spread throughout the country very quickly without resistance (reinforced in some instances by the official prohibitions on the part of the Communist ideology, which was resented by the majority of the people).

The burden of stress was felt upon the *family*. Many family problems have been reflected not only in the high divorce rate, but also in the increasing frequency of psychiatric problems amongst children. Such problems include criminal behavior, functional disorders, substance abuse—especially glue sniffing, which is manifested by children living in disadvantaged areas and coming from disorganized families. The behavior problems are aggravated by the fact that psychiatric and mental health services as well as social services are underdeveloped.

Therefore, the helping professions have low prestige, and their members are extremist in their views. Biological and narrow administrative stances (e.g., preferences for criminalization, administrative solutions, etc.) are widespread among them. The availability of professional help is inadequate, while voluntary helping agencies and self-help structures are lacking. This may also be due to the prevailing attitudes in the original and slowly changing culture. There are rapid developments, however, in this field, especially in Budapest. In the capital, a certain "psychoboom" can be observed. Training in psychotherapy and self-awareness techniques, and encounter methods is increasing and professional help is becoming more accessible for paying clients.

Concerning other forms of *mental illness* and psychopathology, there are probably few differences between Hungary and countries of similar size and socioeconomic conditions. Mental disease due to arteriosclerosis and neurologic disorganization of the brain is probably more frequent in the country because of an adverse morbidity and mortality situation (due to unhealthy diet, widespread drinking and smoking, and poor medical care). *Psychosomatic* symptoms are also frequent and are treated predominantly within the framework of organic medicine, without taking into consideration psychological factors involved. As a result, such cases need longer treatment and have poorer prognosis than elsewhere. Schizophrenia and borderline syndrome are probably as numerous as in other countries. Formerly, as historical studies show, delusions of grandeur were common in psychiatric wards, and patients referred to actual historical persons (e.g., patients believed themselves to be kings, aristocrats, or the children of kings and aristocrats, famous persons, etc.). Now these delusions are almost absent. It is debatable whether the content of delusions has disappeared because of the early and effective psychopharma-cological treatment or are absent because of the changed structure of psychiatric morbidity.

In more severe disturbances, it is worth mentioning that *stigmatization* is still strong. Mentally ill persons such as chronic schizophrenics are not easily accepted in families and communities, and there are no supporting voluntary organizations for the chronic mentally ill. This stigmatization and rejection can be caused by economic problems (e.g., housing shortages) but can be conditioned also by sociocultural processes (e.g., increased competition among the population, increased individualization, etc.).

A country's mental health culture is also reflected in the network, structures, and atmosphere of the mental health services. In this respect Hungary is an underdeveloped country. There are two larger mental hospitals, several general hospital departments, with 100 to 200 beds, and around eighty smaller units in hospitals. There are five university departments, one of them the Psychiatric Clinic of the Postgraduate Medical University where the authors work. The number of outpatient services is relatively small, around 120 at the present time, and there is great need of development in this field. Private practice among mental health professionals is increasing because of the social changes of the last few years, and we are expecting a rapid expansion in the near future, as well as a certain emergence of the "psychoboom" which manifested itself in the seventies in Western countries, the burgeoning of the new schools of psychotherapy, New Age, and so on.

REFERENCES

Akiskal, H. S. (1985), Interaction of biological and psychologic factors in the origin of depressive disorders. *Acta Psychiat. Scand.*, 319(Suppl.):131–139.

Zonda, T., Rihmer, Z., & Lester, D. (1992), Social correlates of deviant behavior in Hungary. *European J. Psychiat.*, 6:236–238.

—

PART VII

Minorities and Ethnic Groups in Britain, New Zealand, and North America

22.

Mental Illness Among American Indians and Alaska Natives

Philip D. Somervell,
Spero M. Manson,
and James H. Shore

INTRODUCTION

American Indians and Alaska Natives number approximately 1.4 million as of the 1980 census. They are the fastest-growing minority group in the United States. Among Alaska Natives are included Alaskan Indians (of two different culture groups) as well as Aleuts and Eskimos. The Eskimos may be further divided into at least two language groups. The definition of an Indian or Native used for census purposes is self-identification, although various membership criteria (e.g., in terms of "blood quantum") are employed by different tribes, and for eligibility for specific government services. Part of this population resides on Indian reservations (land set aside for certain tribes or groups of tribes, with limited legal and political sovereignty). However, some 60 percent now live in urban, non-reservation areas. These designations may be too simplistic, since many individuals primarily live in cities, yet also consider a reservation community as their home.

The term *American Indians and Alaska Natives* glosses over the fact that the tribes included under this rubric have never been unified politically or culturally, nor have they ever shared a common language. From nine to seventeen distinct culture areas or regions have been identified across the geographic distribution of this population, depending upon the criteria applied in terms of differences (often fundamental differences) in language, social organization, religious practice, and ecological relationships. At present, over 250 tribes are officially recognized by the U.S. Federal government. The differences between Eskimos, Aleuts, and Indians, although significant, are no greater than the differences between some Indian tribes.

The current life experiences of all of these people cannot be understood in isolation from their history of conquest and subsequent political subjugation. In fact, this experience provides some of the most striking commonalities shared by the different groups. In the contiguous states, it included the elimination of the subsistence bases, relocation onto usually small areas of land (generally the poorest), and, in the nineteenth century, forced migrations, such as the now infamous Trail of Tears in which the Five Civilized Tribes (Choctaw, Cherokee, Chickasaw, Creek and Seminole) were expelled from the Southeast to reservations in an unfamiliar region hundreds of miles away. Alaska followed a somewhat different pattern, since Alaska Natives were not forcibly relocated. Yet, even there, the history of contact has arguably had similar long-term effects. Economic exploitation, as well as past policies of forced assimilation and devaluing of Indian and Alaska Native cultures, have contributed to an apparently high prevalence of demoralization and to severe identity problems among young people.

Today, in some Native communities, the distinct cultural identity which may persist is not immediately visible to an outsider. In others, many members speak their native language by preference and traditional observances and customs are still widely practiced. The deliberate revival of native traditions is also to be seen. Although the numbers of Indians and Alaska Natives in the professions and in business are increasing, in general this is an extremely low-income, highly stressed population. There is evidence that it suffers from high rates of mental as well as physical health problems.

DESCRIPTIVE EPIDEMIOLOGY OF MENTAL DISORDERS

Although there are some population-based data on alcohol and drug use in these populations (at least on adolescents), there are virtually no such data on other mental disorders defined according to current diagnostic systems, nor on the co-occurrence of other mental disorders with substance abuse. Such data have been available even on majority-culture populations for only ten years. Unfortunately, the studies which collected these data were not designed to sample large enough numbers of American Indians and Alaska Natives, nor to deal with the cross-cultural issues involved in studying them. The older literature on mental illness (dating from some two decades ago) is scanty. Furthermore, the interpretation of these data, and comparison with non-Native communities, is problematic, for methodologic reasons including the sampling methods and/or the use of DSM-II diagnostic criteria, which are considerably more subjective as well as substantively different from the more recent DSM-III (APA, 1980) and DSM-III-R (APA, 1987) systems. However, this literature, anecdotal evidence, and the impressions of service providers and community members all suggest that American Indians and Alaska Natives are at least as heavily impacted by the entire range of mental disorders as any other North American group, if not significantly more so.

Shore, Kinzie, and Hampson (1973) in a quota sample from a small Northwest Coast Indian village (N = 100), found an overall prevalence of definite and probable psychiatric disturbance (DSM-II diagnoses) of 69 percent, even when alcoholism was excluded. In discussing the implications, they point out that much lower prevalence rates (23%, 40%, 45%, and 57%) had been reported from other studies using similar methods in South Africa, two sites in Nigeria, and Nova Scotia. Lower rates of disorder have been reported (Sampath, 1974; Murphy and Hughes, 1965) in two different Eskimo communities. Kinzie, Leung, Boehnlein, Matsunaga, Johnson, Manson, Shore, Heinz, and Williams (1991) in a resurvey of the Northwest Coast community studied by Shore et al., found alcohol use disorders (using DSM-III-R criteria, APA, 1987) still the most common. Among other disorders, the most common were major depression (2.2% among men, 4.7% among women) and posttraumatic stress disorder (4.4% among men). As discussed below, however, the sampling methods used by both the original survey and the resurvey of this village limit their interpretability.

The most extensive literature on Indian and Native mental health has been related to alcohol abuse or dependence (Brod, 1975; Heath, 1989). "Binge" drinking generally appears to be more typical of Indian drinkers than is a steady daily pattern of drinking. There has been some discussion in the literature about social and cultural functions which drinking may serve in certain tribes (Brod, 1975); however, the consequences are increasingly acknowledged by Indian and Native communities as a serious problem. Not all Indian communities experience high rates of alcohol abuse or dependence, but for some these constitute a veritable epidemic and are undoubtedly the most devastating of their public health problems. Shore et al. (1973) reported a prevalence of habitual excessive drinking of 27 percent and of episodic excessive drinking of 4 percent in the Northwest Coast village which they studied. The 1991 resurvey (Kinzie et al., 1991) found a large difference between lifetime rates of alcohol dependence (72.9% for men, 31.0% for women) and the point prevalence (current prevalence) of the same disorders (32.8% and 6.2%, respectively). This is consistent with anecdotal reports that many Native persons who drink excessively in their youth give up this behavior in later life. For alcohol *abuse*, however, there was virtually no difference between lifetime and current prevalence (the point prevalence was 3.6% among men and 0.8% among women). As evidence of the severity of the problem in Indian and Native populations, investigators have reported extremely high mortality rates for causes attributable directly or indirectly to alcohol consumption, including medical complications of alcoholism as well as accidental injuries and suicide (Forbes and Van Der Hyde, 1988; Kraus and Buffler, 1979; May, 1987).

There is some evidence that the prevalence of depressive disorders in this population is higher than in other groups, and that co-occurrence of major depression with alcoholism is common as well (Manson, Shore, and Bloom, 1985; Manson, Shore, Bloom, Keepers, and Neligh, 1987). Among the older generation of studies which constitute the bulk of the population-based data,

Shore, Kinzie, Hampson et al. (1973) report a prevalence of depressive psychoneurosis of 8 percent. With respect to other specific disorders, there is less evidence, and it is rather fragmentary. Sampath (1974) found a prevalence of neuroses of 11.6 percent (among which depression was "the commonest") in a Canadian Eskimo community, which he compared with the 0.2 to 5.2 percent reported in other United States populations. By contrast, Murphy and Hughes (1965) observed rates in their Alaskan Eskimo sample comparable to those of the general population. Foulks and Katz (1973) reported the *treated* prevalence of anxiety neurosis in five Alaska Native culture groups to be nearly as high as the prevalence of depression, and for some groups much higher, which is consistent with the work of Shore et al. (1973). A wide range of (DSM-II) psychoses, neuroses, and personality disorders was found by these investigators. The recent work of Kinzie et al. (1991) which is unique to our knowledge in using DSM-III-R criteria in a population-based sample, also supports the importance of major depression (point prevalence rates of 2.2% among men, 4.7% among women). The latter also found 4.4 percent of the men to suffer from posttraumatic stress disorder. There is recent evidence that panic disorder is seen with more than negligible frequency in several tribes (Neligh, Baron, Braun, and Czarnecki, submitted), although prevalence rates have been estimated only by Kinzie et al. (1991), who found a prevalence rate of 0.6 percent in the village which they studied.

Unfortunately, none of the population-based research summarized above used probability sampling. Except for Sampath, who studied virtually 100 percent of the adult population of a community, samples of convenience of one kind or another (sometimes with age and sex quotas) have been employed. Thus, the potential for selection bias in the results cannot be discounted. The small size of the samples (related to studying very small communities) may also have led to instability in estimating the prevalence of rare disorders. For example, it is difficult to know what to make of the apparently very high prevalence rate of schizophrenia of 4.4 percent in Kinzie et al.'s sample of 131 persons. Unfortunately, these limitations apply to nearly all of the published research on mental disorders among Native people: that which does not use convenience sampling in the general population relies instead on treatment samples, an approach which is even more problematic for drawing inferences about populations.

The abuse of virtually all drugs other than alcohol also appears to be a substantial problem, especially among youth (Beauvais and LaBoeuff, 1985; Beauvais, Oetting, and Edwards, 1985a,b; Oetting, Beauvais, and Edwards, 1988). The use of inhalants such as gasoline or paint thinner is of particular concern, since these substances are very toxic and are thought to produce serious neuropsychological sequelae. The prevalence of inhalant use among Indians at ages 12 to 17 is almost twice as high as U.S. averages (Oetting and Goldstein, 1979).

Suicide rates among Indians and Natives vary greatly between tribes and over time. In these groups, suicide is primarily a phenomenon of the young, and especially of young adult and adolescent males (Berlin, 1987; May, 1987). May (1987) cites Indian Health Service data which show age-specific suicide rates, for ages 10 to 24, some 2.3 to 2.8 times as high as overall U.S. rates, and certain communities have at times experienced much higher rates, as well as clusters of suicides. Similarly, high mortality rates for accidental injury have been cited as indicating high rates of "parasuicide" or quasi-suicidal behavior (May, 1987). The great majority of suicides seem to involve alcohol drinking immediately prior to the act (Berlin, 1987). These patterns appear to be of recent (postcontact) origin. For example, accounts of precontact Inuit (Eskimo) culture include descriptions of suicides. These, however, were not the impulsive and often alcohol-related acts, deeply distressing to the community, which occur today. Instead, they more often involved old people motivated by physical infirmity. Other motives also came into play which (in cultural context) were rational and generally altruistic. Such suicides, which were deliberately planned (and sometimes assisted by family members) were apparently viewed by the community as reasonable and even praiseworthy (Leighton and Hughes, 1955).

THE QUESTION OF INDIGENOUS FORMS OF ILLNESS

The identification and classification of diseases constitute a distinctly culture-bound process. Kleinman has developed the concept of the "explanatory model" by which any illness episode experienced by an individual is defined and given meaning, e.g., as representing some "disease" recognized by the individual or those around him. Such a model implies a classification system for diseases, with beliefs about some or all of the following: type of symptoms, mode of onset and timing of symptoms, etiology, pathophysiology, course (including severity and type of sick role) and appropriate treatment. The explanatory model is a function of the culture in which it is grounded, even in Western psychiatry. In other cultures, disorders (sometimes referred to as indigenous or culture-bound disorders) may be defined and recognized which seem to have no precise counterpart in current psychiatric nosologies.

As with other cultural groups, indigenous psychiatric syndromes have been reported among American Indians and Alaska Natives. It remains unclear how and whether these correspond to, or overlap with, the categories of DSM-III-R or other "Western" classifications. Marano (1982), in discussing one purported indigenous disorder, windigo psychosis, concluded that the voluminous literature on it is based entirely on folktales, indirect evidence, and subsequent reinterpretations. One better documented disorder which may have environmental or dietary causes is *pibloqtoq*, or "arctic hysteria." Some more general categories which have been used for disorders seen in different tribes are soul loss, spirit intrusion, syndromes related to the breaking of religious or social prohibitions, and ghost sickness; but there are great variations among the belief systems of different tribes.

The term *emic* has been used to refer to the point of view internal to the culture being studied, as distinct from the *etic* frame of reference of any external, purportedly universal "scientific" system of thought. A unique attempt to examine psychological symptoms and disorders from both perspectives was reported by Manson et al. (1985), focusing on major depression and indigenous disorders among the Hopi of Arizona. Five emic categories of illness, each associated with a cluster of cognitive, affective, and behavioral states, were identified by Hopi informants. None of these indigenous disorders were associated with all of the DSM-III major depression symptoms. The one indigenous disorder which was associated with dysphoria of two weeks' duration (a crucial DSM-III criterion for major depression) was *not* associated with the greatest number of other DSM-III depression symptoms. In fact, certain individual symptoms defined by DSM-III required modification in order to be meaningful in this population. Feeling guilty, sinful, or shameful (lumped together as one symptom in DSM-III) differed in their correlations with indigenous categories of disorder; the same was found in the case of slowness of thoughts and mixed-up thinking. Even if it is assumed that the underlying disorder is the same for all peoples, the expression of symptoms, as well as their perceived significance, was specific to that culture.

A number of tribes, such as the Navajo and the Sioux, have maintained both well-developed belief systems regarding physical and mental disorders, and well-defined traditional treatment modalities for them. These are used in various ways apart from or in combination with Western medical systems. Guilmet (1984) has described the "hierarchy of resort" among the relatively acculturated Puyallup; Kunitz and Levy (1981) have described the ways in which Navajo healing practices are used alongside Western methods, with neither system changing the other. The Navajo healing system, which is defined as sacred rather than merely utilitarian, is used to remove causes, not to alleviate symptoms; conversely, the Western medical system may be used for symptom relief.

In various tribal groups, attempts to bring Indian or Native healers into the Western medical system or to foster collaboration between the two have had mixed success. Issues of credibility and acceptance by the community of specific healers, communication between the medical and the traditional practitioner, acceptable ways to consult and refer, and acceptable ways to reimburse are only some of the potential pitfalls of such collaboration, but there have been some notable successes. For the vast majority of tribes, these issues have not been studied.

Several approaches to therapy based on traditional methods have been used in the context of modern treatment programs, with Indian people of varied backgrounds: the four circles (for analysis of relationships in one's life); the talking circle (as a form of group therapy); and the sweat lodge (a healing and cleansing ceremony) (Manson, Walker, and Kivlahan, 1987). Jilek (1977) describes how a different tradition, that of the spirit dance, has been revived among certain Northwest Coast tribal groups with a new, psychotherapeutic purpose. At the same time, a caveat may be in order: individual Native people differ greatly in their level of interest in and identification with traditional practices. One cannot assume that these are appropriate for all.

EXISTING TREATMENT SYSTEMS

Treatment systems providing mental health services to Indians and Alaska Natives include private agencies and practitioners, the Bureau of Indian Affairs (BIA—a Federal agency within the Department of Interior), urban Indian health programs, tribal health departments, and the Indian Health Service (IHS—a Federal agency within the Public Health Service). The BIA provides educational and social services, and employs mental health professionals and paraprofessionals; however, their function is largely limited to referral. The IHS is responsible for providing comprehensive health services on the reservations, and almost certainly delivers the majority of mental health treatment. In addition, the IHS purchases contract services, mainly for inpatient care. However, according to a 1986 report of the Congressional Office of Technology Assessment, "mental health services are regarded by Indians and IHS area office staff as relatively unavailable in most IHS areas ... [as are] alcohol treatment and prevention programs" (p. 108).

Reservation communities are legally empowered to assume responsibility for health care and many other services, as a result of a law passed in 1975, but tribal-based health care programs appear to make up a much smaller part of the mental health delivery system at present. It has been pointed out that there are a variety of reasons for a limited utilization of this power, including lack of experience, attitudes of suspicion regarding the motives and commitment of the Federal government, and other political and economic concerns (and disagreements) of Federal and tribal governments. A number of cities have private nonprofit Indian service agencies, some of which offer mental health services; some of these programs receive funding from the IHS. In general, however, urban Indians who need publicly funded health care encounter a fragmented array of services (most not targeted specifically for Indians) which can be difficult to negotiate. Among public services not aimed specifically at Indians and Natives, the Federal community mental health centers (CMHCs), although established to provide services to high-risk populations, appear to be much less used by Indians and Natives than by other ethnic groups.

SERVICE UTILIZATION

Utilization patterns for Indians and Alaska Natives suggest that mental disorders, including alcohol abuse and dependence, do not receive treatment in proportion to the magnitude of their impact on this population. The U.S. Office of Technology Assessment (US Congress, 1986) provides cause-specific rates for Indians and Alaska Natives from Fiscal Year 1984, comparing these with data from calendar year 1989 for all races in United States short-stay, non-Federal hospitals. The discharge rates for mental disorders are lower for Indians and Natives than for all races (57 per 10,000 compared with 72 per 10,000). By contrast, from 1980 to 1982, the ratio of deaths from homicide was approximately 2, and the ratio for suicide rates was 1.7. Indians and Natives did have higher discharge rates for certain alcohol disorders, but primarily for alcoholic psychosis (10.1 compared to 2.3). Indian/Native discharge rates were *equal* to U.S. all races for nondependent alcohol abuse (3.4 per 10,000), and somewhat higher for dependence (23.3 compared to 16.7) (page 107). By contrast, the *mortality* rates for the most clearly alcohol-linked causes (cirrhosis/liver disease) were over four times the rate for all races (page 98). Among outpatient Indian Health Service encounters in 1984, mental health issues were not among the eight specific causes nor the ten leading diagnostic categories of causes. By contrast, for American Indians, from 1980 to 1982, homicide and suicide were the eighth and ninth leading causes of death, respectively, and liver disease/cirrhosis was the fourth. The low hospitalization rates may be due to the lack of IHS hospitals in some areas and a relative lack of funds for contract health care. In urban areas, the American Indian Health Care Association

(AIHCA) (Hograbe, 1989) estimates that in Arizona, some two-thirds of urban Indians have no health insurance, and in Boston, 87 percent. Geographical barriers (defined as more than 30 minutes travel time) are also cited as a reason for nonutilization in some cities.

PAST AND FUTURE RESEARCH

The political climate for research on mental health issues with Indian people has undergone changes, starting in the 1960s, when increasing resistance to research *on* (rather than *by* or *for*) Indian people made itself known. At issue was the often exploitative stance of academic researchers, who might glean material for academic advancement without benefit accruing to the Indian communities (often without the Indian people even receiving a copy of the final report). Another concern has been that reports about mental illness and alcohol consumption might reinforce such stereotypes as the "drunken Indian" (Deloria, 1969).

Collaborative models of research with communities have been suggested, and the now larger number of Indian mental health professionals and researchers has increased the feasibility and acceptance of research activities more responsive to community needs and desires. The political and ethical issues which arise can nevertheless be complicated. In the United States, research activities are funded largely by the Federal Alcohol, Drug and Mental Health Administration, and there is a national minority mental health research center specifically for American Indian and Alaska Native populations; the Indian Health Service also funds a more limited amount of intramural and extramural research.

The lack of well-validated assessment methods for research with Indians has hindered all substantive research on psychopathology. It should not be assumed that instruments of known reliability and validity in the majority culture will perform in the same way for these culturally distinct populations. The development of such methods and instruments is essential for investigation of the distribution and course of mental disorders and their etiology, and for evaluation of the effectiveness of treatment and prevention strategies. There has been very little work in this area to date. The performance of the Center for Epidemiologic Studies Depression Scale (CES-D), a widely used self-report instrument, in Indian samples has recently been investigated (Baron, Manson, Ackerson, and Brenneman, 1991; Manson, Ackerson, Dick, Baron, and Fleming, 1991; Beals, Manson, Keane, and Dick, 1991). This work demonstrates that its dimensional structure is different for this special population. The research of Manson et al. (1985) with the depression section of the Diagnostic Interview Schedule (DIS) has improved our understanding of the limitations of this type of instrument in one specific tribe, but represents only a first step in the search for more valid tools.

Another methodologic issue which has never been satisfactorily resolved in research with Native communities is that of sampling methods in epidemiologic studies. The collection of epidemiologic data requires the use of probability sampling methods if the results are to have much credibility, yet studies in these communities have instead used various convenience sampling approaches. In the past, this has resulted largely from legitimate concerns about community acceptance of the research. Nevertheless, it will be extremely important to move beyond these limitations if epidemiologic methods are to be used to investigate the etiology, and ultimately the prevention, of mental health problems.

There are important substantive questions concerning how effective treatment services can best be delivered to these people, particularly where (as in Alaska and parts of the Southwest) they live in relatively remote and isolated places. Research to guide the prevention and treatment of substance abuse is an especially high priority. Suicide prevention is another area of the highest priority; suicides among young people have been devastating to the small and close-knit communities in which many Indian and Native people live. Psychopharmacologic research is yet a third area which merits attention, particularly since clinical impressions suggest differences in the effectiveness of psychopharmacologic agents, and the severity of side-effects, among Indian patients.

The above discussion of mental illness among American Indians and Alaska Natives, brief as it is, barely touches upon the potential contributions to mental *health* contained within Native

cultures, as, for example, reflected in indigenous healing traditions. It is hoped that those who work with these communities
will take these strengths into account as well.

REFERENCES

American Psychiatric Association (1980), *Diagnostic and Statistical Manual of Mental Disorders*, 3rd ed. (DSM-III). Washington, DC: American Psychiatric Press.
—— (1987), *Diagnostic and Statistical Manual of Mental Disorders*, 3rd
ed. (DSM-III-R). Washington, DC: American Psychiatric Press.
Baron, A. E., Manson, S. M., Ackerson, L. M., & Brenneman, D. L.
(1991), Depression symptomatology in older American Indians
with chronic disease. In: *Screening for Depression in Primary Care*, ed.
C. Attkisson & J. Zich. New York: Routledge, Chapman & Hall.
Beals, J., Manson, S. M., Keane, E. M., & Dick, R. W. (1991), The factorial
structure of the Center for Epidemiologic Studies Depression Scale
(CES-D) among American Indian college students. Submitted
for publication.
Beauvais, F., & LaBoeuff, S. (1985), Drug and alcohol abuse intervention
in American Indian communities. *Internat. J. Addictions*,
20:139–171.
—— Oetting, E. R., & Edwards, R. W. (1985a), Trends in drug use of
Indian adolescents living on reservations. *Amer. J. Drug & Alcohol
Abuse*, 11:209–229.
—— —— —— (1985b), Trends in the use of inhalants among
American Indian adolescents. *White Cloud J.*, 3:3–11.
Berlin, I. (1987), Suicide among American Indian adolescents: An over-
view. *Suicide & Life-Threat. Behav.*, 17:218–232.
Brod, T. M. (1975), Alcoholism as a mental health problem of Native
Americans. A review of the literature. *Arch. Gen. Psychiat.*,
32:1385–1391.
Deloria, V. (1969), *Custer Died for Your Sins, An Indian Manifesto*. New
York: Avon Books.
Forbes, N., & Van Der Hyde, V. (1988), Suicide in Alaska from
1978–1985: Updated data from state files. *Amer. Ind. & Alaska Na-
tive Ment. Health Res.*, 1:36–55.
Foulks, E. F., & Katz, S. (1973), The mental health of Alaskan Natives.
Acta Psychiat. Scand., 49:91–96.
Guilmet, G. (1984), Health care and health care seeking strategies
among Puyallup Indians. *Cult., Med., & Psychiatry*, 8:349–369.

Heath, D. B. (1989), American Indians and Alcohol. Epidemiological and sociocultural relevance. In: *Alcohol Use Among U.A. Ethnic Minorities*, ed. D. L. Spiegler, D. A. Tate, S. S. Aitken, & C. M. Christian. NIAAA Research Monograph No. 18. DHHS Publication No. (ADM) 89-1435. Rockville, MD: National Institute on Alcohol Abuse and Alcoholism.

Hograbe, R. (1989), Barriers to mainstream health care experienced by urban American Indians. St. Paul, MN: American Indian Health Care Association (245 East St. Paul St., Suite 499, St. Paul, MN 55101).

Jilek, W. G. (1977), A quest for identity: Therapeutic aspects of the Salish Indian Guardian Spirit Ceremonial. *J. Operat. Psychiat.*, 8:46–51.

Kinzie, J. D., Leung, P. K., Boehnlein, J., Matsunaga, D., Johnson, R., Manson, S., Shore, J. H., Heinz, J., & Williams M. (1991), Psychiatric epidemiology of an Indian village: A 19-year replication study. *J. Nerv. & Ment. Disorders*, 180:33–39.

Kraus, R., & Buffler, P. (1979), Sociocultural stress and the American Native in Alaska: An analysis of the changing patterns of psychiatric illness and alcohol abuse among Alaska Natives. *Cult., Med., & Psychiat.*, 3:111–151.

Kunitz, S. J., & Levy, J. E. (1981), Navajos. In: *Ethnicity and Medical Care*, ed. A. Harwood. Cambridge, MA: Harvard University Press.

Leighton, A. H., & Hughes, C. C. (1955), Notes on Eskimo patterns of suicide. *SW J. Anthropol.*, 11:327–338.

Manson, S. M., Ackerson, L. M., Dick, R. W., Baron, A. E., & Fleming, C. M. (1991), Depressive symptoms among American Indian adolescents: Psychometic characteristics of the Center for Epidemiologic Studies Depression Scale (CES-D). *Psycholog. Assess.*, 2:231–237.

———— Shore, J. H., & Bloom, J. D. (1985), The depressive experience in American Indian communities: A challenge for psychiatric theory and diagnosis. In: *Culture and Depression*, ed. A. Kleinman & B. Good. Berkeley, CA: University of California Press.

———— ———— ———— Keepers, G. K., & Neligh, G. (1987), Alcohol abuse and major affective disorders: Advances in epidemiologic research among American Indians. In: *The Epidemiology of Alcohol Use and Abuse Among U.S. Ethnic Minority Groups*, ed. D. Spiegler. National Institute on Alcohol Abuse and Alcoholism Monograph Series. Washington, DC: U.S. Government Printing Office.

———— Walker, R. D., & Kivlahan, D. R. (1987), Psychiatric assessment and treament of American Indians and Alaska Natives. *Hosp. & Commun. Psychiat.*, 38:165–173.

Marano, L. (1982), Windigo psychosis: The anatomy of an emic/etic confusion. *Current Anthropol.*, 23:385–412.

May, P. A. (1987), Suicide and self-destruction among American Indian youths. *Amer. Ind. & Alaska Native Ment. Health Res.*, 1:52–69.

Murphy, J. M., & Hughes, C. C. (1965), The use of psychophysiological symptoms as indicators of disorder among Eskimos. In: *Approaches to Cross-Cultural Psychiatry*, ed. J. M. Murphy & A. H. Leighton. Ithaca, NY: Cornell University Press.

Neligh, G., Baron, A. E., Braun, P., & Czarnecki, M. (Submitted for publication), Panic disorder among American Indians: Programs for its detection and treatment.

Oetting, E., Beauvais, F., & Edwards, R. W. (1988), Alcohol and Indian youth: Social and psychological correlates and prevention. *J. Drug Issues*, 18:87–101.

——— Goldstein, G. S. (1979), Drug use among Native American adolescents. In: *Youth Drug Abuse*, ed. G. Beschner & A. Friedman. Lexington, MA: Lexington Books.

Sampath, H. M. (1974), Prevalence of psychiatric disorders in a Southern Baffin Island Eskimo settlement. *Can. Psychiatric Assn. J.*, 19:363–367.

Shore, J. H., Kinzie, J. D., & Hampson, J. L. (1973), Psychiatric epidemiology of an Indian village. *Psychiatry*, 36:70–81.

U.S. Congress, Office of Technology Assessment (1986), *Indian Health Care* OTA-H-290. Washington, DC: U.S. Government Printing Office, April.

23.

Mental Health Patterns for the New Zealand Maori

Mason H. Durie

Although New Zealand is a predominantly Western nation, sharing similar mental health problems with other Western countries, 12 percent of the population of 3.1 million is Maori. They are the indigenous people of New Zealand whose ancestors arrived in a series of epic voyages, from elsewhere in the Pacific, some six or seven centuries ago.

The Maori population is a relatively youthful one, 34 percent of the total 403,185 (1986 census) being under the age of 15 years (Royal Commission, Report I, 1988a). Although a tribal society, Maori people now predominantly live in urban areas, a major shift occurring from rural areas after 1945. With that shift came considerable tribal and family alienation and with its attendant social upheaval. On all indicators of social well-being, Maori people fare poorly. Income levels are significantly lower than for non-Maori, 68 percent of Maori children being born into families who are in the lowest two quintiles of income distribution (Social Monitoring Group, 1989). Lower standards of educational achievement for Maori children are well documented (Benton,

Acknowledgments. Esther Tinirau, for preparation of the manuscript; the Department of Maori Studies, Massey University, for advice and collation of information.

1988). Maori unemployment is almost three times that of non-Maoris and is especially high among 25-year-olds and those associated with agriculture, forestry, and fishing. High Maori imprisonment rates are a further source of concern, the Maori male imprisonment rate of 186 per 10,000 being 13.8 times greater than the non-Maori equivalent (Royal Commission, Report II, 1988b).

Mortality and morbidity statistics show similar disparities for almost all categories of illness. Nearly twice as many Maori infants die from Sudden Infant Death Syndrome (SIDS) than non-Maori; at ages 25 to 64 years, total death rates for Maori women are twice that of non-Maori women; only 34 percent of Maori deaths occur at ages 65 years and over compared to 71 percent of non-Maori deaths (Pomare and deBoer, 1988). Life expectancy at birth is 7 years shorter for Maori males and 8.5 years shorter for Maori females compared to the non-Maori population.

TRADITIONAL ATTITUDES TOWARD MENTAL HEALTH

A characteristic of the traditional (and pre-European) Maori health system was its integrated nature. Mental health as separate from physical health had little traditional meaning, although the influence of *taha wairua* (spirituality) and *taha hinengaro* (cognition, emotions) was recognized as having a profound effect on human behavior and well-being (Durie, 1985). Indeed, Maori theories of health depended on a strong belief in the power of the mind and vulnerability to a number of deities (Durie, 1984).

In understanding Maori views of human behavior, including sickness behavior, the concept of *tapu* is critical. Maori society recognized two complementary states: *tapu* and *noa*. A person, article, building, or area was regarded as *tapu* if it had been declared "special," requiring respect, often avoidance, and a cautious approach. It was an effective social sanction which guided not only interpersonal interactions but also relationships with the environment. A breach of *tapu*, in which a person wittingly or unwittingly failed to treat a *tapu* object or person with sufficient respect, invariably led to misery, and sometimes to death. A violation of the laws of *tapu* was considered a major cause of illness.

In contrast to *tapu*, was the state of *noa*. A *noa* object could be approached freely without fear of misfortune though caution was necessary to keep *tapu* and *noa* objects apart. Food was a *noa* object. Sometimes, particularly after the advent of Western culture, *tapu* and *noa* were erroneously linked with gender, men being supposedly more able to deal with *tapu* states than women, who were associated with *noa*.

Tapu was not necessarily a permanent state, rather it was conferred by particular reasons, usually to ensure the maintenance of tribal integrity and personal safety. By the same token, it could be removed when no longer appropriate or necessary.

The conferring or removal of *tapu* depended on a *tohunga*, a leader skilled in tribal lore with a wide repertoire of ancient incantations and rituals. In many respects the *tohunga* was a combination of priest, physician, and judge, a skilled observer of human nature and astute about the politics of tribal society (Durie, 1977).

Two classification systems were used in the understanding of illness. One was based on etiology and distinguished between accidents (e.g., *mate taua*) and *mate atua* (i.e., illnesses for which there were no obvious external causes). (*Mate atua* translates literally as an illness of the Gods, an indication of spiritual origins.) The other classification was based on symptom clusters, recognizing several discrete syndromes including *wairangi* or *porangi*, insanity. *Tapu* was a major etiological factor for all *mate atua*, and in their diagnostic routines *tohunga* conducted a thorough investigation to determine the circumstances of a breach of *tapu* so that appropriate amends could be made. Another, related, causative factor of *mate atua* was *makutu*. A person or family who had committed an offense could be rendered distraught in either physical or mental terms, by the incantations of a *tohunga*, often from a distance. The victim might have transgressed while visiting another area or might have given serious offense within the family or tribal context. In any event, *makutu* produced a serious state of disability which, without intervention from another *tohunga*, could lead to death.

Mental illness (*wairangi, porangi*) was a subset of the wider *mate atua* classification and as such tended to be explained as an infringement of the laws of *tapu* or of the sensitivities of powerful others whose retaliation could produce derangement even without a physical confrontation. Although there was a spiritual basis to the condition, it was also closely linked with accepted social values and often suggested a departure from community norms either by the patient or the wider family. Individual and family distinctions were not sharp, the health of one being regarded as a symptom of the other.

COLONIZATION

By 1840, when, after the signing of the Treaty of Waitangi, New Zealand was annexed by Great Britain, traditional Maori society had already undergone marked change as a result of contact with missionaries, whalers, and settlers from Great Britain, the United States, and France. New social and economic systems rapidly supplanted the old, and with them came the good and bad influences of Western culture. Inevitably there was conflict and a series of land wars in the 1860s left many tribes in impoverished circumstances as the new settler government asserted itself, paving the way for more English immigrants and the creation of a predominantly Western society. Despite the Treaty of Waitangi, which had guaranteed to the Maori people a measure of control over their own properties and destiny, policies of assimilation were rapidly introduced offering little room for effective Maori participation in law making or the perpetuation of Maori social organization (Walker, 1990).

Health policies failed to recognize Maori views or preferences and indeed saw those views as decidedly counterproductive. The Tohunga Suppression Act (1907) outlawed native healers forcing the *tohunga* underground and discounting their extensive methodology and substantial following. Deaths from tuberculosis were cited as the main reason for outlawing the *tohunga* (M. Pomare, 1916), but the effect was to totally denigrate Maori views of health and mental illness.

Health professionals trained in Western medicine replaced tribal elders as leaders in health, increasingly relegating Maori people to passive consumer roles within a set of values and expectations which were culturally alien and only superficially accepted.

Over the past two decades, however, the significance of cultural factors to health has been reassessed. Maori groups throughout the country have expressed skepticism at the diagnostic categories and treatment methods used in contemporary psychiatric settings (National Mental Health Consortium, 1989), and have reaffirmed confidence in some traditional views on illness and healing (Rolleston, 1989). While there is general recognition that Western medicine has much to offer Maori people, there is a parallel observation that it is limited in many respects and that the concepts of *tapu, noa, makutu,* and the role of the *tohunga* provide a residual reality for many Maori people, including those living in urban situations.

CONTEMPORARY MANIFESTATIONS OF MENTAL ILLNESS

Maori people did not figure prominently in mental illness statistics until relatively recent times and there was even a suggestion that the incidence of psychosis was less, a conclusion based on lower rates of hospital admission (Beaglehole, 1939). But current admission rates could well suggest the opposite (Sachdev, 1989).

Since 1962 Maori admissions to psychiatric hospitals have increased substantially. Whereas prior to 1960 non-Maori hospital admission rates were higher than those for Maoris, by 1974 the situation had reversed, with Maori rates exceeding non-Maori except for the elderly.[1]

In order to compare Maori and non-Maori rates it is necessary to look at age-specific rates because of the different age structures of the two populations.

Table 23.1 shows that in general over this period, the average rate of first admissions to inpatient psychiatric care for Maori has been highest in the 20 to 29 year age group. This age group has had an average yearly first admission rate of 285 per 100,000 compared with a non-Maori rate of 220 per 100,000.

---

[1]Maori and non-Maori health statistics are subject to the same requirements and are kept by the same agency. Prior to 1970 Maori had a lower reporting rate for mental illness. Since 1974 the reverse has been true. Outside hospital, Maori more frequently come to the attention of police and similar authorities (possibly because there is less opportunity for other sources of help).

TABLE 23.1
First Admissions: Age Specific Rates Maori and non-Maori

| | | \
Rates per 100,000 population | | | | | | |
|------|----------|------|------|------|------|------|------|------|
| | | 0− | 10− | 20− | 30− | 40− | 50− | 60+ |
| 1962 | Maori | 44 | 170 | 223 | 164 | 154 | 180 | 104 |
| | non-Maori | 33 | 86 | 207 | 248 | 247 | 214 | 360 |
| 1968 | Maori | 46 | 215 | 356 | 140 | 146 | 126 | 100 |
| | non-Maori | 28 | 145 | 259 | 249 | 246 | 185 | 266 |
| 1974 | Maori | 30 | 191 | 344 | 296 | 227 | 202 | 222 |
| | non-Maori | 29 | 130 | 241 | 200 | 204 | 193 | 222 |
| 1980 | Maori | 17 | 133 | 341 | 226 | 175 | 99 | 168 |
| | non-Maori | 23 | 96 | 222 | 476 | 173 | 156 | 206 |
| 1986 | Maori | 9 | 216 | 533 | 244 | 128 | 62 | 122 |
| | non-Maori | 15 | 109 | 228 | 163 | 117 | 98 | 146 |
| 1987 | Maori | 15 | 170 | 393 | 253 | 117 | 103 | 51 |
| | non-Maori | 13 | 111 | 218 | 149 | 127 | 98 | 149 |

Source: Department of Health, New Zealand, in Sachdev, P.S., "Psychiatrict Illness in the New Zealand Maori," *Australia and NZ J. Psychiat.*, 1989: 23:529–541; and *Mental Health Data,* 1987.

It is difficult to determine accurately the prevalence of mental illness among Maori people as there has been no serious attempt to record the extent of psychiatric disorders within a Maori community using either Western or Maori diagnostic criteria. Such information as there is comes from data on hospital admissions, though for a variety of reasons even that is likely to underrepresent Maori illness.

First, if the family feels that a disturbed state is related to *makutu* or some infringement of *tapu*, then, regardless of severity, strenuous efforts will be made to resist hospitalization. Second, communities may have differing levels of tolerance. Households accustomed to high levels of stress and, for socioeconomic reasons less inclined to seek professional advice, especially if class and ethnic barriers prevail, may simply accept abnormal behavior as the norm.

Third, for other reasons Maori patients may never reach hospital. Using conventional criteria several studies have shown that Maori inmates in institutions other than hospitals have disproportionately high levels of mental illness particularly in prisons (Roper, 1989), but also in Child Health Camps[2] where Maori

---

[2]Child Health Camps are similar to holiday camps for children with health problems. They are voluntary and are not part of the juvenile court system. In earlier years they

admission rates remain high (Hancock, 1984). Insofar as most hospital admissions depend on referral from community health services, hospital statistics will have limited reliability in estimating community prevalence rates as long as Maori patients have less recourse to primary health care facilities, or mask psychological symptoms in the presence of their general practitioner or present with different symptoms, not immediately associated with mental illness.

The source of referral to a psychiatric facility suggests differing patterns for Maori and non-Maori. Table 23.2 summarizes by ethnic groups referrals for first admissions to psychiatric hospitals for 1987. Of concern are the relatively high numbers of Maori and Pacific Island patients referred by a law enforcement agency (Mental Health Foundation, 1988). Maori patients accounted for over 26 percent of all patients in that category and over one-fifth of all Maori first admissions were from the courts or police. It suggests a late stage of intervention and poses further questions about the quality and accessibility of community services.

Table 23.3 which lists first admission diagnoses for the five years 1893 to 1987 shows that alcohol dependence or abuse was by far the leading reason for inpatient care during this period.

There is evidence that both schizophrenia and alcohol dependence are overrepresented in Maori admissions, but it is difficult to conclude that prevalence rates are in fact excessive. The higher figures may reflect reduced levels of care within the community, underutilization of primary health care facilities, or more frequent resort to the committal of Maori patients.

Although the disorders which result in Maori people being admitted to psychiatric hospitals are said to be similar in form to those in the non-Maori population (Social Monitoring Group, 1987) four categories are of particular concern.

Suicide

Maori suicide rates remain lower than non-Maori rates but the gap appears to be closing (Robinson, 1988). Apart from *whakamo-mori* (suicide by widows during bereavement) there is little evidence that suicide was extensively practiced in traditional Maori

---

were for children who were malnourished. Now there is a great proportion of children with mental health problems. Children stay at the camps for about six weeks.

TABLE 23.2
First Admissions: Source of Referral by Ethnic Groups
1987

Source of Referral	Maori (n = 540)	Pacific Islander (n = 87)	Other (n = 3,724)
	%	%	%
Self and/or relative	14	9	12
Private psychiatrist	0.1	-	2
Other medical practitioner	26	22	30
Non-psychiatric hospital unit	13	15	13
Geriatric unit	-	-	1
Psychiatric unit of general hospital	2	1	3
Inpatient sector of psychiatric care	1	1	1
Outpatient sector of psychiatric care	10	14	13
Day patient sector of psychiatric care	-	1	1
Law enforcement agency	22	28	8
Nonmedical agency	12	5	12
Domiciliary nursing service	1	3	1
Unknown	1	1	2

Source: National Health Statistics Centre, Mental Health Data 1987, Department of Health, New Zealand.

society, so that reports of suicide among young Maori in recent times (*mate taurekareka*) have provoked considerable discussion and alarm in some Maori communities. While the numbers are not large they suggest a changing pattern. In the years 1973 to 1984 the number of suicides for Maori males was 47 in the first six years and 67 in the second six years; an increase of 43 percent; and for Maori females it was 14 in the first six years and 22 in the second six years, an increase of 57 percent. During this period there has also been a steady increase in suicides amongst non-Maori males from 173 in 1973 to 280 in 1984. Suicides amongst non-Maori females revealed no clear trend varying between 78 and 100. In times of economic hardship, an increase in the number of deaths due to suicide might be expected. This has certainly been the case in the 15- to 24-year-old group where there has

TABLE 23.3
First Admissions: Short List Diagnoses
1983-1987

FIRST ADMISSIONS (Maori) Percentages

Short list diagnoses	1983	1984	1985	1986	1987
Senile and pre-senile organic					
psychotic conditions	1	4	.8	.9	.2
Alcoholic psychoses	.2	7	.4	.4	.8
Drug psychoses	1	2	1	2	2
Other organic psychotic					
conditions	2	1	2	.6	1
Schizophrenic psychoses	12	10	11	11	9
Affective psychoses	6	7	9	6	1
Paranoid states	.2	.4	1	1	1
Other psychoses	5	5	6	4	7
Neurotic depression and other					
depressive disorders	12	10	12	12	9
Other neurotic disorders	3	2	.8	.6	.2
Alcohol dependence or abuse	30	32	28	25	27
Drug dependence or abuse	3	5	6	13	9
Other personality disorders	6	7	5	4	6
Stress and adjustment					
reactions	10	8	9	9	9
Non-psychotic disorders of					
childhood and adolescence	.2	.4	–	–	.4
Non-psychotic mental disorders					
following brain damage	.2	.4	.4	.5	.4
Conditions associated with					
physical disorders	.2	–	.1	–	.2
Mental retardation	3	3	.7	1	2
No psychiatric diagnosis	5	5	6	9	8
	100	100	100	100	100
n=	557	579	653	650	540

Source: National Health Statistics Centre, Mental Health Data 1987, Department of Health, New Zealand.

been an increase in both the Maori and non-Maori rates with a 2.5 percent increase in young Maori male suicides occurring in the decade to 1980 to 1984 (Pomare and deBoer, 1988). Given the rapid economic, social, and cultural changes confronting Maori society, the removal of social restraints such as *tapu* and the diminishing authority of tribal elders without clear or meaningful substitutes, the emergence of suicidal behavior is not surprising,

adding to the high death toll resulting from motor vehicle accidents among Maori males in the 15- to 24-year age group.

Depression and Other Stress-Related Reactions

These disorders hardly featured in 1970 but have emerged as the
most important causes of mental illness in females, and among
the Maori community are thought to be associated with obesity,
alcohol and drug abuse, and poor physical health. In a major
study of Maori women involving 1177 respondents (Murchie,
1984) depression was highlighted as the most significant symptom
for young women and a major cause of distress for older women.
It was linked with the availability of tribal supports; five in every
ten young women (n = 298) being at high risk through tribal
supports not being readily accessible and four in every ten middle-
aged women (n = 268) being similarly jeopardized. Mature
women (n = 211) were most secure, six in any ten living in or
close to their own tribal area.

Despite the increasing incidence of anorexia nervosa in New
Zealand (Social Monitoring Group, 1989) the condition does not
appear to be prevalent to any degree among Maori women nor
has there been any reported increase in bulimia. On the other
hand, between the ages of 20 and 64 years, Maori people are on
average both heavier and more obese than non-Maoris. It has
been estimated that three-quarters of Maori women are over-
weight and nearly half are obese (Pomare and deBoer, 1988).[3]

Forensic Psychiatry

The Psychiatric Report illustrates the high numbers of Maori patients in the forensic sector, represented mainly by patients re-
manded by the courts for psychiatric examination as well as
special patients transferred from prison to hospital under special

---

[3]A larger body frame (not necessarily obesity) is valued and there is no great emphasis
on thinness as aesthetically desirable. If anything Maori people (and other Polynesians)
tend to regard slenderness as a sign of poor health.

TABLE 23.4
Total Special and Remand Patients Admitted to Psychiatric Hospitals
During the Years 1980–1986 and the Percentages of These Admissions
Identified as Maori

Year	Total Admissions	Maori		
		% Total Admissions	% Remands	% Special Patients
1980	414	32	27	45
1981	442	26	21	40.5
1982	425	30	26	40
1983	390	31.5	26	47
1984	298	29.5	27.5	37
1985	255	28	24.5	42
1986	149	36	31	67

Source: Psychiatric Report, 1988.

status following involvement with the criminal justice system. Maori inclusion in those categories is shown in Table 23.4.

Because of the "open-door" policy of psychiatric hospitals and a reluctance to admit patients who might require excessive security, there has been an overall reduction in admission rates for remand and special patients, less, however, for Maori than other groups. Whilst Maori comprise 12 percent of the general population they accounted for 67 percent of special patient admissions in 1986.

There are several aspects to the situation requiring further investigation. Are psychiatric symptoms in Maori patients masked by a behavioral overlay which leads to prison rather than medical intervention? Does the Maori offender react adversely to imprisonment as suggested in the Psychiatric Report? Is entry into the health system biased against Maori patients diminishing the chances of early detection and treatment of mental health problems?

Mate Maori

Reference has already been made to *mate Maori*, an affliction said to be a type of *mate atua* related to spiritual causes, and requiring the intervention of a *tohunga*. In the 1984 Rapuora study one in every five women respondents said they would go to a Maori traditional healer if they had a *mate Maori* though not all knew who might be an appropriate healer, nor did one in five women know what *mate Maori* was.

The term refers essentially to a state of ill-health attributable to an infringement of *tapu* or the infliction of a *makutu*. The prevalence of *mate Maori* has never been estimated although there are published accounts of the condition and its management (Palmer, 1954; Gluckman, 1976). It may take several forms, physical or mental, and various illnesses, not necessarily atypical in presentation, may be ascribed to it. Thus there is no single clinical presentation and psychiatrists need to be alert to the possibility of *mate Maori* when obtaining a history. Most families will be reluctant to discuss *mate Maori* in a hospital or clinic setting fearing ridicule or, perhaps more importantly, being pressured to choose between psychiatric and Maori approaches. In fact one need not exclude the other, cooperation between traditional Maori healers and health professionals being more acceptable now to both groups.

While *mate Maori* applies to physical as well as mental illnesses, increasingly it has become a focus to explain emotional and psychiatric disorders. The author has had the experience of several patients presenting with severe psychomotor retardation, depression, high levels of anxiety, insomnia, and withdrawal not dissimilar from a depressive psychosis except in the suddenness of onset. In each case there was a history of a very recent stay in the territory of another tribe and concern on the part of the family that a *makutu* had emanated from that tribe for some indiscretion. Intervention by a *tohunga* from the patient's tribe led to a rapid resolution of symptoms in most cases.

Treatment by a *tohunga* involves the family as well as the patient and may include *karakia* (prayers, incantations), immersion in *wai tapu* (water from a special stream), some act of restitution, the use of herbs and *whakamanawa* (reassurance, support). Many *tohunga* distinguish between Maori and Pakeha (i.e., non-Maori) components of the disorder and advise patients to seek medical treatment if there is some aspect that they cannot heal. It is not unusual for Maori patients to accept psychiatric and *tohunga* treatment concurrently, nor does there appear to be any sound reason why that dual approach should not occur.

CONCLUSIONS

Socioeconomic disparities are thought to account for the increase in mental illness among Maori people but attention must also be given to those particular cultural factors which contribute to the genesis and understanding of mental disorder. Psychiatry in New Zealand has, to some extent, begun to face that challenge both by encouraging greater Maori participation and by attempting to match progress in psychiatry with progress in Maori social, economic, and cultural development.

Four approaches have been advocated to ensure greater Maori participation in psychiatric services:

Workforce Development

Maori involvement in the mental health professions has been extremely low in all disciplines (Abbott and Durie, 1987), a situation which many groups are attempting to rectify both by providing incentives, including scholarships for Maori recruits into training programs, as well as by adding a Maori perspective to some courses, again in order to provide Maori students with a greater sense of relevance and balance.

Policy Development

Area health boards, which administer public mental health services, have appointed Maori board members and have been encouraged to formalize links with appropriate Maori communities (Ministerial Advisory Committee, 1990). In some areas representative regional Maori health councils have been established expressly to ensure that health services are appropriate to Maori people, and accessible both in cultural and economic terms.

Special Units

Aware of the reduced emphasis placed on spirituality and other cultural values within treatment settings, Maori groups, often Maori staff members, have been successful in establishing three Maori units for Maori patients. Located in psychiatric hospital grounds these units attempt to provide appropriate conventional psychiatric treatment which incorporates Maori values including visits from *tohunga* and the use of *karakia* as an integral part of the treatment program (Rankin, 1986).

Biculturalism

Over the past five years, state agencies in New Zealand have accepted a need to develop greater understanding of Maori culture, language, and society, largely as a consequence of a report prepared for the Department of Social Welfare which alleged institutionalized racism in many welfare institutions (Ministerial Advisory Committee, 1984). Although the parameters of biculturalism remain somewhat obscure, psychiatric services have made major advances in educating staff and modifying existing programs so that Maori values might find suitable expression in an otherwise alien environment. The rationale for biculturalism comes from Maori/non-Maori disparities in health standards as well as from the Treaty of Waitangi which laid the foundation for a partnership between Maori tribes and the state (Durie, 1989). Opinion is divided as to whether biculturalism, within a predominantly Western institution, can flourish in a meaningful way or whether it simply creates a misleading impression of the acceptance of Maori culture without any major concessions to Maori input in decision making.

Psychiatric services, like other social services, have had to assess the impact of tribal development and cultural reassertion on both diagnostic and treatment processes. Most have responded with some movements toward biculturalism, less often toward the establishment of special Maori units or the appointment of Maori liaison workers. In turn, some tribes have developed strong and useful links with psychiatric services accepting their general approach but supplementing them with tribal expertise and knowledge.

Not all tribes, however, are so ready to accept the premises upon which modern psychiatry is based, maintaining that fundamental philosophical differences prevent any real amalgamation of their approaches and advocating instead a greater reliance on traditional treatments. To them psychiatry is seen as an agent of oppression, a vestige of colonization that applies culturally inappropriate classifications and treatments to situations that are better explained and managed within tribal understandings of individual behavior. While that stance may not represent a majority view, it does raise questions about the degree to which Maori cultural views might be incorporated into modern psychiatric practice without diminishing the ethos of either.

REFERENCES

Abbott, M. W., & Durie, M. H. (1987), A whiter shade of pale: Taha Maori and professional psychology training. *NZ J. Psychol.*, 16:58–71.

Beaglehole, E. (1939), Culture and psychosis in New Zealand. *J. Polynesian Soc.*, 48:144–155.

Benton, R. (1988), *How Fair is New Zealand Education*, Vol. 2. Paper for Royal Commission on Social Policy. Wellington, NZ: NZCER.

Durie, M. H. (1977), Maori attitudes to sickness, doctors and hospitals. *NZ Med. J.*, 86:483–485.

——— (1984), Te Taha Hinengaro. An integrated approach to mental health. *Community Ment. Health in NZ*, 1:4–11.

——— (1985), A Maori perspective of health. *Soc. Sc. Med.*, 20:483–486.

——— (1989), The treaty of Waitangi and health care. *NZ Med. J.*, 102:283–285.

Gluckman, L. K. (1976), *Tangiwai Medical History of New Zealand Prior to 1860*. Auckland: Whitcoulls.

Hancock, M. (1984), *Children's Health, Tomorrow's Wealth*. Report of the Committee to Review the Children's Health Camp Movement, Wellington.

Mental Health Foundation of New Zealand (1988), Submission to the Royal Commission on Social Policy.

Ministerial Advisory Committee on Maori Health (1990), *Maori Health*

Policy: Guidelines for Area Health Boards. Wellington: Department of Health.

Ministerial Advisory Committee on a Maori Perspective for the Department of Social Welfare (1984), *Puao-te-ata-tu.* Wellington: Department of Social Welfare.

Murchie, E., Ed. (1984), *Rapuora: Health and Maori Women.* Wellington: The Maori Women's Welfare League Inc.

National Mental Health Consortium (1989), *The Tangata Whenua Report, the Consumer Report, the Consortium Report.* Departments of Health and Social Welfare, Wellington.

Palmer, G. Blake (1954), Tohungaism and Makutu. *J. Polynesian Soc.,* 63:147–163.

Pomare, E., & deBoer, G. (1988), *Hauora: Maori Standards of Health.* Special Report Series 78. Wellington: Department of Health.

Pomare, M. (1916), The Maori. In: *Transactions of the Eighth Session of the Australasian Medical Congress.* Melbourne, Australia.

Rankin, J. F. A. (1986), Whaiora: A Maori cultural therapy unit. *Community Ment. Health NZ,* 3:38–47.

Robinson, J. (1988), Maori futures: The paths ahead. Paper prepared for the Royal Commission on Social Policy.

Rolleston, S. (1989), *He Kohikohinga: A Maori Health Knowledge Base.* Wellington: Department of Health.

Roper, J. (Chairman). Prison Review (1989), *Te Ara Hou: The New Way.* Report of the Ministerial Committee of Inquiry into the Prisons System, Wellington.

Royal Commission on Social Policy (1988a), *The April Report I.* Wellington: Royal Commission on Social Policy.

———— (1988b), *The April Report II.* Wellington: Royal Commission on Social Policy.

Sachdev, P. S. (1989), Psychiatric illness in the New Zealand Maori. *Austral. & NZ J. Psychiatry,* 23:529–541.

Social Monitoring Group (1987), *Care and Control, the Role of Institutions in New Zealand.* Report No. 2. Wellington: New Zealand Planning Council.

———— (1989), *From Birth to Death II: The Second Overview Report.* Wellington: New Zealand Planning Council.

Walker, R. (1990), *Ka Whawhai Tonu Matou: Struggle Without End.* Auckland, NZ: Penguin.

24.

Mental Health Among Minorities and Immigrants in Britain

Raymond Cochrane

In addition to the problems which beset cross-cultural psychiatry everywhere, a special problem in Britain has been the confounding of minority ethnic status and cultural differences with immigration. Until very recently a very high proportion of the nonwhite minority groups in Britain, especially adults, were also first-generation migrants, therefore any differences observed between the mental health of such minorities and that of the white majority could not be attributed unambiguously to any one, or any combination of the following variables: (1) cultural/ethnic differences; (2) selection (positive or negative) for migration; (3) the process of migration/culture shock; (4) the experience of being an immigrant in a hostile society. In addition there were the other problems associated with the depressed socioeconomic structure found in first-generation immigrant groups almost everywhere.

In fact Britain has always been a center for migration. Historically many more people have left Britain to settle elsewhere in the world, and fewer, but still substantial numbers of people have come from elsewhere to live in Britain. Since the Second World War, however, there have been some changes in the patterns of inmigration to Britain which have affected the way in which

347

immigration is regarded. First, an increased proportion of immigrants were nonwhite and, therefore, more visible than the previous waves of Irish, Jewish, and European immigrants that occurred in this century. Second, some of the newer immigrants came from very different religiocultural backgrounds to those of the host society and, what is more, some of these groups have shown no desire to abandon their culture of origin and to become homogenized into the dominant Anglo culture. Third, perhaps as a result of the fact that many post-World War II immigrants came from societies which had previously been subjected to British imperialism, prejudice, racism, and discrimination against them became widespread.

One manifestation of this prejudice was the automatic equation of immigration into Britain with social problems. An assumption was readily made that immigrants would place great demands on the welfare and health services of the receiving country, both absolutely and disproportionately to their numbers in the population. Considerable concern was generated about the mental health of those involved (Littlewood and Lipsedge, 1982).

Perhaps the most extreme, and in many ways misleading, expression of this concern appeared in 1978 in a booklet published by the British Commission for Racial Equality (CRE) entitled: *Aspects of Mental Health in a Multi-Cultural Society.* Based on a few early studies of mental illness rates among West Indian and Asian immigrants, which were methodologically simplistic if not unsound, the CRE perpetuated the myth that immigrants pay a heavy psychological price in terms of mental illness for going to live in Britain. This booklet listed the following as being groups at special risk of mental illness: immigrant adolescents, second generation immigrants, Muslim women, Sikh women, Hindu women, West Indian women, West Indian men, Asian men, the elderly—in other words almost everyone who was not native born white British.

Assessing the mental health of immigrants has always posed a problem for epidemiologists for a number of reasons, and it has, therefore, been difficult to compare the mental health of immigrants with that of the native born. In early studies, for example in America (Odegaard, 1932; Malzberg, 1955), Scandinavia (Eitinger, 1959; Astrup and Odegaard, 1960), and Australia

(Krupinski, Schaechter, and Cade, 1965; Krupinski and Stoller, 1965) the general consensus was that immigrants faired poorly compared to the native born when it came to mental health, at least when measured by psychiatric hospital admission figures. Very few early studies put forward a positive view of the mental health of immigrants in their new country of settlement (Murphy, 1965).

A similar trend appeared in Britain, where the majority of early studies indicated that those who had originated in the Caribbean (Pinsent, 1963; Kiev, 1963, 1964; Gordon, 1965; Hemsi, 1967), and those born on the Indian subcontinent (Hashmi, 1968; Bagley, 1969; Pinto, 1974) suffered excess psychiatric morbidity in comparison with the native born. These earlier studies, however, were criticized on a number of methodological grounds such as the way in which "Asian" and "black" immigrants were poorly differentiated; and for failing to take into account the large demographic differences that inevitably exist between native and immigrant populations in terms of their sex ratios, age structure, social class composition, and rural–urban disposition patterns (Cochrane, 1983).

More recent studies on Caribbean migrants using regional hospital admission statistics (Carpenter and Brockington, 1980; Dean, Walsh, Downing, and Shelley, 1981), or case registers (Rwegellera, 1977) still show a higher overall rate of admission compared to the native born. With Asians the picture is somewhat less clear. While Carpenter and Brockington's (1980) study in Manchester showed that Asians had a higher rate of first admissions compared with the native born, Dean et al.'s (1981) study in southeastern England found significantly higher rates of psychiatric admissions for Indians, but lower rates for Pakistanis. Both studies used data for first admissions only, however, while Carpenter and Brockington also fail to differentiate between Indians and Pakistanis. As both these studies are small scale, it is difficult to generalize from their findings.

The most reliable data on the mental health of immigrants to Britain comes from two analyses of all mental hospital admissions for the whole of England that occurred in the two census years 1971 and 1981 (Cochrane, 1977; Cochrane and Bal, 1989). These studies showed that, overall, the foreign born had a higher

TABLE 24.1
**Rates of Admission to Mental Hospitals for All Diagnoses in England in
1981 by Country of Birth (adapted from Cochrane and Bal, 1989)**

Country of Birth	Rates per 100,000 population			
	Male		Female	
	First	subsequent	First	subsequent
England	95	225	127	358
Ireland	272	751	269	898
India	84	226	97	234
Pakistan[1]	70	146	106	123
Caribbean	111	391	105	484
Hong Kong	47	96	87	116

[1] Includes Bangladesh

rate of mental hospital admission than did the native born in
both 1971 and 1981. However, this bald statistic conceals more
than it reveals. A subset of the data from the more recent of these
studies is included in Table 24.1.

What is clear from these data is that it is the (white) Irish-
born migrants to Britain who have by far the highest rates of
mental hospital admissions of any immigrant group. Because they
are also the largest minority group (567,000 people or 1.24% of
the total population of England in 1981) they heavily inflated the
overall figure for the foreign born. In general Asian-born migrants to Britain, who constituted smaller groupings (Indian
born, 0.83%; Pakistani, 0.49%; Hong Kong Chinese, 0.11%) had
lower rates of mental hospital admissions than did the native
born. Those people born in the Caribbean but living in England
in 1981 (0.64% of the total population) had somewhat higher
rates than the native born but nowhere near the rates found for
the Irish born. The relatively good mental health of the Asian-
born population of England has been confirmed in community
surveys (Cochrane and Stopes-Roe, 1977, 1981). It is, of course,
possible to examine these figures from a variety of perspectives.
Table 24.2 includes a breakdown of admission rates by selected
diagnostic categories.

Leaving aside the Irish, who tend to show relatively high rates

TABLE 24.2
Rates of All Mental Hospital Admissions for Selected Diagnosis per
100,000 Population in England, 1981, Country of Birth (adapted from
Cochrane and Bal, 1989)

Country of birth	Schizophrenia and Paranoia		Depression[1]		Neuroses[2]		Alcohol Abuse[3]	
	Male	Female	Male	Female	Male	Female	Male	Female
England	61	58	79	166	28	56	38	18
Ireland	158	174	197	410	62	111	332	133
India	77	89	68	118	22	27	73	8
Pakistan[4]	94	32	68	96	15	47	6	1
Caribbean	359	235	65	152	6	25	27	9
Hong Kong	65	50	12	75	16	29	4	8

[1]Affective psychoses and depressive disorders
[2]Includes "neurotic depression"
[3]Alcohol psychosis, alcohol dependence, and nondependent abuse of alcohol
[4]Includes Bangladesh

for all disorders, the nonwhite immigrant populations of Britain consistently show higher rates of admission for schizophrenia and lower rates of admission for depression and neuroses. The high rate of admissions for alcohol-related disorders exhibited by Indian-born men is likely to be accounted for by the drinking habits of older Sikh men in England (Cochrane and Bal, 1990).

The most surprising data in Table 24.2 are undoubtedly the enormously elevated rates of admission for schizophrenia found for the Caribbean born. They are surprising for two reasons: First, they indicate that a very large proportion of all admissions for this group are for this disorder (52% for males and 40% for females compared to 19% and 12% respectively for the native born). Second, other evidence seems to suggest that schizophrenia is the one major mental illness that is least variable in its incidence across location and culture (WHO, 1979; Leff, 1981; Sartorius, Jablensky, Korten, Emberg, Anker, Cooper, and Day, 1986).

Although the Cochrane and Bal (1989) analysis is based on the largest data set, other researchers in Britain have consistently reached the same conclusions (Gordon, 1965; Twefik and Okasha, 1965; Hemsi, 1967; Bagley, 1971; Littlewood and Lipsedge, 1978; Carpenter and Brockington, 1980; Giggs, 1986;

McGovern and Cope, 1987; Harrison, Owens, Holton, Neilson, and Boot, 1988). At least two of these studies (Harrison et al., 1988; McGovern and Cope, 1987) have shown that the same pattern holds for those of Afro-Caribbean origin who were born in Britain (i.e., the second generation) and, indeed, may even be more exaggerated.

More detailed analysis of the repeatedly confirmed finding that Afro-Caribbeans in England have very high treated prevalence rates for schizophrenia, show that the phenomenon is particularly marked for young (< 35 years old) men, where the black to white ratio reaches 6 to 1 but falls back to about 2 to 1 in the older age groups (Cochrane and Bal, 1987). There have been many attempts to explain this gross overrepresentation of Afro-Caribbeans among those being treated for schizophrenia in Britain. In the past decade my colleagues and I have examined six possible explanations (Cochrane and Bal, 1987, 1988, 1989).

1. The "ethnic density" hypothesis suggests that there is an inverse correlation between the incidence of schizophrenia in a particular ethnic group and the size of that group relative to the total population. An analysis of the rates of schizophrenia in minority ethnic groups of different sizes in England revealed no support for this hypothesis (in fact the correlations between rates of schizophrenia and relative size of the population were positive and significant for males—not negative as predicted). A second tack, that of correlating rates of schizophrenia with the relative size of the Afro-Caribbean population in different regions of England, also yielded no support at all for the ethnic density hypothesis.

2. Could demographic differences between blacks and whites in England account for the differences in rates of schizophrenia? For example, it has often been demonstrated that social class and marital status are related to relative risk of schizophrenia (with lower social status and being never married associated with higher risk). In fact single status is much more likely to be a consequence than a cause of schizophrenia, so, even if there were a difference between ethnic groups in marital patterns, this in itself could not be used to explain the different prevalence of schizophrenia. The same causal argument has been made for the link between low social status and high rates of schizophrenia,

but it is less overwhelming. It is true that Afro-Caribbeans in England are overrepresented in the socioeconomic groups most vulnerable to schizophrenia, but the black to white relativity in rates of schizophrenia is far greater than the manual to nonmanual social class ratio. Even if some adjustment to rates were to be made to allow for social class differentials between the majority white and the minority Afro-Caribbean communities, most of the Afro-Caribbean excess in treated prevalence of schizophrenia would remain to be explained.

3. Perhaps there is a high rate of schizophrenia in the West Indies and the migrants from there to Britain reflect this. If migrants are a roughly representative selection of the population of the home country, and this population as a whole has a particularly high incidence of schizophrenia, then it would be expected that, after migration, they might show a higher rate than the population they join. This argument has been used to explain the higher than expected rates of schizophrenia and alcohol-related problems of the Irish in Britain (Walsh, 1971; Cochrane and Stopes-Roe, 1979). However, available evidence seems to indicate that the incidence of schizophrenia in the Caribbean is about the same as it is in Britain (Royes, 1962; Littlewood and Lipsedge, 1982), thus ruling out this particular explanation.

4. Could schizophrenia predispose people to migrate? This, of course, was the explanation offered in one of the very first systematic studies of migration and schizophrenia conducted by Odegaard (1932). He concluded that the high rate of schizophrenia he observed among Norwegian immigrants to the United States was because "many maladjusted schizophrenic personalities choose emigration as the best solution to social defeats and adversities in the old country" (p. 203). Cochrane and Bal (1988) pointed out that this hypothesis does not sit very well with the circumstances of West Indian migration to Britain. The overwhelming majority of migrants from the Caribbean came to Britain to seek work and gain economic improvement, and accounts of the careers and work habits of West Indians in Britain show a pattern of stable employment and slow but sure economic advance (Walvin, 1984). It seems inherently unlikely that people with typical premorbid signs of schizophrenia such as social withdrawal, passivity, and lack of adaptability would also display the

ambition, energy, and enterprise necessary to migrate from the West Indies to Britain in search of work.

5. Possibly the stress associated with migration and the culture shock and racist environment encountered on settling in Britain produced adverse psychological reactions in immigrants. This was the causal explanation advanced by the Commission for Racial Equality (1976) in the dubious analysis of the mental health of immigrants to which reference has already been made. Again this hypothesis is inherently implausible for two reasons. First, those disorders which are usually considered to be most stress-related are not found at higher rates in the black communities in England. Indeed, the treated prevalence rates for neuroses and depression are substantially lower in the West Indian born population than in the native born. Of all the major disorders, we might expect rates of schizophrenia to be the least responsive to stress, but it is this disorder which is most strongly related to migration and minority status—at least for Afro-Caribbeans in Britain. Second, all of the stresses, difficulties, and traumas surrounding migration and living in an undeniably racist society are also experienced by other nonwhite minority groups. Yet it is the case that the Indian, Pakistani, and Chinese communities in Britain do not exhibit the same phenomenally high rate of schizophrenia as do Afro-Caribbeans.

6. Possible misdiagnosis by hospital psychiatrists has been put forward as an explanation for the racial differentials in treated prevalence of schizophrenia. It is widely recognized that the diagnosis of schizophrenia in clinical settings is problematical to say the least (Cooper, Kendall, Gurland, Sharpe, Copeland, and Simon, 1972; Kendall, 1975), and a high proportion of those initially diagnosed as schizophrenic subsequently have that diagnosis changed (Joyce, 1984). What is more important is the evidence that black patients are much more likely to have an initial diagnosis of schizophrenia, which is subsequently changed, than are white patients (Jones and Gray, 1986; Neighbors, Jackson, Campbell, and Williams, 1989). In the United States Mukherjee, Shukla, Woodle, Rosen, and Olarte (1983) found that the presence of auditory hallucinations in young black patients, which were eventually attributed to bipolar affective disorder, had often led to an initial misdiagnosis of schizophrenia. Auditory hallucinations

were found significantly more often in black nonschizophrenic patients than in white nonschizophrenic patients, which could go some way toward explaining the overrepresentation of blacks with a diagnosis of schizophrenia in the United States.

In Britain two studies by Littlewood and Lipsedge (1981a, b) have shown that the West Indian born were much more likely to be misdiagnosed as schizophrenic than were white patients. Littlewood and Lipsedge suggest that a significant proportion of Afro-Caribbean patients diagnosed as schizophrenic are, in fact, experiencing an acute psychotic episode or an acute paranoid reaction. Carpenter and Brockington (1980) also found that the apparent excess of schizophrenics in their black patients compared to their matched white patients was almost entirely accounted for by those with delusions of persecution and who were, therefore, according to these authors, not suffering from "true schizophrenia."

This same hypothesis has been suggested by Rack (1982), who uses the term *psychogenic psychoses* to label a condition which has some features similar to schizophrenia but which differs in that it is much shorter lived and has a much better prognosis than does true schizophrenia.

Why should this disorder (i.e., acute psychotic reaction or psychogenic psychosis) be much more likely to be misdiagnosed as schizophrenia in the Afro-Caribbean population of Britain than in any other group? The answers that have been offered are only tentative but they seemed to add up to a convincing picture: First, hallucinations and even delusions are often taken to be indicative of schizophrenia in patients of Western European origin, and this assumption usually turns out to be justified. However, this is not necessarily the case for people from other cultural backgrounds (Rack, 1982, p. 124). Second, cultural differences between the backgrounds of patients and psychiatrists may lead to misinterpretation of thought processes as disordered or delusional when, in fact, they are not necessarily pathological if viewed in their appropriate cultural context. It is interesting to note in this context the very large numbers of Indian- and Pakistani-born psychiatrists in British hospitals compared to the very small number of Afro-Caribbean psychiatrists. Perhaps this helps explain why Asian patients are less likely to be "misdiagnosed" than are Afro-Caribbean patients.

The misdiagnosis explanation is the one that has been most favored by those who have pursued this subject (Cochrane, 1983; Littlewood and Lipsedge, 1982; Rack, 1982). This is due not only, or even mainly, to the empirical evidence supporting it, but because as a hypothesis it avoids the very uncomfortable overtones of explanations which may be interpreted as indicating genetic differences between blacks and whites, or suggesting that there might be pathological aspects of black community organization, culture, history, or personality. Those of a liberal frame of mind feel more at ease blaming psychiatry and psychiatrists than pointing to possible racial differences. Unfortunately, studies by Harrison and his coworkers (1988) have made the misdiagnosis hypothesis less tenable. Having found a very high rate of diagnosed schizophrenia among the Afro-Caribbean population of Nottingham, England (about twelve times greater than for the whole population of that city), Harrison et al. set about applying increasingly restrictive diagnostic criteria to both the Afro-Caribbean and general population patients (the latter group including some black patients). The results are contained in Table 24.3. It is immediately evident that there is an overwhelmingly similar proportion of Afro-Caribbean and general population patients diagnosed as schizophrenic at all levels of certainty. So while there remains a doubt over the reliability of the diagnosis of schizophrenia (for less than 40% of the total sample was the diagnosis "certain"), Harrison's study undermines the suggestion that more black people are misdiagnosed than are patients from other ethnic groups.

Perhaps the most profitable direction for future research to explore is to adapt the hypothesis put forward by Melvin Kohn twenty years ago (Kohn, 1968, 1972) to explain the social class/schizophrenia relationship. Kohn suggested that it was necessary for three independent factors to coincide in an individual for schizophrenia to appear: genetic predisposition, high levels of stress, and values related to "conceptions of reality" which are produced by the day-to-day experiences of the family and the individual in their contact with others and the institutions of society. Repeated exposure to discrimination and consequent lack of

TABLE 24.3
Applying Increasing Restrictive Definitions of Schizophrenia Based on
ICD-9 Coding for Certainty of Schizophrenia (adapted from Harrison
et al., 1988)

Certainty Coding	Cumulative Frequency (%)	
	Afro-Caribbean	General population*
N=	42	99
Certain	38	37
Very Likely	67	67
Probable	74	78
Possible	86	89
Not schizophrenia	14	11

*Includes some minority ethnic group patients.

instrumental efficacy can produce an external locus of control,
lowered self-esteem, helplessness, "and a fatalistic belief that one
is at the mercy of forces and people beyond one's control . . ."
(Kohn, 1972, p. 300). This orientation is antipathetic to an effective response to stress which is, in any case, likely to be greater
in a disadvantaged minority. Where these factors impinge on a
person with a genetic predisposition, then schizophrenia will be
manifested. Thus two populations with identical genetic vulnerability may show different rates of schizophrenia depending on
their exposure to the other variables in Kohn's equation.

REFERENCES

Astrup, C., & Odegaard, O. (1960), Internal migration and mental dis-
     ease in Norway. *Psychiat. Quart.*, (suppl.) 34:116–130.
Bagley, C. (1969), A survey of problems reported by Indian and Pakistani
     immigrants in Britain. *Race*, 9:65–78.
———— (1971), The social aetiology of schizophrenia in immigrant
     groups. *Internat. J. Soc. Psychiat.*, 17:292–304.
Carpenter, L., & Brockington, I. F. (1980), A study of mental illness in
     Asians, West Indians and Africans living in Manchester. *Brit. J.
     Psychiat.*, 137:201–210.
Cochrane, R. (1977), Mental illness in immigrants to England and

Wales: An analysis of mental hospital admissions in 1971. *Soc. Psychiat.*, 12:25–35.

——— (1983), *The Social Creation of Mental Illness.* London: Longmans.

——— Bal, S. S. (1987), Migration and schizophrenia: An examination of five hypotheses. *Soc. Psychiat.*, 22:181–191.

——— ——— (1988), Ethnic density is unrelated to incidence of schizophrenia. *Brit. J. Psychiat.*, 153:363–366.

——— ——— (1989), Mental hospital admission rates of immigrants to England: A comparison of 1971 and 1981. *Soc. Psychiat. & Psychiat. Epidemiol.*, 24:2–12.

——— ——— (1990), Patterns of alcohol consumption by Sikh, Hindu and Muslim men in the West Midlands. *Brit. J. Addict.*, 85:759–769.

——— Stopes-Roe, M. (1977), Psychological and social adjustment of Asian immigrants to Britain: A community survey. *Soc. Psychiat.*, 12:195–206.

——— ——— (1979), Psychological disturbance in Ireland, in England and in Irish emigrants to England: A comparative study. *Econ. & Soc. Rev.*, 10:301–320.

——— ——— (1981), Psychological symptom levels in Indian immigrants to England: A comparison with native English. *Psycholog. Med.*, 11:319–322.

Commission for Racial Equality (1976), *Aspects of Mental Health in a Multicultural Society.* London: CRE.

Cooper, J. E., Kendall, R. E., Gurland, B. J., Sharpe, L., Copeland, J. R. M., & Simon, R. (1972), *Psychiatric Diagnosis in New York and London.* Maudsley Monograph Series No. 20. London: Oxford University Press.

Dean, G., Walsh, D., Downing, H., & Shelley, E. (1981), First admissions of native born and immigrants to psychiatric hospital in South East England, 1976. *Brit. J. Psychiat.*, 139:506–512.

Eitinger, L. (1959), The incidence of mental disease among refugees in Norway. *J. Ment. Sci.*, 105:326–380.

Giggs, J. (1986), Ethnic status and mental illness in urban areas. In: *Health, Race and Ethnicity*, ed. T. Rathwell & D. Phillips. London: Croom Helm.

Gordon, E. B. (1965), Mentally ill West Indian immigrants. *Brit. J. Psychiat.*, 111:877–887.

Harrison, G., Owens, D., Holton, A., Neilson, D., & Boot, D. (1988), A prospective study of severe mental disorder in Afro-Caribbean patients. *Psycholog. Med.*, 18:643–657.

Hashmi, F. (1968), Community psychiatric problems among Birmingham immigrants. *Brit. J. Soc. Psychiat.*, 2:196–201.

Hemsi, L. K. (1967), Psychiatric morbidity of West Indian immigrants. *Soc. Psychiat.*, 2:95–100.

Jones, B. E., & Gray, B. A. (1986), Problems in diagnosing schizophrenia and affective disorders among blacks. *Hosp. & Commun. Psychiat.*, 37:61–65.

Joyce, P. R. (1984), Age of onset in bipolar affective disorder and misdiagnosis as schizophrenia. *Psycholog. Med.*, 14:145–149.

Kendall, R. E. (1975), *The Role of Diagnosis in Psychiatry.* Oxford: Blackwell.

Kiev, A. (1963), Beliefs and delusions of West Indian immigrants to London. *Brit. J. Psychiat.*, 109:356–363.

——— (1964), Psychiatric illness among West Indians in London. *Race*, 9:48–51.

Kohn, M. L. (1968), Social class and schizophrenia: A critical review. In: *The Transmission of Schizophrenia*, ed. D. Rosenthal & S. S. Kety. Oxford: Pergamon Press.

——— (1972), Class, family and schizophrenia: A reformulation. *Soc. Forces*, 50:295–304.

Krupinski, J., Schaechter, F., & Cade, J. F. L. (1965), Factors influencing the incidence of mental disorders among immigrants. *Med. J. Australia*, 2:269–274.

——— Stoller, A. (1965), Incidence of mental disorders in Victoria according to country of birth. *Med. J. Australia*, 2:265–269.

Leff, J. (1981), *Psychiatry Around the Globe: A Transcultural View.* Geneva: Marcel Dekker.

Littlewood, R., & Lipsedge, M. (1978), Migration, ethnicity and diagnosis. *Psychiatrica Clinica* (Basel), 11:15–22.

——— ——— (1981a), Some social and phenomenological characteristics of psychotic immigrants. *Psycholog. Med.*, 11:289–302.

——— ——— (1981b), Acute psychotic reactions in Caribbean born patients. *Psycholog. Med.*, 11:303–318.

——— ——— (1982), *Aliens and Alienists.* Harmondsworth, Middlesex: Penguin Books.

Malzberg, B. (1955), Mental disease among native and foreign-born white populations of New York State 1939–41. *Ment. Hyg.*, 39:545–555.

McGovern, D., & Cope, R. V. (1987), First psychiatric admission rates of first and second generation Afro-Caribbeans. *Soc. Psychiat.*, 22:139–149.

Mukherjee, S., Shukla, S., Woodle, J., Rosen, A. M., & Olarte, S. (1983), Misdiagnosis of schizophrenia in bipolar patients—A multi-ethnic comparison. *Amer. Psychiat.*, 140:1571–1572.

Murphy, H. B. M. (1965), Migration and major mental disorders: A reappraisal. In: *Mobility and Mental Health*, ed. M. B. Kantor. Springfield, IL: Charles C Thomas.

Neighbors, H. W., Jackson, J. S., Campbell, L., & Williams, D. (1989), The influence of racial factors on psychiatric diagnosis: A review and suggestions for research. *Commun. Ment. Health J.*, 25:301–311.

Odegaard, O. (1932), Emigration and insanity. *Acta Psychiat. Neurol.*, 4(suppl.):1–206.

Pinsent, R. F. N. (1963), Morbidity in an immigrant population. *Lancet*, 1:437–448.

Pinto, R. (1974), A comparison of illness patterns in Asian and English patients. *Ind. Psychiat.*, 16:203–210.

Rack, P. (1982), *Race, Culture and Mental Disorder*. London: Tavistock.

Royes, K. (1962), The incidence and features of psychosis in a Caribbean community. *Soc. Psychiat.*, 2:1121–1125.

Rwegellera, G. G. C. (1977), Psychiatric morbidity among West Africans and West Indians living in London. *Psycholog. Med.*, 7:317–321.

Sartorius, N., Jablensky, A., Korten, A., Emberg, G., Anker, M., Cooper, J. E., & Day, R. (1986), Early manifestations and first-contact incidence of schizophrenia in different cultures. *Psycholog. Med.*, 16:909–928.

Twefik, G. L., & Okasha, A. (1965), Psychosis and immigration. *Postgrad. Med. J.*, 41:603–612.

Walsh, D. (1971), Patients in Irish psychiatric hospitals in 1963—A comparison with England and Wales. *Brit. J. Psychiat.*, 118:617–620.

Walvin, J. (1984), *Passage to Britain*. Harmondsworth, Middlesex: Penguin Books.

World Health Organization (1979), *Schizophrenia: An International Follow-Up Study*. Chichester, U.K.: Wiley.

Name Index

Abbott, M. W., 343
Abe, Y., 5
Abramson, J. H., 131
Ackerknecht, E., 250
Ackerson, L. M., 326
Adachi, J., 25
Adasal, R., 170
Aggarwal, A. K., 18–19, 58, 120
Aguirre Beltrán, G., 232
Ahyi, R. G., 101, 107
Ajmany, S., 117
Akimoto, H., 5
Akiskal, H. S., 307
Al-Issa, I., 26, 33, 36
Allen, E. A., 222
Alleyne, E., 217
Alonso-Fernandez, F., 286
Alterwain, P., 241
Ames, D., 193
an der Heiden, W., 257, 258
Ananth, J., 124
Andrade, A., 99t
Andrews, G., 187
Angelo-Khatar, M., 24
Anker, M., 15, 351
Anthony, J. C., 150
Apter, A., 139
Arafa, M., 59, 60
Arieli, A., 139
Arnon, A., 131
Arora, U., 120
Artner, K., 262
Arya, O. P., 12
Ashour, A., 57
Astrup, C., 348
Asuni, T., 19, 88
Atcho, A., 105
Auslander, G. K., 143
Austin, G., 189, 197
Aviram, U., 131, 134

Bagley, C., 349, 351
Bal, S. S., 221, 224, 349–350, 351–352, 353
Baldwin, B. A., 31
Bales, R. F., 23
Banerjee, G., 117, 119, 120
Bannister, D., 57
Barilar, E., 236–237
Barnaby, D. M., 224
Baron, A. E., 319, 326
Bar-On, R., 143
Barrett, L. E., 220
Barry, III, H. 23, 24, 26
Bashaar, T., 55
Basker, E., 138
Basoglu, M., 176
Bauer, M., 252
Bayat, A. H., 172, 174
Beaglehole, E., 335
Beals, J., 326
Beaubrun, M. H., 223
Beauvais, F., 320
Bedi, H., 16
Beiser, M., 28, 29, 36
Belknap, I., 10
Bell, C. C., 31
Ben-Arie, O., 24, 76, 77
Benedict, P. K., 5
Ben-Ezer, G., 139
Ben-Shaul, R., 137, 138
Benton, R., 331–332
Berah, M., 193
Beran, B., 138
Berlin, I., 320
Bernadr, P., 61
Berne, C., 94
Berne, E., 6
Bertelsen, A., 275, 276
Bespali de Consens, Y., 240–244
Betts, K., 188

Subject Index

373